THE COMPLETE BOOK OF KETONES

A Practical Guide to Ketogenic Diets and Ketone Supplements

by MARY T. NEWPORT, M.D.

Foreword by Theodore VanItallie, M.D.

Graphics by Joanna Newport Rand

TURNER PUBLISHING COMPANY

Turner Publishing Company
Nashville, Tennessee
www.turnerpublishing.com

The Complete Book of Ketones: A Practical Guide to Ketogenic Diets and Ketone Supplements

Cover design: Maddie Cothren
Book design: Tim Holtz

Library of Congress Cataloging-in-Publication Data Upon Request

9781684421602 Paperback
9781684421619 Hardback
9781684421626 eBook

Printed in the United States of America
· 18 19 20 10 9 8 7 6 5 4 3 2 1

DEDICATION

This is dedicated to the memory of Steven Jerry Newport, my best friend and husband of forty-three years, who made it possible for me to be both a mother and a doctor. He said taking care of our girls was the best job he ever had. He was an active, intelligent, and creative person, helpful in every way to everyone, and one of the most pleasant people you could ever meet. He was well aware of the toll Alzheimer's disease was taking on him and fully embraced the idea of ketones as an alternative fuel for the brain. He was a willing and eager participant in his reprieve from the disease, first by taking ketogenic medium-chain triglycerides and coconut oil, then a ketone ester in a pilot study of one patient. We were given at least three extra good years with Steve, thanks to ketogenic therapies.

Steve lost his battle with Alzheimer's disease and Lewy body dementia on January 2, 2016. This book represents his legacy to the world.

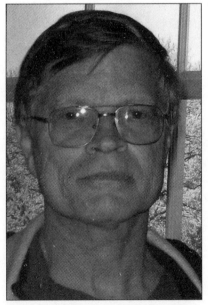

Steven Jerry Newport—1950 to 2016.

CONTENTS

FOREWORD

Dr. Mary T. Newport, author of this invaluable compilation of up-to-date information about ketogenic diets and supplements, could not have foreseen how seriously her life would be affected by her untimely confrontation with a wholly unexpected adversary—Alzheimer's disease-induced dementia (ADd). In the space of a few months, her existence as a busy neonatologist and homemaker was transformed. And in the subsequent course of her courageous campaign against this implacable neurodegenerative disorder, she became a model of initiative and perseverance. These qualities were her strongest weapons in the fight to save her beloved husband, Steve, from rapidly evolving dementia. During this protracted battle, she found a treatment approach—not a cure—that worked surprisingly well for Steve for almost four years.

Sadly, misfortune challenged her at a time when she should have been allowed to continue to enjoy her marriage to Steve unimpeded. It was his generosity of spirit that enabled her to attend medical school, while he was content to stay at home and care for their young children.

But fate intervened. In 2001, at age 51, Steve Newport, in the midst of a promising career as an accountant, developed early-onset dementia (which post-mortem studies disclosed was caused by a virulent combination of Alzheimer's disease with a condition known as Lewy body dementia). Deterioration of his memory and cognitive skills progressed with alarming speed, and by 2006 he was unable to function in his job and had to give up driving. As his illness continued to progress, he became progressively more confused and disoriented and eventually was unable to carry out simple household chores or self-care without assistance.

The collective experience and professional knowledge of Mary's Newport's medical colleagues had no promising treatments to suggest. Steve's situation soon reached a point where most spouses would have thrown up their hands and accepted palliative care as the only humane intervention possible.

But *surrender* is not in Mary Newport's lexicon. By will alone, she forced herself to conduct a systematic search of the medical literature, hunting for any evidence of a treatment approach that might counter the process that was inexorably destroying brain functions that had made Steve such an admirable human being. As her mission progressed, Mary found her first glimmer of hope in the writings of Dr. Richard L. Veech, a Harvard Medical School graduate who went on to take graduate training in biochemistry at Britain's University of Oxford. There Veech earned the doctor of philosophy degree (DPhil) for studies carried out under the tutelage of Sir Hans Krebs, discoverer of the famed "Krebs cycle." After Oxford, Veech joined the intramural research staff at the National Institutes of Health and founded the Laboratory of Metabolic Control, which, at age eighty-two, he still heads.

Krebs had an interest in ketone body metabolism, which was transmitted to Veech. But the principal ketone bodies, D betahydroxybutyrate (D-βOHB) and acetoacetate (AcAc) did not come into their own scientifically until 1966–67. That's when a group of clinical scientists working under the leadership of Dr. George F. Cahill Jr. at Harvard's Peter Bent Brigham Hospital discovered the importance of ketone bodies for brain function and human survival. These investigators found that, contrary to the belief of earlier scientists, the ketones produced in abundance by the liver during fasting are far from being potentially dangerous waste by-products of a starving organism. Rather, they serve as the brain's primary alternative fuel when its usual fuel, glucose, is in short supply. Unlike the fatty acids from which they are derived, ketone bodies can cross the blood-brain barrier (BBB), after which they are readily metabolized by the brain's parenchymal cells and neuronal structures.

The extra ketones manufactured during periods of starvation have been found to alleviate the brain's destructive dependence on glucose derived from the breakdown of the body's stores of essential protein. Thus, it gradually became clear to knowledgeable scientists that the ketone body "safety net" is the outcome of an evolutionarily determined adaptation designed to prolong and save the lives of starving mammals, humans included. As a result of the original observations by Cahill and his co-workers, ketone bodies, derived from the body's fat stores, became recognized as a life-prolonging and lifesaving fuel for individuals whose sources of dietary energy were cut off by famine or other interruptions, including politically- or religiously-motivated fasting.

As a consequence of her desperate literature search, Dr. Newport came across several articles that gave reason to hope that placing Steve on a ketogenic diet and/or feeding him coconut oil-derived medium-chain triglyceride (MCT) supplements known to raise blood ketone levels to a modest degree would provide his brain with sufficient energy from D-βOHB and AcAc to rescue his failing brain function. Although the precise reason why this approach is often effective is not entirely clear, the rationale for trying it is scientifically sound. As reported by Stephen Cunnane and his co-workers at the University of Sherbrooke in Quebec, as well as by several other investigators, incontrovertible evidence exists that, in general, elderly individuals and patients with classical late onset Alzheimer's dementia are unable to use the brain's normal fuel, glucose, with normal efficiency. This reduction in brain glucose uptake is thought to give rise to "hypometabolism" (reflecting a degree of energy shortage) occurring in brain structures involved in memory and cognition. Over time such hypometabolism tends to worsen and appears to be associated with progressive cognitive impairment. On the other hand, the same subjects whose cognition-associated brain areas show an appreciable reduction in glucose uptake (as manifested by a diminution of the cerebral metabolic rate of glucose, or CMRgluc) appear able to metabolize D-βOHB and AcAc normally.

The work of two scientists, Dr. Richard L. Veech (referred to above) and Dr. Samuel Henderson, particularly influenced Mary Newport at this stage of her quest. In 2004, Henderson was among the first scientists to test the hypothesis that raising the blood ketone body concentrations well above their usual low levels (≤ 0.2 mM) would improve cognitive function in elderly individuals, including some in an early stage of Alzheimer dementia. Veech and his associate, Dr. Yoshihiro Kashiwaya, a neurologist and talented Japanese scientist, had found that ketone bodies added to tissue-culture models of Alzheimer disease and Parkinson disease blocked progression of the both disorders. Such findings strongly suggested that ketone body preparations, such as ketone esters, should undergo clinical trials to test their therapeutic efficacy in clinical versions of both neurodegenerative conditions. While Dr. Newport was obviously not in a position to conduct randomized placebo-controlled double-blind clinical trials of a ketogenic diet or the effect of ketone-body food supplements, she was able to test whether induction of various degrees of ketosis in her husband would have any beneficial effect on the downhill course of his illness.

Between 2004 and 2008, Steve's mini-mental state examination (MMSE), a commonly used test of cognitive status, declined from 23 (already well below the more acceptable 26 to 30 range) to 12—a seriously low level. Brain magnetic resonance imaging studies in 2008 showed involutional changes consistent with Alzheimer's disease.

It was at this point that Mary Newport played her last therapeutic card. She started Steve on about two tablespoonfuls of coconut oil (CO) per day, to which increasing quantities of medium-chain triglyceride (MCT) were gradually added[1]. When ingested, MCT's content of medium-chain fatty acids (MCFA [consisting of *caproic* (6 carbons), *caprylic* (8 carbons), and *decanoic* (10 carbons) had been known since the 1960s to cause the liver to increase its ketone body output and significantly raise ketone body levels in the blood circulation. Eventually, Steve was consuming about 5½ ounces of a 4:3 mixture of MCT:CO per day, divided into three or four servings. This dietary treatment was associated with dramatic improvement in Steve's personality, mood, and tremor. During the ensuing two and a half months, his MMSE rose from 12 to a high of 20. Several other standard tests of Steve's cognition also showed changes for the better. In the year that followed, he showed improvements in gait, social participation, word finding, and recall of recent events. During the two-year period of MCT:CO treatment, his MRI failed to show any morphologic changes indicative of further brain deterioration.

The gratifying clinical change associated with his MCT:CO treatment was nullified when Steve was placed on the drug, *semagacestat*, a presumed inhibitor of gamma secretase, an enzyme believed to promote accumulation in the brain of amyloid-beta (Aβ), the principal ingredient in the Aβ plaques that Alois Alzheimer found in the brains of his first two dementia patients. For many years, Aβ has been suspected

---

1   This foreword's description of Steve's response to coconut oil, MCT, and ketone monoester (KME) has been taken (sometimes directly) from the scientific report of these therapies published in 2014 in *Alzheimer's & Dementia*, official journal of the Alzheimer Association. Dr. Mary Newport is first author and Dr. Richard Veech is the senior author.

of being a major contributor to Alzheimer's development; however, its precise role in the disease's initiation and progression has yet to be fully worked out.

Steve's alarming clinical deterioration—thought to result from semagacestat-induced collateral damage to other proteins affecting neurocognitive function—persisted after the drug was stopped. Thus, Steve's condition gradually worsened, and his wife again found herself searching for new treatments that might increase blood ketone values to substantially higher levels than the ~ 0.5 mM concentration attainable with MCT:CO mixtures.

This time, she learned from Veech that a new ketone ester, known as *ketone monoester* (KME), which he and his co-workers had discovered and were manufacturing on a laboratory scale, was a safe and potent ketone-raising agent that could be taken by mouth. It was determined by Dr. Veech and his associates that Steve Newport would be the first patient with advanced dementia caused by Alzheimer's disease to receive the world's limited supply of the KME.

Thus Steve was started at home on orally administered KME. During the first two days on this novel treatment, Steve received 21.5 g three times a day. Thirty minutes of video that Mary took two to three hours after the first dose of KME disclosed a marked improvement in mood and the ability to recite and write out the complete alphabet, which he had been unable to do for many months. "The next morning, he spontaneously chose clothes and dressed himself—also a new development. On the third day of KME treatment, when his KME intake was increased to three 28.7 g servings/day, he began to initiate and complete many other activities without prompting or assistance."

As described in their publication by Newport et al. (2014), other changes for the better associated with Steve's adherence to the KME regimen included the following: "Showering, shaving, brushing teeth, finding his way around the house, choosing and ordering food from a menu, and distributing utensils from the dishwasher. . . . Abstract thinking, insight, and a subtle sense of humor returned to his conversation. In his own assessment of his response to KME, he stated that he felt 'good,' and had 'more energy,' and was 'happier.' He found it 'easier to do things'—which coincided with the caregiver's observations."

After six to eight weeks of taking 28.7g of the KME three times daily (he also continued to take some MCT:CO), he began to exhibit improvement in memory retrieval, spontaneously discussing events that occurred up to a week earlier. The greatest improvements in performance—namely, in conversation and interpersonal interaction—were observed at the higher "post-dose" D-βOHB blood levels.

Needless to say, Steve's caregivers welcomed the physical, cognitive, and behavioral changes that occurred while Steve was ingesting the Veech KME. One hour after he swallowed a 25g serving of KME, Steve's whole blood D-βOHB levels rose to levels ranging from 3.0 to 5.5 mM, approximately ten times the blood concentrations obtained after consumption of 20g of MCT alone. Two hours after KME ingestion, D-βOHB concentrations had fallen to values ranging from 2 to 4 mM. Associated with this striking increase in the blood D-βOHB level was a dramatic enhancement of daily activity performance that expressed itself in more fluent conversation and more lively interpersonal interaction. These improvements seemed to track, to a degree, blood ketone concentrations, with the quality of conversation and interaction, for example, declining as D-βOHB levels fell toward baseline.

These observations suggest that, despite the brain atrophy that becomes more marked as dementia progresses, there remain neurons and synapses that seem to be in a hibernation-like state, but which awaken when exposed to the new source of energy provided by the availability of ketone bodies. The rapidity of Steve's response to his first feeding of KME and the relationship of the quality of this response to the increased blood concentration of D-βOHB induced by the KME suggest that there is an ongoing dynamic relationship between the status of the brain's energy metabolism—especially the availability of fuel—and the organism's performance in a number of domains, including cognition.

For more than three and a half years from when Steve first started taking coconut oil/medium-chain triglyceride on May 21, 2008, he remained greatly improved, and his life became much healthier and happier than it had been before the ketogenic regimen was initiated. However, in January 2012, his physical state and his dementia worsened. Several events contributed to this downhill course. Among them, a fall resulted in a serious head injury followed by a full-body seizure, after which he temporarily stopped breathing. He also had a dramatically adverse response to several tranquilizers unwittingly given him during a stay in the hospital. He began to have hallucinations (which commonly occur in patients with Lewy body dementia). From that point on, he had increasingly frequent bouts of sleep apnea and required supplementary oxygen. On December 19, 2015, his breathing further deteriorated, and he became barely responsive, dying on January 2, 2016.

Dr. Mary Newport, author of this comprehensive *arbeit* describing the saga of her husband's dementia and her valiant efforts to rescue him from this seemingly untreatable condition, deserves strong commendation for creating what she calls Steve Newport's "legacy to the world." Dr. Newport is a practicing physician, and yet she had the insight and initiative to tackle a medical challenge that, to date, has defeated the efforts of numerous professional research scientists to discover and develop even partly effective treatment and prevention strategies. She is the first physician to administer and study the effect of a ketone ester in a patient with severe dementia of long duration. This practical guide to the nutritional prevention and management of Alzheimer's disease represents another phase of her battle against this monstrous illness.

It is ironic that the professional scientists who are in a position to fund clinical trials that can test the implications of the pilot and pre-clinical studies carried out, for example, by Richard Veech, the world's foremost ketone-body pioneer and NIH veteran, and by others like Stephen Cunnane and his team at Sherbrooke University, Quebec, do not seem to have grasped the potential of ketone body therapy for Alzheimer's dementia and many other medical conditions. Today's cadre of neuroscientists can surely benefit from emulating the enlightened example set by Mary Newport. With the help of an open mind, there is much of importance to be learned from the published experience of even one man: Steve Newport.

ACKNOWLEDGEMENTS

As I was writing this book, it occurred to me that it would be much more interesting to share the history of ketone research through the eyes of the people who have lived it, and so I want to acknowledge and thank the following individuals for their important work in ketone research, implementation, awareness and advocacy, and their willingness to let me interview them and to review the write-ups of their many interesting stories: Richard L. Veech, MD, DPhil, Theodore B. VanItallie, MD, Sami Hashim, MD, Thomas Seyfried, PhD, Stephen Cunnane, PhD, Dominic D'Agostino, PhD, Russell Swerdlow, MD, George Yu, MD, Angela Poff, PhD, Jacob Wilson, PhD, Ryan Lowery, PhD, Jim Abrahams, Beth Zupec-Kania, RDN, CD, Miriam Kalamian, EdM, MS, CNS, and two patients who were willing to give up their privacy to share their compelling responses to ketogenic therapies, William Curtis and Joe Prata, along with his wife Carol Henry Prata.

I also wish to acknowledge:

My daughter Joanna Newport Rand who spent countless hours typing up references and creating numerous graphics for the book, as well as the many hours she and her husband Forrest spent helping me take care of Steve. They never hesitated for a second to come to my rescue when I called.

My daughter Julie DiPalo for helping with the list of resources and for her love and support.

My sister Angela Bertke for the countless hours she worked to increase awareness among the older population of ketones as an alternative fuel for the brain, and she and her husband John Bertke for their help with proofreading, commenting on content, encouragement, love, and support.

The Pruvit Ventures company for taking awareness of the power of ketones to a whole new level though their dedication to education, and the many thousands of ketone messengers they have launched, who are now spreading the good news around the world. Todd King for his work in providing us with Dr. Veech's ketone ester and for carefully proofreading my book.

Turner Publishing and the many people involved in helping me carry on my husband Steve Newport's legacy by sharing the message of ketones with the world.

STEVE'S EMERGENCE FROM ALZHEIMER'S AWAKENS A MESSENGER FOR KETONES IN ME

"A discovery is said to be an accident
meeting a prepared mind."
—Albert Szent-Gyorgyi

I remember the exact moment I became a messenger for ketones. It happened quite by accident late on the evening of May 19, 2008, when I first read the words, "Ketones are an alternative fuel for the brain." Up to that point, as a physician, I mainly thought of ketones as a dangerous product of life-threatening diabetic ketoacidosis and vaguely recalled from freshman biochemistry in medical school that ketones are produced from the breakdown of fat during starvation and on certain low-carbohydrate, high-fat diets. But this was the first time I'd heard of ketones in the context of a potential therapeutic for disease. At that moment, I was provided with an idea that changed the course of my husband's early-onset Alzheimer's disease for the better.

I will tell you up front that this story does not have a happy ending. Steve lost his battle with Alzheimer's on January 2, 2016. The story does, however, have a happy middle.

My husband, Steve Newport, and I grew up in Cincinnati, Ohio, and we met at Good Samaritan Hospital, where I was working after school as a nurses' aide and Steve was working in the housekeeping department to pay for college. We fell in love and were married before I started medical school; I was just twenty years old. Steve was as an accountant, and I became a neonatologist, a physician who cares for sick and premature newborns. As we approached the end of my training, we struggled with how we could welcome children into our lives, given that Steve would work long hours, and I could expect to be called away from home for emergencies day and night. After careful thought, Steve announced that he would like to work from home to be there for our children and, not long after, Julie and then Joanna were born. Steve's selflessness made it possible for me to fulfill my dreams to be a doctor and mother, and he took great care of all of us. He often said with a big smile that taking care of our girls was the best job he ever had.

Steve is not someone you would ever expect to have developed Alzheimer's disease. He was outgoing and friendly, active and physically fit, constantly working in the yard or kayaking more than a mile to islands off the coast of Florida. He read novel after novel and loved to travel. He had to have the latest and fastest computer and, when he wasn't working on it, he was playing on it. He could design letter-perfect, complex accounting forms and documents. But in 2001, when he was just fifty-one years old, Steve began to make large payroll mistakes and miss appointments for the children, even when I reminded him thirty minutes before it was time to leave. He started to hang reminder notes to himself on a long strand of tape that hung in the doorway to his office, but still he would forget. At first, I thought he was going through a mid-life crisis or had simply lost interest. But then he began to forget whether he had been to the bank and post office and would misplace important mail. This was clearly not normal, and I worried that something serious was going on. He was also quite depressed at that time, so we went to a neuropsychiatrist, who mentioned dementia as a possibility but attributed these problems to his depression. Looking back, it was probably the other way around—he was depressed because he knew he wasn't functioning as well as he used to. The doctor started Steve on an antidepressant but, over the next year, it became obvious that he was getting worse.

In 2003 we moved about an hour north from Dunedin to Spring Hill, Florida, so that I could open a new neonatal intensive care unit. It soon became apparent that Steve was becoming more confused. Spring Hill is a small town with just a few major roads, but he could not remember which street he was driving on or in which direction, and he was no longer able to read a map. He began to spend endless hours in the garage looking for "something" and, at the end of the day, he would no longer remember what he was looking for but still would be looking. This behavior was not normal, so I made an appointment for Steve with a neurologist who specialized in Alzheimer's disease. He performed a complete evaluation with cognitive testing, an EEG, an MRI, and blood work to rule out known causes of memory impairment, and concluded that Steve had some type of dementia, which was quite a shock to us. Six months later, as Steve's memory continued to worsen, he was diagnosed with probable early-onset Alzheimer's disease. By then, he was only fifty-four, and I was fifty-two. We had been married for thirty-two years at that point and looked forward to living out our golden years together, but this cruel diagnosis abruptly changed everything. He was started on Aricept, the only medication approved at that time for Alzheimer's. We saw no obvious change but kept him on it, since we were told the drug could slow the progress of the disease.

So many things that happened made no sense. In spite of working and playing on his computer for hours every day, Steve gradually lost his accounting skills, beginning with the more complex annual reports, and then the quarterly reports and payroll and, by 2006, he could no longer remember how to use a mouse or turn on his computer, use a calculator, or even perform simple math. One evening, as I watched for Steve to appear with his truck in the driveway, he called to say that he had missed a turn when following our daughter in her car and had ended up on the opposite coast of Florida. He reluctantly gave up his keys for the safety of himself and others. His behavior became stranger and stranger. For instance, instead of cutting the grass, he would take his lawn tractor apart, and the pieces would go missing. Our world was truly upside-down.

Later that year, I began to consider the role of nutrition in Alzheimer's disease and read everything I could get my hands on. I was convinced that what we eat has something to do with the disease and its progression after I came across a study published in a medical journal reporting that people with Alzheimer's who followed a diet that most closely adhered to a Mediterranean diet lived an average four years longer than those who ate a diet least similar to the Mediterranean diet (Scarmeas, 2007). Until then, our family had fully embraced what I call the "convenience-food diet," consisting largely of packaged frozen dinners and frequent trips to fast food restaurants. During four years of medical school, I received only three hours of education on nutrition in one afternoon.

Until I began to research the connection between nutrition and Alzheimer's, I had bought into the "lipid heart hypothesis" espoused by the United States Department of Agriculture (USDA) and the American Heart Association (AHA) and, therefore, believed that a low-fat diet was the way to go. (*Lipid,* loosely, is another word for "fat.") In spite of drinking skimmed milk, taking the skin off the chicken, cutting the fat off the meat, and using non-stick oil sprays instead of real oil to cook with, in early 2006, I was grossly overweight and on the verge of diabetes. Since I was not supposed to eat fat, my diet was made up mostly of carbohydrates, and I was constantly hungry, typically craving more carbs immediately after eating. After I read every book I could find on nutrition and various types of diets, as well as published medical studies on those same diets, we transitioned to a whole-food Mediterranean-type diet, stressing more fish, eggs, and other healthy proteins, different colors of vegetables and fruits, small portions of whole grain rice and breads, olive oil, butter, avocados, and nuts. After I learned that there was a going to be a clinical trial for the use of 900 milligrams of docosahexaenoic acid (the omega-3 fat DHA) to determine if it would improve memory and cognition in people with Alzheimer's, I added this to our diet. I lost a lot of weight along with my sugar cravings; however, Steve continued to get worse. It was hard to know what impact, if any, these dietary changes had for Steve.

Alzheimer's has a way of sneaking up on you as it slowly, but surely, robs your loved ones of everything they once could do, so that they have to be helped through even the most basic everyday tasks. If they do not die of something else in the meantime, eventually they become bedbound and have to be fed, bathed, and dressed. In the end, they forget how to chew and swallow and can inhale food and develop aspiration pneumonia. People sometimes opt for a feeding tube at this point, but the bowel eventually stops functioning, so this helps only temporarily. Caregivers are often woefully unprepared and do not know what is coming. Presently, no good system is in place to mentor caregivers about what to expect and how to deal with it. As the disease progresses, just when you think the situation cannot get any worse, it does, and you feel as if you are helplessly falling into the deep end of a pool unable to swim and wondering how you will stay afloat. This disease not only takes the victim on a terrible journey, but it also hijacks the lives of his or her loved ones as well. Until you live through it yourself, whether as the victim or as a family caregiver, you cannot imagine how truly horrible it is.

Steve was the love of my life and my best friend. He had taken great care of our daughters and me, but as the disease progressed, I became his caregiver. Many people with Alzheimer's seem oblivious to their condition, but Steve was well aware that he had Alzheimer's: he knew what he had been able to do before and what he could not do now. This was frustrating and depressing for him.

By spring 2008, Steve was on a downward spiral, and I worried we would not have much more time together. By then, not only did he have trouble staying on task, but he also could no longer read or even write a simple sentence, and he had developed physical symptoms as well. He had a tremor in his jaw when he tried to talk and in his hand when he tried to eat. He could no longer pick up his feet and run; instead he walked with a slow, stiff gait. He used to whistle the most wonderful medleys, and now he would get stuck on the same eight notes, like a continuous loop, from the Johnny Cash song "I Walk the Line." He whistled it over and over, so many times that I thought I would go out of my mind. In the morning, he was very sluggish, barely spoke, and had trouble remembering how to fill a glass with water from the refrigerator dispenser. I had to stay with him when he took a shower and shaved, I helped him pick out his clothes and get dressed, and I tied his shoes for him. He could no longer put a simple meal together for himself, and our daughter Joanna would stay with him while I was working to make sure he ate and didn't get into trouble.

I was always on the lookout for clinical trials—maybe Steve would be one of the first fortunate people to receive the drug that would cure Alzheimer's—but these trials were few and far between and, much to our distress, he failed to qualify because he had a history of depression. This made no sense to me: Wouldn't anyone who had Alzheimer's and was aware of it be depressed, as Steve was? Finally, in May 2008, a new clinical trial became available in our area for an intravenous vaccine called bapineuzumab, which would remove beta-amyloid plaques from the brain. In the earlier part of the twentieth century, Dr. Alois Alzheimer discovered that some people with dementia had a buildup of plaques and tangles in their brains; this form of dementia was named after him in the 1970s. Billions of research dollars have been poured into learning more about these plaques and tangles and into the development of drugs to remove them, since many researchers think they may be the cause of Alzheimer's. Still, the reason why this buildup occurs in the first place remains far from clear. The great hope has been that removal of this unwanted, brain-toxic debris would bring about improvement in memory and cognition and would save people from dying of Alzheimer's.

Arriving at an Alzheimer's research center with hope and excitement on May 9, 2008, Steve screened for the clinical trial but did not qualify. We were deeply disappointed, but the doctor told us we could return in a couple of weeks, and he could try again. In the meantime, another clinical trial became available for a different oral drug, semagacestat, which would help reduce further buildup of beta-amyloid plaque.

Steve was scheduled to screen for the clinical trials two days in a row, on May 20 and 21, 2008. Knowing that he could not enter two different clinical trials at the same time, I got on the internet on the evening of May 19 to look for information about the risks and benefits of the two new drugs being used in the trials. Purely by chance, I came across a press release about three promising treatments for Alzheimer's disease. One of the treatments was a prescription "medical food," called AC-1202, whose developers were working toward getting it recognized by the Food and Drug Administration (FDA), though it would not be available for another year. In their pilot study, first reported in 2004 (the year Steve was diagnosed), they tested people with mild to moderate Alzheimer's disease on two different occasions: before and after taking placebo on one day, and before and after taking AC-1202 on another day. To maintain objectivity, neither the patient nor the testers knew which substance the patients had taken on which day. (This testing process is called a "double-blind" study and is considered the gold standard for clinical drug trials.) After just a single dose of AC-1202, nearly half of the people had significantly better scores on the tests than when they were given the placebo (Reger, 2004).

The press release did not say what AC-1202 was or how it worked, but I was determined to learn more. I found the website www.freepatentsonline.com, which lists every United States patent application. Here I found the very lengthy renewal of the patent application

(Henderson, U.S. Patent #20080009467) for the medical food AC-1202, which was originally filed in 2000, the year before Steve began to have obvious symptoms. For the first time, I read about an aspect of Alzheimer's disease that I was not aware of: Some researchers consider Alzheimer's disease a type of diabetes of the brain, a problem of insulin resistance and insulin deficiency in the brain that is present at least ten to twenty years before symptoms appear. For people who eat a typical higher-carbohydrate Western diet, glucose is the primary fuel for the brain. Glucose drives a series of chemical reactions that results in production of adenosine triphosphate (ATP), which is required for nearly all of our cells to carry out their functions. For example, to flex your bicep muscle, every muscle fiber involved in that action requires ATP to contract. ATP is required again to allow the muscle to relax. We make an extraordinary amount of ATP, many kilograms on a daily basis, to carry out the numerous functions of our many different types of cells, a process called metabolism.

The brain is especially active and complex and, even though it represents only about 2 percent of our total body weight, the brain requires 20 to 25 percent of the calories we burn. ATP is needed for the neurons (brain cells) to communicate with each other and numerous other functions. Neurons require insulin and functioning insulin receptors to allow glucose to cross through the cell membrane and enter mitochondria, the miniscule factories in the cell where ATP is produced. Alzheimer's cases show a deficiency of an enzyme complex called pyruvate dehydrogenase (PDH), which is involved in the pathway between glucose and the making of ATP, as well as deficiencies of the proteins GLUT 1 and GLUT 3, which help glucose cross the blood-brain barrier and enter neurons (Simpson, 1994). It seems that there is a conspiracy against getting glucose into the brains of people with Alzheimer's disease.

A group at Brown University led by Suzanne de la Monte, PhD., performed autopsies on the brains of people who died with Alzheimer's and did not also have type 1 or type 2 diabetes. They found insulin deficiency and insulin resistance in the areas of the brain affected by Alzheimer's and coined the term "type 3 diabetes" to describe Alzheimer's disease (de la Monte, 2005). They then looked at brains at all stages of Alzheimer's and found that this problem with insulin worsens and spreads throughout the brain until it is very severe at the last stage of Alzheimer's (de la Monte, 2008).

Dr. de la Monte suggested that treatments for type 2 diabetes might benefit people with Alzheimer's. However, a different, profound idea emerged from the lab of another researcher. In the mid-1990s, Richard L. Veech, then with the National Institutes of Health in Bethesda, Maryland, began to focus on the ketones produced in the human body during starvation, looking at how ketones work and whether ketones might be useful to treat disease. He and his associates discovered that the ketone betahydroxybutyrate increases the work output of the heart while using less oxygen than when glucose is used (Sato, 1995). They learned that this ketone mimics many of the effects of insulin when glucose and insulin levels are low. In May 2000, they reported that betahydroxybutyrate protects neurons from toxins that cause Alzheimer's and Parkinson's diseases and suggested that ketones could provide alternative fuel to neurons and effectively bypass the lack of glucose uptake that occurs with these diseases (Kashiwaya, 2000). In the mid-1990s, Veech was already developing and had filed a patent for a ketone ester that could be used to treat Alzheimer's and many other diseases (World Intellectual Property Organization/1998/041200). He and others published hypothesis papers about the therapeutic implications of ketones beginning in 2001 (Veech, 2001; Cahill, 2003; VanItallie, 2003; Veech 2004).

Also, in May 2000, another researcher, Samuel Henderson, whose mother had died from Alzheimer's, filed the patent application I was now reading. He had the brilliant idea that the mild increase in ketones that occurs when medium-chain triglyceride (MCT) oil is consumed could provide alternative fuel to the brain and might be adequate to improve the memory and cognition in people with Alzheimer's disease. My mind lit up with excitement at that moment. As a neonatologist, I was very familiar with MCT oil because in the late 1970s and early 1980s we began adding it to the feedings of our very tiny premature newborns; it was easily absorbed, well-tolerated, and helped the babies grow faster. Eventually, formula companies developed formulas specifically for premature infants, adding MCT oil to the recipe to mimic human breast milk, which has a fat content that contains 10 to 17 percent medium-chain triglycerides. I also learned from the patent application that MCT oil is extracted from coconut oil and palm kernel oil. At that moment, an idea came to me about how I might be able to help Steve.

It was now 1:00 a.m. Steve was scheduled to screen for the first clinical trial at 9:00 a.m. that morning, so I did not have time to do anything about my idea. We went for the screening, and Steve scored only fourteen out of thirty points on the mini-mental status exam (MMSE), too low to qualify for the trial. We were bitterly disappointed. The doctor asked Steve to draw a clock, a standard test for Alzheimer's, and he drew a few small random circles and four numbers, not at all organized like a clock (see Figure Intro.1). The doctor advised me that Steve was on the verge of severe Alzheimer's. While I knew this in my heart, it was still a shock to hear those words. On the way home, I thought, "What do we have to lose?" and we went out of our way to pick up some coconut oil at a health food store. I did not know then that MCT oil was also available over-the-counter through the internet.

I found the fatty acid composition of coconut oil on the United States Department of Agriculture (USDA) food composition website https://ndb.nal.usda.gov/ndb and calculated what I believed to be the amount of

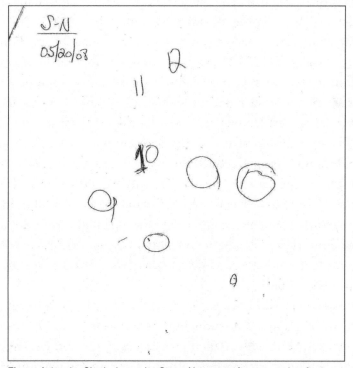

Figure Intro.1. Clock drawn by Steve Newport after screening for a clinical trial the day before starting coconut oil.

coconut oil it would take to equal the MCT content of the medical food AC-1202. In the medical food, the only active ingredient is tricaprylic acid, the medium-chain triglyceride also called C8, and the dosage was 20 grams. I figured that 35 grams of coconut oil, equivalent to 7 teaspoons, would be needed to provide this amount of MCTs. I was considering all the MCTs called C6, C8, C10, and C12 in my calculation.

The following morning, I mixed the teaspoons of coconut oil into some oatmeal, which Steve ate without hesitation. We drove to Tampa for the second clinical trial screening, and this time he gained four points on the MMSE test and qualified for the trial! We were elated. At that moment, I did not know if it was really the coconut oil, just good luck, or prayers but I decided to continue with this idea. Thereafter, I added seven level teaspoons of coconut oil to Steve's breakfast every morning and began cooking with coconut oil for other meals, finding every recipe I could get my hands on. We soon discovered coconut milk, which is mainly coconut oil, and flaked coconut. Fortunately, we liked the fragrance of coconut very much. My thinking at that point was that his brain needed ketones around the clock—a single dose of MCT in the morning, as studied in the AC-1202 clinical trial, with ketone levels peaking after just one and a half hours, didn't seem adequate to carry the brain through an entire twenty-four-hour period.

Within just a few days, it was obvious that Steve was improving in many ways. He was more energetic and talkative in the morning and could finish his sentences. He began to whistle his medleys and make jokes again. The animation returned to his face, and the jaw tremor was gone. The hand tremor disappeared after he had his first serving of coconut oil in the morning. He could fill up his glass with water from the refrigerator dispenser. He said it was as if the light switch had come on in his brain the day he started taking coconut oil and the fog lifted. Steve said he felt as if he had a future, and his depression lifted very quickly. By the fifth day, we looked at each other and said that our life had changed for the better. I got my husband back!

I contacted Dr. Veech when I learned that he was the world expert on ketones and asked him if he thought the ketones from eating coconut oil could help someone with Alzheimer's improve. He said Dr. Henderson had contacted him years earlier with the same question about MCT oil and related that he had told Henderson that he did not believe the levels of ketones would be adequate. I did not tell Veech what I was doing at that point, but I knew that coconut oil had helped Steve.

Two weeks after starting coconut oil, Steve drew another clock. This time, the clock was a large full circle with all the numbers around it and many extra lines, probably hands of the clock, messy, but a huge improvement from the day before taking coconut oil (See Figure Intro.2). I called Veech and faxed him the two clocks. He said this was quite "unexpected," sent me articles on his ketone studies, and had several other ketones researchers call me. They were all quite excited because this was the first person they were aware of with Alzheimer's who had responded to ketones as an alternative fuel for the brain. One was George Cahill, who first reported that ketone levels become very elevated during starvation in 1967 (Owen, 1967). The others were Theodore VanItallie and Sami Hashim, MD, who reported that MCT oil is converted to ketones in the liver in 1966 (Bergen, 1966).

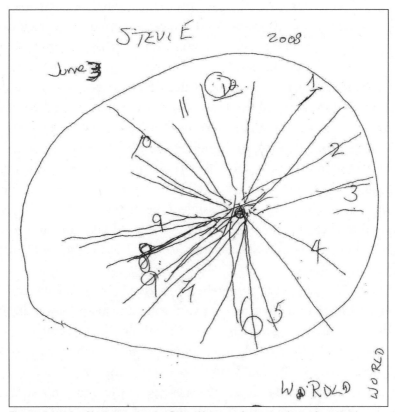

Figure Intro.2. Clock drawing by Steve Newport fourteen days after starting coconut oil.

When Steve drew this second clock, I became overwhelmed with the idea that if Steve had improved, other people with Alzheimer's might improve as well. I had a secret that I could not contain when more than 30 million people with Alzheimer's around the world needed this information. I became a messenger for ketones as an alternative fuel for the brain, starting with a letter-writing campaign. I wrote letters to former Supreme Court justice Sandra Day O'Connor, whose husband had Alzheimer's, the Alzheimer's Association, politicians, and the major news outlets, requesting that they make the public aware of this and complete clinical trials urgently, so that the millions with Alzheimer's could benefit as soon as possible. There was no response.

Six weeks after starting coconut oil, we made a trip home to visit our families in Cincinnati. Many family members remarked that Steve did not seem lost and confused compared to the previous year. He now remembered names of our nieces and his brothers-in-law; he participated in conversations, laughed, and joked. I showed everyone the two clocks he had drawn the day before and two weeks after starting coconut oil. They were amazed and confirmed that Steve's remarkable improvement was not a figment of my imagination. I decided to attend the Alzheimer's Association International Conference and wrote an article called, "What if There Was a Cure for Alzheimer's and No One Knew" and requested a table in the exhibit hall at the conference to distribute the article, which I included with the application. Five thousand Alzheimer's researchers from all over the world would be attending the conference, and we hoped to reach as many of them as possible. One or more of them might be inspired to study ketones, and many more could take this information back to their communities. I arranged to have 1,500 copies of the article printed in Chicago.

Three days before the conference, I received an email from the Alzheimer's Association advising me that they had reviewed my application again and were denying the table, even though they had accepted payment for it previously. No amount of pleading by email could convince them otherwise. They said I could attend the conference but could not pass out the articles. My plan to get the message out in a big way suffered a major setback. We went to Chicago anyway, I attended the conference, and I spoke to as many researchers as I could about ketones and Steve's experience. We passed out articles in Grant Park, left them in health food stores, and I slipped as many as I could to researchers who seemed interested. When we got home, I decided to go the grassroots route, sending the article out via the internet to everyone I knew and talking with health food store owners, who were happy to keep stacks of the articles to pass out to their customers.

Soon invitations came along to speak in local health food stores and at the hospital where I worked. When our regional newspaper ran a story about what had happened, along with a photo of us and Steve's clocks, including a third even more improved clock, the news went viral. (See Photo Intro.1.)

In the meantime, Dr. Veech asked us to arrange for a blood draw to measure Steve's ketone levels, first on a day when he took two servings of coconut oil (35 grams/2 tablespoons each) and then after one dose of pure C8 MCT oil (20 grams/4 teaspoons). The ketone levels were lower and peaked at three hours with coconut oil but were higher and peaked at ninety minutes with MCT oil. With MCT oil, the ketone levels were already back to baseline at three hours (See Figures Intro.3 and Intro.4).

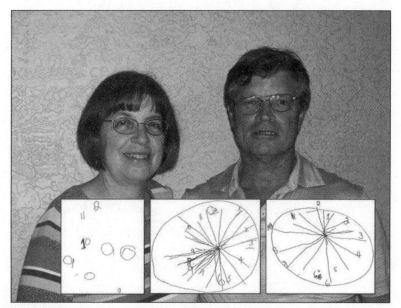

Photo Intro.1. Steve and Mary Newport with clocks drawn by Steve the day before starting coconut oil and fourteen and thirty-seven days after starting it.

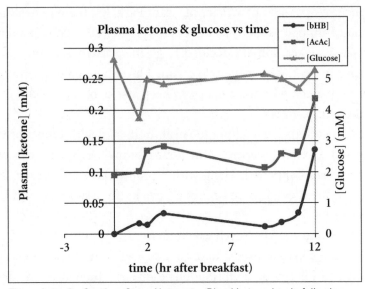

Figure Intro.3. Caption: Steve Newport—Blood ketone levels following two doses of coconut oil, 35 grams (2 tablespoons) per dose.

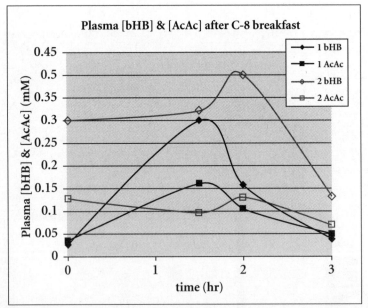

Figure Intro.4. Caption: Blood ketone levels for Steve Newport (lower line) and FO (upper line) after taking 20 grams (4 tablespoons) of tricaprylic acid (C8).

Veech suggested that I give Steve only MCT oil and forget the coconut oil, however, I was reluctant to do that, since he had responded so well to coconut oil alone in the very beginning. I thought coconut oil could conceivably contain one or more nutrients that might enhance the effect of the medium-chain triglycerides or be beneficial in some other way.

I began to give Steve both MCT oil and coconut oil, at first separately, but then I noticed that if I combined the oils, the mixture stayed liquid at room temperature. I experimented with various proportions of the oils and found that a 4:3 ratio of MCT oil to coconut oil worked particularly well for several reasons. Most important, however, Steve continued to improve. He screened again for another clinical trial, and his MMSE score increased further from a score of 18 on May 21, 2008, to a score of 20 (out of 30 points) on July 27, 2008. His gait normalized, and he was able to pick up his feet and run again. His tremors were essentially gone, and his speech was more fluent. When he took pure C8 MCT oil alone, he would sometimes have diarrhea, but he tolerated the mixture of the oils very well. Coconut oil is solid at 75° F (24° C) and below and, even if melted first, tends to chunk up as soon as it touches anything cold. This 4:3 mixture of MCT and coconut oil is liquid at room temperature, can be stored at room temperature, and does not harden when added to cold foods, making it very versatile. It can be added to many different foods such as coffee, tea, smoothies, yogurt, cottage cheese, ricotta, salad and other vegetables, soup, or chili. It also can be used to cook on the stove at low to medium-low heat or mixed into foods to bake at 350° F (177° C) or below. I soon began to add soy lecithin to emulsify the mixture, which breaks lipid globules down so that they can be digested more easily. At the same time lecithin contains phospholipids, such as phosphatidylcholine, that are abundant in the brain and important to brain function. The 4:3 ratio also reduces the heavier long-chain saturated fats from coconut oil to less than 10 percent of the total fats. Steve very slowly increased his intake of coconut oil and the MCT/coconut oil mixture to 11 tablespoons (165 ml) per day divided into four servings, and at the same time, greatly reduced his intake of bread, pasta, rice and fruit, effectively placing him on a ketogenic diet.

By the end of July 2008, Steve qualified for both clinical trials, and we were given a choice of the two drugs: the intravenous vaccine bapineuzumab or the oral medication semagacestat. We chose the oral medication since the clinical trial was a crossover study, meaning that if he was on placebo initially, he would be placed on the study drug at about twelve to fourteen months into the study. I advised the researcher of our dietary intervention and Steve's response to it. This group participated in a clinical trial of the MCT oil medical food AC-1202 (Axona®), and they were well aware of the scientific basis, but they did not believe it would interfere with the results of their study and accepted Steve anyway. This was a miracle for us . . . at last there was hope! We later learned that he was on the placebo during the initial twelve to fourteen months, and he had considerable testing during that time. During the first year in the trial, he had a net improvement of six points on the seventy-five point Alzheimer's Disease Assessment Scale-Cognitive and improved by fourteen points on the seventy-eight point Activities of Daily Living test (a lower score is better). We could clearly see these results in his day-to-day functioning. The only thing that could account for this improvement was the dietary intervention with coconut oil and MCT oil.

By three to four months after starting coconut oil (and then adding MCT oil), Steve was taking at least two tablespoons per serving three times a day. One day, he announced that he could read again and, for the first time, could explain why he was unable to read for the past couple of years. He explained that the words would "go into little boxes, like pixels" and jump around on the page. But that had stopped now, and he could actually read again. By nine months after coconut oil, he would talk about events that occurred several weeks before and could recall what he had read earlier in the day and tell me about it. Invitations to speak at health food stores and assisted living facilities became more frequent, and Steve came along, answering questions and engaging with members of the audience after the presentations. Steve improved so much that he yearned to go back to work and became a volunteer in the warehouse of the hospital where I worked, putting stickers onto supplies and helping with deliveries to the various nursing units. I am so grateful to Chuck and the other staff who supervised Steve and gave him so much encouragement. A photo of Steve working in the warehouse accompanied a second article on Steve's response to ketones, published by our regional newspaper, the *St. Petersburg Times* (now the *Tampa Bay Times*) in the fall of 2009 (See Photo Intro.2).

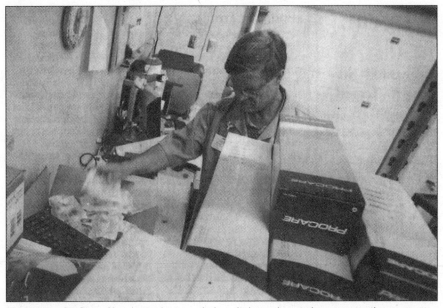

Photo Intro.2. Steve Newport volunteers in hospital supply warehouse more than one year after starting coconut and MCT oil.

DR. VEECH'S KETONE ESTER TO THE RESCUE

During the second half of 2009, Steve's improvement seemed to level off, but then around February and March of 2010, some new problems emerged. By this time, we were quite sure that he was on the study drug semagacestat—his hair was growing out in a light gold color, a common side effect of the drug. He began to have a problem with wound healing, bleeding, and fainting shortly before we were to travel to Greece where I was to give an oral presentation on Steve's case report. With mixed feelings, we made the very difficult decision to withdraw Steve from the study.

We received a phone call several months after withdrawing from the study advising us that the semagacestat clinical trial was discontinued because the drug was found to cause *accelerated worsening of the disease* (Doody, 2013). This explained some of the changes we saw that spring. The irony is that Steve qualified for the trial, thanks to coconut oil, only to be placed on a drug that would make his Alzheimer's disease worse, not better. He was fortunate to be on the placebo for at least the first twelve of the eighteen months he was in the study. This story would be very different (and I would not be writing this at all) if he had been placed on the clinical trial drug at the beginning of the study.

Further compounding the apparent damage from semagacestat, which manifested as deterioration of his ability to do everyday tasks, Steve's father died in March 2010, sending him back into depression. In addition, he developed a respiratory infection accompanied by an outbreak of fever blisters (herpes simplex virus 1), which we had rarely seen after he started taking coconut oil two years earlier. He had frequent prolonged outbreaks before starting coconut oil, and research supports the possibility that this virus may cause Alzheimer's in some people (Itzhaki, 2008). In addition to worsening depression, he once again began to require help from me with step-by-step instruction for showering, dressing, and shaving. If left to his own devices, he would put on mismatched clothes, often inside out or backward. He lost interest in yard work and helping with housework. He was sometimes lost in the house, and, worse, he began to wander from home, looking for his brothers who he thought were just over the hill, when, in reality, they lived more than 900 miles away. His volunteer work at the hospital was no longer possible. One day we were looking in the mirror together, and he told me that I looked like myself, and that he looked like himself from the neck down, but that the face in the mirror was not his own . . . very startling. This gradually evolved into him seeing his recently deceased father when he looked in the mirror and, later, him becoming distressed when he caught images in windows darkened by the night. He talked to his "father" in the mirror and to people on the television screen. After improving so much, it was heartbreaking to see so much decline over just a few months.

But then Dr. Veech came to our rescue. We had maintained close contact throughout this nearly two-year period; I learned so much from him. Toxicity testing had already been completed on his ketone ester (Clarke, 2012) but funding for mass production and clinical testing was not forthcoming. This particular ketone ester is a combination of the ketone betahydroxybutyrate with butanediol. After consumption and absorption, these two molecules split apart and the butanediol is converted to more betahydroxybutyrate . . . genius! Veech was able to make just enough ketone ester in his lab to complete his work and help one person. After learning of Steve's deterioration, he chose Steve for a pilot study of one person using his ketone ester. In my wildest dreams, I never imagined this would really happen. The day the package of ketone ester arrived on our doorstep was one of the happiest days of our lives. Not only did the ketone ester turn Steve's condition around again, but the ester gave us twenty more months of relative stability before the next serious setback occurred.

The main drawback to the ketone ester in its raw form is the breathtaking "jet fuel" taste, even when diluted. But Steve was determined to give it a go—he was still so well aware of his disease—and he consented with full cooperation and anticipation. Veech believed 150 grams per day would be most beneficial to someone with Alzheimer's, however, the supply was very limited, so we started with 65 grams divided into three daily doses. Beginning about two hours after knocking back the very first dose, Steve's mood became euphoric, and he was very talkative. He was determined to say and write out the entire alphabet, which he had been unable to do for several months. After trying repeatedly for twenty minutes, he succeeded in both speaking and writing out the alphabet. Trying over and over for twenty minutes to complete this task was amazing in and of itself. He pulled the name of his first-grade teacher out of thin air, blaming her for his self-proclaimed atrocious handwriting. The next morning, it was apparent that he was able to "do things" again. He showered, shaved, picked out his clothes, and dressed himself without prompting.

After several days, the dose of the ketone ester was increased to 85 grams per day divided into three doses. I tried many ways to disguise the overpowering taste of the ketone ester. I was determined to find something sugar-free, however, everything without sugar added bitterness, making the taste even worse. I found that orange or cranberry Soda Stream concentrate provided a relatively good cover-up for the taste. It bothered me immensely that we had to add sugar to the ester to make it drinkable. As it turns out, this may have been somewhat fortuitous, since, in a recent study of athletic performance and the ketone ester, performance was improved if glucose was added as well (Cox, 2016).

Over the next days to weeks through the spring and summer of 2010, Steve resumed activities such as yard work, washing dishes, and vacuuming, and he was able to choose food from a menu. Abstract thinking, a sense of humor, and insight returned to his conversation. He brought up events that happened a week or so earlier. He told me that he felt "good," that he was "happier," and that he found it "easier to do things," all of which aligned with my observations. To be clear, we continued plenty of MCT and coconut oil throughout this time, along with the ketone ester. After the first twenty months, there were sometimes weeks or a few months where the supply of the ketone ester was low, and Steve would take much less to stretch out the supply until it was available again.

We measured Steve's betahydroxybutyrate (BHB) level periodically and at various doses using a Precision Xtra ketone monitor (See Figure Intro.5) and also measured his glucose level with another monitor at the same time. With a dose of 25 grams, his BHB level peaked at 3 millimoles per liter (mmol/L) one hour later and was back to baseline three to four hours later. At 50 grams, the BHB level reached 7 mmol/L, much higher than the 4 to 5 mmol/L level that Veech believes is needed to provide benefit. Another interesting observation was that Steve's glucose level would drop from the 90–100 milligrams per deciliter (mg/dL) range to the 70–80 mg/dL range

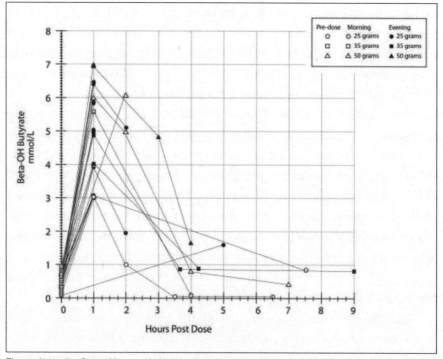

Figure Intro.5. Steve Newport's betahydroxybutyrate levels with Precision Xtra at various doses of ketone ester.

after taking the ketone ester, regardless of what he had eaten after taking it and in spite of flavoring with the sugary Soda Stream concentrate to disguise the taste. I often wonder how many type 2 diabetics could benefit from taking the ketone ester and potentially no longer require insulin and/ or oral medications.

Steve's case report while taking medium-chain triglycerides and then receiving Veech's ketone ester was published in the journal *Alzheimer's and Dementia* in January 2015 and can be printed out for free from PubMed.gov. I am very proud to be first author on this report with Dr. Richard Veech, Dr. Theodore VanItallie, Dr. Yoshiro Kashiwaya, and Todd King (Newport, 2015). Our daughter Joanna Newport Rand designed the mitochondria figure in the article demonstrating the entry of glucose and ketones into the metabolic pathway that produces ATP (See Figure Intro.6).

For more than three and a half years from when Steve began taking coconut oil in mid-2008, life was much better than it had been the year before he started taking coconut oil. His condition began to decline again

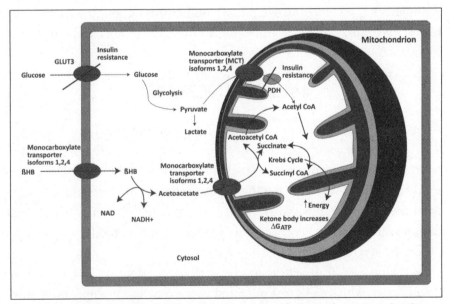

Figure Intro.6. When there is insulin resistance or other blocks to glucose entering the mitochondria, ketones can bypass this blockade by using monocarboxylate transporters to enter the mitochondria and fuel the tricarboxylic acid (TCA) cycle to make adenosine triphosphate (ATP).]

in January 2012 related to serious side effects of medications and, later, seizures, which are common in the later stages of Alzheimer's, and he was admitted to the hospital twice over the next two years. Still, with the help of caregivers, we managed to keep him at home rather than placing him in assisted living. After all, Steve had stayed home by choice to take care of me and our children; I owed so much to him. How could I put him in assisted living? The end started one morning in December 2015 when he began to breathe rapidly and became barely responsive. He hung in there long enough for his mother and sister to come from Cincinnati and say their goodbyes. In the early evening of January 2, 2016, his breathing suddenly slowed. As we held him, Steve took his last breath to a very meaningful and fitting song, "Hymn for the Departed," by Dave Thomas Jr.

Steve lived with Alzheimer's for fifteen years from the time we first noticed his symptoms. The average lifespan after diagnosis is seven years. We were grateful to have at least three to four extra good years, thanks to ketones as an alternative fuel for his brain. Steve donated his brain to the Florida Brain Bank, for study in a clinical trial for dementia. We felt a sense of closure when an autopsy revealed that, yes, he did have end-stage Alzheimer's disease. He also had Lewy bodies throughout the limbic system of his brain, which accounted for his unusual tremors and sensitivity to medications.

A MESSENGER FOR KETONES

After Steve's improvement from coconut oil became obvious, I became a lonely messenger for the idea of ketones as an alternative fuel for the brain. I passed out copies of the article I had written and talked to whoever would listen. Thanks to my family, Steve's excellent caregivers, the internet, print media, radio show hosts, podcasters, and *The 700 Club* (which had done a segment about Steve's positive reaction to coconut oil), the message picked up steam.

A major part of my effort has been to draw attention to Dr. Veech's ketone ester, which has great potential to prevent and possibly even cure Alzheimer's disease in the earlier stages; however, it lacks funding for mass production and clinical testing. With Dr. Veech's encouragement, I decided to write a book. The first edition of that book, *Alzheimer's Disease: What if There Was a Cure? The Story of Ketones*, was released in the fall of 2011, with the second edition published in 2013.

As I learned more about the serious problem of eating too much sugar and the many benefits of low-carbohydrate eating, it was time to write a second book, *The Coconut Oil and Low-Carb Solution for Alzheimer's, Parkinson's and Other Diseases* (Turner Publishing, 2015). The main point of the second book is to offer a practical guide to reducing sugar in the diet using a whole foods approach and combining that with coconut and MCT oil to increase ketones as alternative fuel for the brain. This is not a strict ketogenic diet but teaches people how to plan out their diets so that they eat adequate protein, healthy fats, and aim for carbohydrates intake of less than 60 grams per day, mainly as vegetables, berries, and small portions of whole grains.

The development of ketone salts in the lab of Dominic D'Agostino, PhD at University of South Florida (USF), has taken awareness of the potential benefits of "ketosis" (elevated ketones) to a whole new level. I first met D'Agostino in 2009. Steve's story struck a chord for him because he was studying the possibility of using a ketogenic diet to prevent seizures in Navy SEALs during exposure to 100 percent oxygen when they deep dive. We became friends and co-messengers for ketones. (See Chapter 5 for more about D'Agostino's work, and Chapters 7 and 10 for more about ketone salts.)

Invitations to speak stemming from the translations of my books have taken me to places I never dreamed I would see, including Japan, Germany, France, Singapore, Thailand, Australia, and New Zealand, to name a few. With each trip, I have the opportunity to introduce a new culture to the idea of ketones as an alternative fuel for the brain through the simple dietary interventions of coconut oil and MCT oil. For some of these populations, coconut has been a staple in their diet for generations. For others, using coconut oil is a new idea.

This book, *The Complete Book of Ketones: A Practical Guide to Ketogenic Diets and Ketone Supplements*, provides a broad range of information about the history of ketone research, what ketones do, ketogenic diets, exogenous ketone supplements and other strategies to enhance ketosis. As awareness of the potential benefits of ketosis increases, the scientific research in this area has been growing exponentially. The potential applications of ketosis are so diverse that this lifestyle change can help a person lose weight, can bring about improvement in a variety of medical conditions, and can even enhance sports performance, since fat, from which ketones are produced, can supply a nearly endless source of fuel for the serious endurance athlete. This book is intended for people who are interested in learning more about the many potential benefits of ketosis, including parents of children and teens, as well as adults of all ages who are overweight or dealing with pre-diabetes or type 2 diabetes, people with inflammatory conditions or neurodegenerative diseases, athletes ranging from weekend warriors to elite professionals, and the larger group of people who just want to improve their overall general health and well-being.

This book reviews the scientific basis and evidence for each of the potential benefits of ketones and provides anecdotes and testimonials of individuals who have personally experienced these benefits for themselves or their loved ones. The book explores several strategies for increasing ketone levels from mild to maximum, pointing to a spectrum of low-carbohydrate and ketogenic diets, the use of special foods such as coconut and MCT oil, and other ketogenic substances and supplements, such as ketone salts and ketone esters. It also takes a look at the way exercise can enhance the state of ketosis.

It is possible to implement these strategies separately or in combination, and the book gives special attention to consideration of the individual's age and health status. Common concerns and questions about ketogenic diets and exogenous ketone supplements are addressed, such as effects on hydration, blood pressure, electrolyte balance, and worries about diabetic ketoacidosis. The book also touches on the ongoing debate about cholesterol, saturated fats and heart disease. For the science-minded, I've included citations for the scientific articles mentioned. And I've included a section of recipes and a list of resources such as books, articles, helpful organizations, websites, and sources for special ketogenic foods and supplements.

As I travel around the world telling Steve's story, I become emotional when I see his sweet, handsome face on the screen during my presentation. Steve would be thrilled to know how many people have already benefited from his story. He fully embraced the idea of taking coconut and MCT oils and, later, Dr. Veech's ketone ester. Not every spouse or caregiver has such a willing accomplice in the fight against Alzheimer's. The story of ketones is Steve Newport's legacy to the world. I am his messenger.

CHAPTER 1

WHY GO KETO?

"Ketones are a high-energy fuel that nourish the brain."
"Ketones are evolution's survival
mechanism for starvation."
—Theodore VanItallie
(Hosley-Moore, 2008; Nohlgren, 2009)

"Going keto" isn't really a new idea; it's just a new way of saying it. It is very likely that our ancient ancestors throughout most of evolution were in a state of ketosis (that is, they had elevated levels of ketones in their system) much, if not most, of the time because of the many days and weeks when food was scarce, and they relied on their stored fat to survive.

Ketones are an end product of breaking down that stored fat, and they can serve as a fuel for the brain and nearly all of our other organs, except the liver, where ketones are made. The ability to switch from using glucose to using fatty acids and ketones as fuel is likely a major factor in the survival of humans as a species to the modern day. Our large and complex brains require substantial fuel to operate. If we were limited to using glucose for fuel, we would not be able to survive for more than seven to ten days of starvation, since we would break down muscle rapidly and become too weak to breathe within that short time frame. Because we have stored fat and can use fatty acids and ketones for fuel, we can survive for forty to sixty days or even longer depending on how fat we are as long as we have enough water to drink. Long-chain fatty acids can provide fuel for most of our organs in this situation; however, they do not cross the blood-brain barrier very well, so the brain is highly dependent on the availability of ketones to survive.

The best evidence suggests that life appeared on Earth more than 3.5 billion years ago, and the ketone betahydroxybutyrate (BHB) was there at the very beginning, fueling the simplest one-celled organisms that still exist today. If we fast forward rapidly through evolution to the modern day, humans and many other creatures large and small continue to have the ability to use ketones as a powerful, effective and efficient fuel, but most of us are not taking full advantage of the many benefits that a state of ketosis could provide.

A striking difference between human life in ancient times and life now is that most of us have an abundance of food and an overabundance of food choices that our very distant relatives could not begin to imagine. We have something today that our ancient predecessors didn't have—sugar and lots of it! Well, actually, they had a little bit of sugar when they were able to find sugar cane, beets, tubers, berries, seasonal fruits and other starchy foods. But it would take many hours of chewing on a tall stick of fibrous sugar cane to get the same amount of carbohydrate we can knock back in a few minutes from drinking a can of Coca-Cola. Since modern humans as a group tend to eat a lot of sugar, the primary fuel for our brain and other organs on this type of diet is glucose. We do not use our stored fat very much unless we deliberately cut down on food to lose weight, so most of us do not spent much time in ketosis.

Sugar is a big problem in today's world. Rates of diabetes are growing rapidly. The Centers for Disease Control (CDC) reported in 2017 that more than 100 million adults in the United States have diabetes or pre-diabetes, with diabetes at 30.3 million or 9.4 percent and pre-diabetes at 84.1 million or an astonishing 26 percent of Americans. Pre-diabetes can lead to diabetes within five years if not treated. Diabetes stands as the seventh leading cause of death (Alzheimer's is in sixth place) (CDC, 2017). The United States has the highest rate of obesity in the English-speaking world. Between 1960 and 2014, the rate of obesity tripled in U.S. adults and nearly quadrupled in children and adolescents, and the rate of extreme obesity in the United States increased nearly seven-fold. Today, two out of three American adults are considered to be overweight or obese according to the National Health and Nutrition Examination Survey (NHANES). (See Figure 1.1).

Eating more calories than we can burn is the main culprit in the obesity epidemic, but eating the wrong kinds of calories is a big contributor to the problem as well. Food manufacturers and fast food restaurants have become so good at making us want more, that we simply eat more. CDC survey data show that the average intake of food in the United States increased from 2,100 calories per day in 1970 to more than 2,500 calories per day by 2006, and that obese Americans eat 33 percent more

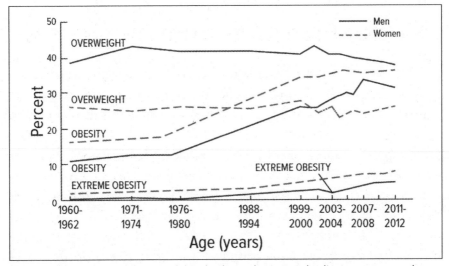

Figure 1.1. Trends in adult overweight, obesity, and extreme obesity among men and women aged 20–74: United States, selected years 1960–1962 through 2011–2012. From https://www.cdc.gov/nchs/data/hestat/obesity_adult_11_12/obesity_adult_11_12.htm

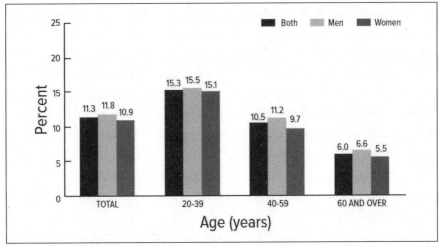

Figure 1.2. Percentage of calories from fast food among adults aged 20 and over, by sex and age, United States 2007–2010. From https://www.cdc.gov/nchs/products/databriefs/db114.htm.

calories from fast food than normal weight Americans (See Figure 1.2). With about 3,500 calories to a pound of body fat, eating that extra 400 calories per day can add another pound every nine days. No wonder so many of us are struggling to get slim and stay slim. This is almost certainly the first time in the history of humans that large populations take in more calories on average than they can possibly burn.

DR. WESTON A. PRICE RECOGNIZES THAT POOR FOOD CAUSES DISEASE

Individuals with great foresight have alerted us along the way that we were heading toward the crisis of obesity and related diseases that we are experiencing now. One of the earliest spokespersonS was dentist Weston A. Price (1870–1948), who recognized that nutritional deficiencies often play a prominent role in disease. He published his seminal book, *Nutrition and Physical Degeneration: A Comparison of Primitive and Modern Diets and Their Effects* in 1939, the culmination of years of travel during which he studied many different cultures throughout the world. He acquired more than 15,000 photographs, 4,000 slides, and many filmstrips in the process. He found that more primitive non-Western populations were nearly free of dental decay and the poorly developed facial structure that comes with crowding of teeth, compared to their Western counterparts, and he provided photographic evidence in his book.

Price was one of the first to recognize that many diseases common in Western cultures, such as dental caries and tuberculosis, were rare in non-Western populations and that people from non-Western societies were acquiring these problems as they abandoned their native diet to adopt a more Western diet. He blamed the heavy reliance in the Western diet on commercially prepared and stored flours, sugars, and processed vegetable fats, which are stripped of vitamins and minerals needed to prevent dental decay and many other diseases. The Weston A. Price Foundation and the Price-Pottenger Nutrition Foundation perpetuate Dr. Price's research, and Price is often considered to be the initiator of the movements of holistic dentistry and medicine.

Nearly a century after Price began to focus on excessive intake of nutrient-poor refined flour (which is mainly carbohydrate) and sugar as a cause of disease, our diet has changed so drastically and the balance of the food scale is leaning so far in the direction of way too much carbohydrate. More people than ever are too large to get weighed on standard scales, and our statistics are flying off the charts with ever-growing epidemics of obesity, diabetes, and metabolic syndrome, which lead to a plethora of chronic conditions.

The rates of Alzheimer's disease and autism have been steadily climbing along with the spread of the sugar-laden, low-fat Western diet throughout the world. Stephan Guyenet, PhD, an obesity researcher, neurobiologist and author of *The Hungry Brain*, graphed the intake of added sugar in the United States over nearly two hundred years using U.S. Department of Agriculture data and U.S. Department of Commerce reports. He found that our intake of added sugar (the sugar we add to foods, not the naturally occurring sugar contained in foods) increased from about 6.3 pounds per person per year in 1822 to 107.7 pounds per person per year by 1999 (See Figure 1.3). In a blog post dated February 18, 2012, Guyenet points out, "In 1822, we ate the amount of added sugar in one 12-ounce can of soda every five days, while today we eat that much sugar every seven hours" (Guyenet, 2012).

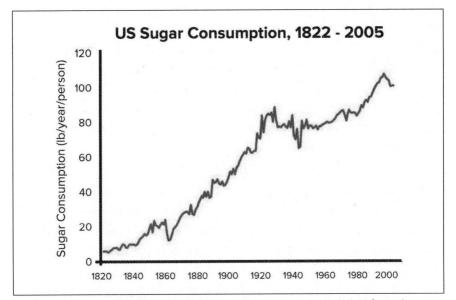

Figure 1.3. The massive increase in added-sugar consumption in the United States between 1820 and 2000. With permission from Stephan Guyenet, PhD from Guyenet, S., Blog Post: "By 2606, the U.S. diet will be 100 percent sugar." *Whole Health Source: Nutrition and Health Science* www.wholehealthsource.blogspot.com, February 18, 2012

"In 1822, we ate the amount of added sugar in
one 12-ounce can of soda every five days,
while today we eat that much sugar every seven hours."
—Stephan Guyenet, PhD (Guyenet, 2012).

In large part, added sugar consists of sucrose, which is also called table sugar, and high-fructose corn syrup. Other sources of excessive sugar intake are refined flours, which are mainly non-fiber carbohydrates. If you are on a typical Western diet, it is very likely that you are eating something made from flour with virtually every meal and snack. Think cereals, pastries, breads, pastas, crackers, and cookies. If you eat white rice, you are getting about 90 percent of the calories from that rice in the form of non-fiber carbs.

Until the last two centuries, table sugar was available only to the wealthiest people, and so it has come very late in our evolutionary development. When we eat table sugar and other simple sugars, our glucose levels increase rapidly and our insulin levels spike shortly thereafter. The hormone insulin is needed to get glucose into our cells for fuel, but it also enables excess glucose to be stored in the form of glycogen. Table sugar is roughly half glucose and half fructose, which is far and away the sweetest of all sugars. This factored into the creation of high-fructose corn syrup (HFCS), which is made very inexpensively from cornstarch and was first marketed to the public around 1970. Consumption of HFCS, which appears in most soft drinks and many processed foods, has taken off from zilch before 1970 to more than 40 pounds per year now for the average person in the United States.

In addition to table sugar and HFCS, other foods that are naturally high in fructose include agave nectar, honey, molasses, maple syrup, fruit, and fruit juices. A surprising fact about fructose is that when we have an adequate supply of glucose stored as glycogen in our liver, the remaining breakdown products of fructose will be redirected to make triglycerides. (See Figure 1.4.) Triglycerides are the primary form taken by the fats in our bodies. The average adult human is about 22 to 30 percent fat and most of our stored fat is in the form of triglycerides. Triglycerides are also present in the bloodstream as a way to transport fats from organs such as the liver to other organs and tissues in the body. A triglyceride consists of three

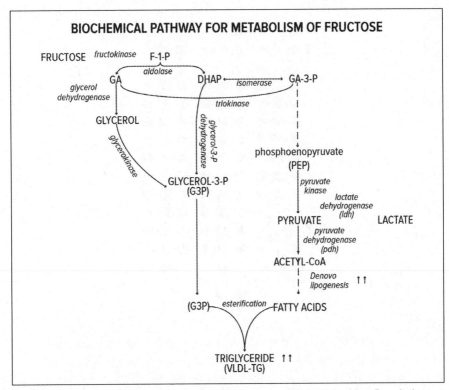

Figure 1.4. Biochemical pathway for conversion of fructose to triglycerides. Permission granted on Wikipedia page by NuFS San Jose State University on https://commons. wikimedia.org/w/index.php?curid=3934560.

fatty acid molecules attached to a glycerol molecule (see Figure 1.5). They are broken down to release the fatty acids for an abundance of important uses in the body; for example, fatty acids and proteins may combine to form the phospholipids that make up every cell membrane in the body and control what goes in and out of the cell. Also, during fasting, starvation or ketogenic diet, triglycerides in our stored fat are broken down into fatty acids, some of which are converted to ketones, which can readily be used by the brain and most other organs as fuel in place of glucose.

Triglycerides are not inherently "bad" but are important and necessary to the structure and function of our organs and tissues. The worry about triglycerides comes into play when levels in the blood are too high. This can result in overproduction of small, dense LDL particles, which induce inflammation and may place us at greater risk of heart disease from atherosclerosis, the abnormal build up of plaque in arteries (Ivanova, 2017).

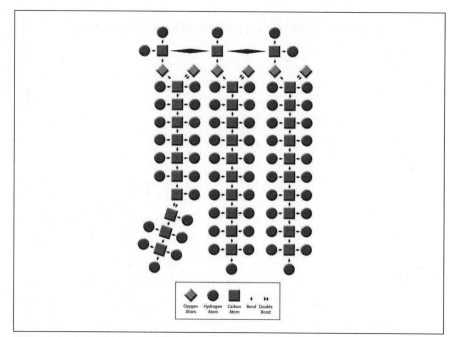

Figure 1.5. A triglyceride consists of three fatty acid molecules attached to a glycerol molecule as the backbone. The positioning of each specific fatty acid on the glycerol backbone can affect the properties of the triglyceride, such as absorption rate from the bowel.

It is a misconception that high triglyceride levels in the blood come strictly from too much fat intake. Very often triglyceride levels become elevated from eating either too much sugar or too many calories; simply cutting down on sugar intake can often bring a person's triglyceride level down. In addition to the obesity and diabetes issues, some other problems related to too much fructose consumption include high blood pressure, gout, and non-alcoholic fatty liver disease.

You can avoid consuming added sugar by looking closely at the list of ingredients in packaged foods and, even better, by focusing on eating whole foods—real unadulterated vegetables and fruits, whole grains, legumes, and nuts, instead of the highly processed packaged versions. A big advantage to eating whole foods is that they contain the naturally occurring forms of vitamins and a host of phytonutrients to support our metabolism as opposed to the synthetic vitamins found in many supplements, white flour, and packaged foods. Many infant formulas and toddler foods even contain synthetic vitamins. How can we be certain these foods contain no hormones, antibiotics, or pesticides when they are not labeled organic? Also, in contrast to the spikes in blood-insulin levels induced by simple sugars, complex sugars, such as those found in whole grains, are digested more slowly, and the insulin level rises more slowly in response. Repeated chronic spikes in glucose and insulin set us up for insulin resistance, which is found in pre-diabetes and type 2 diabetes mellitus (See Figures 1.6 and 1.7).

If you are not convinced yet to give up sodas, sugary fruit juices, and refined flour, here are a few studies that might persuade you. A very large population study published in 2013 made it quite clear that, on average, the more sugar a person eats, the greater is the likelihood of developing diabetes (Basu, 2013). Basu and others completed an analysis of data for 175 countries, collected from 2000 to 2010, comparing food supply data with prevalence of diabetes in each of these countries. The food supply data was published by the United Nations Food and Agricultural Organization to capture availability of total food and specific foods including

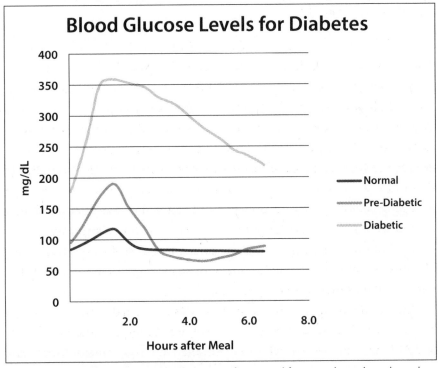

Figure 1.6. Typical response of blood glucose after a meal for normal people and people with pre-diabetes and diabetes. (Graphic by Joanna Newport.)

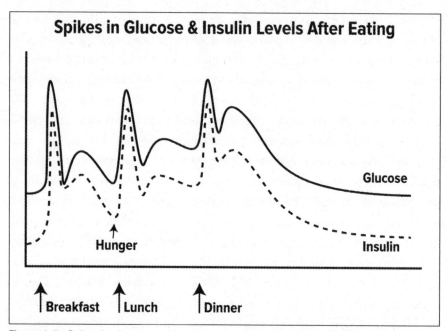

Figure 1.7. Spikes in glucose and insulin occur after eating high-carbohydrate meals. (Graphic by Joanna Newport).

sugars, fibers, fruits, meats, cereals, oils in kilocalories per person per day in each country for each year of the analysis. They used estimates of diabetes prevalence for people ages 20 to 79 years old reported by the International Diabetes Federation. Overall, the prevalence of diabetes increased 27 percent over the ten-year period. They found that an increase in total calories of 150 per person per day in a population related to an increase in prevalence of diabetes of just 0.1 percent, which was not statistically significant. However, an increase of 150 calories per person per day rise in sugar availability (one 12-ounce can of soft drink) was associated with a 1.1 percent rise in diabetes prevalence, which is very significant.

The bottom line is that as sugar became more available to certain populations and annual per capita intake of sugar increased as a result, the rate of diabetes increased proportionately.

The Adult Changes in Thought Study was published in the prestigious *New England Journal of Medicine* in 2013. Researchers studied outcomes of 2,067 men and women who were enrolled at Group Health for at least five years and had at least five measurements of glycated hemoglobin documented. Glycated hemoglobin, often called hemoglobin A1C or

HbA1C, is a measure of glucose contained within red blood cells and provides a three-month average of plasma blood sugar. Over the median follow-up period of 6.8 years, 524 of the subjects developed dementia. The study found that non-diabetics with blood sugars averaging 115 mg/dl (6.4 mm/L) over the preceding five years were more likely (1.18 to 1 odds) to have dementia than those with blood glucose of 100 mg/dl (5.5 mm/L). Diabetics with an average blood glucose of 190 mg/dL (10.5 mm/L) over the preceding five years were much more likely (1.4 to 1 odds) to develop dementia than diabetics with better control and average blood glucose of 160 mg/dl (8.9 mm/L) (Crane, 2013).

A study of brain aging and sweet drinks provides very compelling evidence that excessive sugar intake may increase risk of dementia. Matthew Pase, PhD, and others published a report in which they looked at middle-aged participants (53 to 56 years old) in the Framingham Heart Study to determine if consuming sugary drinks—including sugar-sweetened soft drinks, fruit drinks with added sugar, and 100 percent fruit juice— was associated with signs of pre-clinical Alzheimer's (the point at which Alzheimer's is underway but symptoms are not yet obvious) and vascular injury. Every two years the participants underwent an MRI (4,276 people) and/or neuropsychological testing (3,846 people). Researchers also looked at intake of diet soft drinks for comparison. They found that consumption of one or more sugary drinks per day resulted in lower total brain volume, lower hippocampal volume (hippocampus is an important part of the brain for memory and is also where the process of Alzheimer's disease starts), and worse scores on delayed-recall memory testing (the ability to remember something, such as a list of words, after a distraction). The brain shrinks a little bit each year as we age, but the shrinkage appeared to be accelerated in certain of the study subjects: people who consumed one to two sugary drinks per day experienced the equivalent of 1.6 years of brain aging per year, and people who drank more than two sugary drinks experienced the equivalent of 2.0 years of brain aging per year. The test of delayed-memory recall was equivalent to 5.8 years of brain aging for people who consumed one to two sugary drinks per day, and an astounding 11.0 years of brain aging for those who consumed more than two sugary drinks per day. People who consumed three or more sugary drinks per day experienced 2.6 years of brain aging based on shrinkage of the brain, and 13.0 years of brain aging for the delayed-recall memory test. These data are all compared to people who did not consume sugary beverages (Pase, 2017).

If you are worried about heart disease, which accounts for one in three deaths in the United States, about 800,000 per year, here is another study to think about. The PURE Study, an enormous undertaking, published in *The Lancet* in 2017, was conducted in eighteen countries on five continents worldwide with 135,335 participants who were studied for an average of 7.4 years (Dehghan, 2017). One of their findings relevant here is that higher carbohydrate intake was associated with a higher risk of overall, total mortality. They also found that higher intake of total fat and of each type of fat, including saturated fat, was associated with a *lower than average risk of dying* prematurely and was not associated with a higher risk of heart disease, heart attacks, or heart-related deaths. Higher-saturated fat intake was associated with a lower risk of stroke as well. This flies in the face of what the American Heart Association has preached since the 1960s: that we should eat a low-fat diet, which, more often than not, is a high-carbohydrate diet.

The bottom line is that if you do not want to experience accelerated brain aging and/or die younger than necessary, it is time to give up excessive sugar, sugary soft drinks, and fruit juice, including 100 percent fruit juice.

A number of other studies strongly suggest that changing from a higher-carbohydrate to a lower-carbohydrate diet could be very beneficial to our health. Just one of these studies reports that, when people with type 2 diabetes make the change to a very low-carb, high-fat diet, within a matter of weeks, they begin to see a drop in their fasting blood sugar, hemoglobin A1c (an indication of average glucose levels), a drop in total cholesterol, LDL cholesterol, and triglycerides, as well as improved HDL cholesterol and weight loss (Dashti, 2006). In addition, they are often able to reduce or even eliminate the need for insulin and other glucose-lowering medications, sometimes within two or three weeks.

Eric Westman, MD, one of the authors of *A New Atkins for a New You* (2010) has spent years taking care of people with obesity and type 2 diabetes mellitus, using the very-low-carbohydrate diet as the backbone for disease management. He provides patients with a simple one-page list of foods to avoid and foods to eat. At the beginning of a 2015 article (Feinman, 2015) encouraging the low-carbohydrate diet as the first approach to dietary management of diabetes, Westman is quoted as saying, "At the end of our clinic day, we go home thinking, 'The clinical improvements are so large and so obvious, why don't other doctors understand?' Patients easily grasp carbohydrate restriction: Because carbohydrates in the diet raise the blood glucose, and as diabetes is defined by high blood glucose, it makes sense to lower the carbohydrate in the diet. By reducing the carbohydrate in the diet, we have been able to taper patients off as much as 150 units of insulin per day in eight days, with marked improvement in glycemic control-even normalization of glycemic parameters." In this article, they present twelve points supporting the use of this type of diet, citing numerous studies that support this approach, showing improvements in blood levels and health outcomes. They point out studies showing that carbohydrate has more effect on plasma saturated fat levels than dietary fats do, and that restricting carbohydrates is "the most effective method (other than starvation) of reducing serum triglycerides and increasing high-density lipoproteins [HDL]." They note that even people with type 1 diabetes, which requires insulin injections for life, can reduce how much insulin they need by adhering to a carbohydrate-restricted diet.

Metabolic syndrome is a very common disorder in which a person has at least three of the following symptoms: abdominal obesity, high blood pressure, high fasting blood glucose, high triglycerides, low HDL cholesterol. They are at higher risk of heart disease and diabetes as a result. People with metabolic syndrome who consume a lower-carbohydrate and higher-fat diet while eating the same number of calories often experience dramatic improvement in the signs and symptoms of this condition compared with people who eat a low-fat diet (Volek, 2009).

All the calories in our food come from what are known as the three *macronutrients*: carbohydrate (which includes complex carbs and sugar), protein, and fat. (Calories also come from alcohol, but it's not considered a macronutrient.) An important point related to carbohydrates and sugar is that we have no minimum requirement for their intake in order to survive. Of the three macronutrients, carbohydrate/sugar is unique in this regard. Our bodies need no "essential" carbohydrates to survive or thrive. In order to survive, we *must* consume protein in our diet so we can obtain the eight essential amino acids (required to build proteins in the body), and we *must* consume fat, including the essential omega-3 and omega-6 fatty acids (which have many important functions in cell membranes, in the brain, in metabolism, and as precursors to many hormones). By contrast, if we do not eat any carbohydrate, our body is still able to make the glucose it requires in a few different ways: from specific amino acids that result from protein breakdown (gluconeogenesis, or "making new glucose"); by converting glycogen, which is stored in our liver and muscles, into glucose; and by breaking down triglycerides, which releases fatty acid molecules and a glycerol molecule that can then be converted to glucose through a couple of different chemical pathways (glycolysis or gluconeogenesis). (See Figure 1.8.)

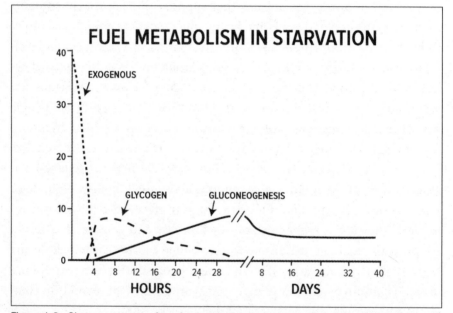

Figure 1.8. Glucose can come from food and drink that we consume, from glycogen stored in muscle and liver, or though glycerol or amino acids converted to glucose through gluconeogenesis. Relative proportions of these three sources from information in Cahill, 2006.

ANOTHER PROBLEM WITH TOO MUCH SUGAR: ADVANCED GLYCATION END-PRODUCTS

Advanced glycation end-products (AGEs) occur when a sugar such as glucose, fructose, or galactose (but not glycerol) binds to a protein or fat. Fructose appears to have ten times the glycation activity of glucose (*McPherson*, 1988). Glycation happens during cooking when sugar is added to protein and/or fats, even at lower temperatures, but is accelerated with higher cooking temperatures over 248°F (120°C). Browning and caramelizing foods are examples of this process, and AGEs are often added by manufacturers to their food products to enhance flavor and color—think pastries and French fries. This process also occurs within the body, starting with sugars in the bloodstream and transforming through a complex multistep process to AGEs. Some (but not all) of these AGEs can be harmful, especially if the levels of glucose in the blood are chronically elevated, resulting in larger amounts of AGEs, as in diabetes.

Proteins and fats that have undergone glycation are altered such that they are no longer shaped normally and may not function normally. These abnormal substances can link together and cause damage to surrounding tissues. AGEs can attach to many different types of cells, interfering with molecular and cellular functions throughout the body. They can also trigger the release of excessive amounts (more than the body can detoxify) of potentially damaging substances, such as hydrogen peroxide, a condition known as oxidative stress. AGEs can damage nearly every type of cell. They can also damage substances that are important to the function of various tissues, including collagen (a component of blood vessel walls, joints, tendons, bones, corneas, and skin) and fibrinogen (which is involved in blood clotting). AGEs can attack myelin, which is a protective covering on nerves, and have even been implicated as carcinogens, which can cause normal cells to convert to cancer cells.

AGEs' pathologic effects include inflammation, leaking of blood vessels, and entrapment and oxidation of LDL in the lining of blood vessels resulting in stiffening and decreased elasticity, also called atherosclerosis or hardening of the arteries. Some of the resulting disease processes include heart disease, heart attacks, strokes, asthma, kidney disease, Alzheimer's disease, cataracts, peripheral neuropathy (burning, tingling, numbness and loss of sensation in hands or feet), arthritis, and complications of diabetes, specifically nephropathy, retinopathy, and neuropathy.

AGEs play a major role in the aging process and are a major factor in the accelerated aging that occurs in people with inadequately controlled diabetes.

THE BENEFITS OF TRANSITIONING FROM A HIGH-CARB, LOW-FAT DIET TO A LOW-CARB, HIGH-FAT DIET

There are numerous potential benefits in reducing sugar intake and choosing foods that do not cause insulin levels to spike. Here are just a few:

- Those relentless carb cravings and constant thoughts about that next meal could go away after just a few days on a low-carb, high-fat diet. The slower rise and fall of blood sugar and insulin levels is much less likely to stimulate hunger than the spikes in blood sugar and insulin that occur after a high-carb meal or snack (Lennerz, 2018; Goodman, 2018).

- If you are not diabetic, you may be able to avoid becoming diabetic (Basu, 2013).

- If you are already pre-diabetic or suffer from type 2 diabetes, you may be able to lower your blood sugar and insulin levels, gradually reverse the problem of insulin resistance, and avoid a multitude of complications that may occur over time such as mental decline, dementia, kidney failure, blindness, and/or amputations related to poor circulation (Feinman, 2015).

- Adults and children who are type 1 diabetics may be able to improve control of their blood sugar and reduce dosages of insulin (Feinman, 2015; Lennerz, 2018).

- You may reduce your risk of certain types of cancer (Makarem, 2018; Sieri, 2015). In general, many types of cancer cells thrive on sugar, and depriving them of sugar could help shrink or kill the tumor and metastases. Human case reports and animal studies showing reduction or elimination of cancerous tumors with ketogenic diets or supplements have lead to clinical trials using a strict ketogenic diet in conjunction with standard treatments that are now in progress (Nebeling, 1995; Zuccoli, 2010; Poff, 2014). Maintaining a low-carbohydrate diet in general could potentially discourage cancerous tumors from forming in the first place. This is detailed in a book by Thomas Seyfried, *Cancer as a Metabolic Disease: On the Origin, Management, and Prevention of Cancer.*

- You may be able to reduce symptoms of diseases caused by inflammation. Chronically high blood sugar levels can result in inflammation through the process of glycation (see discussion of advanced glycation end-products (AGEs) earlier in this chapter), which is a common denominator in many neurodegenerative disorders, including Alzheimer's, Parkinson's, ALS, and autism. Inflammation in blood vessel walls is common in people who have high blood pressure and in people who have had a heart attack or a stroke. Arthritis often involves inflammation of joints and lower blood sugar levels could potentially reduce arthritic pain.
- Reducing sugar in the diet could help you produce healthier, longer-living cells and tissues and ultimately live longer. There will be less AGE formation and therefore less damage to cells and tissues, such as less sagging and wrinkling of skin as we age and our internal organs will benefit as well.
- Too much sugar can increase triglyceride levels substantially and reducing sugar can bring the triglyceride level down. If you drink Coca-Cola, Mountain Dew, Red Bull, or other sweetened sodas or energy drinks and you have a high triglyceride level, consider giving the axe to these drinks. Wean off them one can at a time if you need to. Humans didn't drink soda until the last century and your quality of life as you age could be much better without it.

MY PERSONAL EXPERIENCE

Until about twelve years ago, I listened to the propagators of the "low-fat diet" guidelines and consequently ate what turned out to be a high-carb diet, eating and drinking fat-free milk and milk products, reduced-fat snacks, breads, cereals for breakfast and for an evening snack, crackers, fruit juice every day and plenty of packaged foods and fast foods, with diet cola in between. I believed I was doing the right thing by eating as little fat as possible and mainly trying to control my caloric intake. Vegetables were barely on my radar. As soon as I finished eating a bowl of cereal, I would crave another (carbs taste so good!) and start thinking about my next meal. I was always "on a diet," and my weight went up and down like a yo-yo, becoming heavier and heavier each time I gained it back. At the end of 2005, I was nearly 100 pounds over my ideal weight, pre-diabetic, and quite unhappy that I could not seem to control this aspect of my life. I blamed it on my genes rather than considering that I might just be eating the wrong combination of foods. I was not a food glutton to become that overweight, since I was ever conscious of how many calories I was eating, but I figured out for me that just 250 calories a day (half of a Panera cookie) in either direction was enough to make me lose weight or gain weight.

Also, in 2006, I began to consider that food might play an important role in my husband Steve's early-onset Alzheimer's disease. I began to read and learn intensively about nutrition and a multitude of different options for a healthier diet and losing weight. As mentioned in the introduction, I found a study in which people with Alzheimer's who ate a diet that most resembled the classic Mediterranean diet lived on average four years longer than those who ate a diet that least resembled the Mediterranean (Scarmeas, 2007). The diet stresses whole foods, including whole grains (rather than refined white flour), nuts, avocados, various colors of vegetables, and low-sugar fruits like berries. Olive oil, omega-3 and omega-6 fats became important in our diet as well as well as eggs, chicken, much more seafood, and less beef. I began to look for cage-free eggs and poultry, grass-fed beef, and wild salmon. I learned more about macronutrients (which provide fuel in the form of calories, as discussed above) and micronutrients (vitamins, minerals, and phytochemicals) and began some serious meal planning to ensure we were getting a good balance of them all. This approach greatly reduced our carbohydrate intake since we also ate much smaller portions, choosing fresh or fresh frozen organic vegetables, whole grain breads, oats or rice.

The most amazing part for me of transitioning from a high-carb to a lower-carb, higher-fat diet, was that, around the third day and from that point on, I stopped craving carbs and thinking about my next meal incessantly. I rarely heard my stomach growling from hunger. It was much easier to control my caloric intake, and I managed to lose more than fifty pounds the first year and another forty-five in the next two years. I learned about the problem of muscle loss that often accompanies weight loss and fought it by eating more protein than I was accustomed to and engaging in a combination of weight training and aerobic exercise up to five or six hours per week. As a side benefit, my fasting blood sugar normalized and I was no longer in the pre-diabetic range. While some of the pounds found their way back, as of early 2018, I weigh 60 pounds less than I did twelve years ago, I feel much healthier, and I love the healthy food I eat.

WHY GO KETO?

Right about now, you may be wondering what I mean by "going keto," what ketones actually are, and what the heck a "state of ketosis" is. Good questions. "Going keto" is a popular expression for adopting a ketogenic diet and/or using ketone supplements to increase blood ketones. A "state of ketosis" is a condition in which there is a sustained level of ketones; it implies that the body has switched over from burning carbohydrates to burning fat as the primary fuel. I explain what ketones are and address these ideas in more detail in Chapters 2, 3, 6, and 7.

Up to this point, we primarily have been looking at the benefits of cutting down on sugar in the diet, and there are many. What would compel us to take the next step and adopt a ketogenic diet? The simple answer is that you may be able to experience even greater benefits by achieving a state of ketosis. Perhaps you are looking for improvement in your overall physical and cognitive health and would like to lose some fat, have sharper mental focus, clearer memory, better sleep, better mood, more energy, and relief from aches and pains associated with inflammation. You might be a parent worried that your child is overweight and heading toward a lifetime of diabetes and illness. You might be an endurance athlete hoping to improve your results. Or you or your loved one might have cancer, epilepsy that is not responding well to medications, diabetes, arthritis, Alzheimer's, Parkinson's, or other neurodegenerative disease.

The ketogenic diet is not only a low-carb diet, but, very important, it also is a high-fat diet. We need a certain number of calories to keep our bodies alive and functioning. Remember that calories come from protein, carbohydrate, and fat (and alcohol, which is not under discussion at the moment). The amount of protein we require is fairly straightforward and relatively easy to calculate with the right tools. So, if we cut down on carbs in the diet, those calories will need to be replaced with something else unless we are purely overeating. Healthy fats can fill that calorie gap, with the added benefits of feeling more satisfied when we eat, improving the taste of many foods, and slowing down digestion so that we do not want to eat as often. If the relative proportions of carbohydrate and fat are shifted enough (less carb and more fat), this can become a ketogenic diet, a diet that increases ketone levels, which could benefit overall health and bring about improvement in a variety of different health problems.

The ketogenic diet is not an "all or none" type of diet, since there is a range of ketone levels that are considered to represent "physiologic ketosis," with at least a ten-fold difference between mild ketosis and "deep" ketosis that occurs during prolonged fasting or starvation. Physiologic or physiological ketosis is a level of ketosis that does not result in ketoacidosis, a condition in which ketone levels are extremely high with abnormally low blood pH and requiring medical intervention. (Ketoacidosis is discussed in more detail in Chapters 6, 8, and 10.) The level of ketosis you arrive at will depend on how you manipulate the ratios of fat, carbohydrate, and protein. Basically, while keeping protein at an appropriate amount, the more fat and less carbohydrate you eat, the higher your ketone levels will go. So the ketogenic diet actually represents a spectrum, and we will explore this idea more in Chapter 6. Where you decide to fit on the spectrum will depend on what you hope to achieve.

Another factor that may affect how successful you are in achieving ketosis is how consistent you are with adhering to the diet. The strict, classic ketogenic diet has been used for nearly a century to successfully eliminate or reduce the number of seizures in children with epilepsy who do not respond to medications. (This is discussed in detail in Chapter 4.) In this world of epilepsy, there is a phenomenon known as the "birthday syndrome" in which the family decides to take a break from the strict weighing and measuring of the classic ketogenic diet by allowing the child to have a piece of birthday cake and, unfortunately, a seizure ensues. For the vast majority of us, taking a break from the diet for a meal or even a day or two would not have such dire consequences, but we need to be aware that it could take several days or even a week or longer to get the ketone levels back to the same level. You might think twice about whether taking a break is worth it.

Ketones are molecules of hope for modern-day humans. Ketones are an alternative fuel to glucose for the brain and most other organs, but they also enter other pathways and have many other important effects that we will explore in the upcoming chapters. The "low-fat diet" guidelines of the past few decades moved us in the wrong direction toward obesity, diabetes, and other chronic diseases—a massive public experiment gone awry. Some experts predict that the average lifespan of the younger generation will be lower than that of their parents. It doesn't have to be that way. Getting back to a diet that allows us to use stored fat and ketones as fuel could reverse the unfortunate trends toward obesity and disease that we have witnessed over recent decades.

CHAPTER 2

QUICK START TO A LOW-CARB KETOGENIC DIET

"The greatest discovery of all time is that a person can change his future by changing his attitude."
—Oprah Winfrey

If you are not already on a low-carbohydrate ketogenic diet, you may be anxious to get started, so here are some quick tips to get you on your way while you are learning about the history of the ketogenic diet and what ketones can do for you. There will be more detail later to help you hone in on the type of ketogenic diet that will fit your goals and your lifestyle, as well as some other strategies you can use to enhance the ketogenic effects of the diet. And please note that when we talk about *diet* in this book, I am not necessarily referring to a weight loss diet, though it very well could be. Rather, we are using the word in the broader sense—simply, your personal, habitual eating pattern.

Even if you follow only the tips in this chapter without going any further in adopting the ketogenic lifestyle, you can considerably reduce your carbohydrate intake and begin to enjoy the long-term health benefits of eating less sugar.

SOME CAVEATS BEFORE GETTING STARTED

- It is strongly recommended that you discuss beginning this, or any other significant dietary change, with your physician first. This is particularly true for children, pregnant or breastfeeding mothers, seniors, and people who suffer from chronic diseases and/or are taking medications.

- Do not stop any medications without specific discussion with your physician.
- Do not use coconut oil, or any other oil, if you are allergic to it.
- If you are on insulin or diabetes medication, be sure to monitor your blood sugar closely since some people will experience a drop in blood sugar, particularly when taking larger amounts of coconut or medium-chain triglyceride (MCT) oil or taking an exogenous ketone supplement. (I explain MCT oil and exogenous ketone supplements in more detail in Chapter 7.) Discuss this dietary intervention with your doctor so that your medications can be adjusted if necessary.
- A very-high-fat diet is not for you if you have severe liver disease or liver failure or certain rare enzyme defects involving fat metabolism. In some cases, use of MCT oil could help with certain liver diseases or malabsorption conditions, but always discuss this with your doctor first.
- People who take certain blood thinners such as warfarin (Coumadin, and other trade names) should consult with their physician. A small amount of vitamin K, present in some natural oils, could affect bleeding time and should be monitored closely if you and your physician decide to allow this dietary intervention.

CLEAN OUT YOUR PANTRY AND FRIDGE

If you are like most people, you are on the "see-food" diet: if you see it, you want to eat it. A good way to start any new diet is to look closely in your pantry and your fridge and get rid of the candy, pastries, chips, crackers, cookies, sugary drinks and snacks that tempt you. If you are unsure about whether the food contains sugar, look at the labels. The nutrition facts will list the calories per serving and what constitutes a serving as well as the number of grams and calories per serving for the macronutrients fat, protein, and carbohydrate. The macronutrients are further broken down to list the saturated fat and trans fats, and the carbohydrates are broken down further into fiber, sugar, and sugar alcohols. The most important fact for our purpose here is how much "sugar" is in each serving of the food. We will talk more about the number of grams of sugar and how to work that into your diet in Chapter 6. Next, look at the list of ingredients in the food. Sugar may simply be listed as sugar but could also be listed as glucose, sucrose, dextrose, maltodextrin, lactose, galactose, fructose, high-fructose corn syrup, HFCS, corn syrup, other kinds of syrup, agave, or honey; words ending in "ose" often indicate a sugar but could indicate a sugar alcohol, like sucralose, which is a calorie-free sweetener.

If the packages you remove from your pantry and fridge are intact and the food is within the expiration dates, consider donating them to a food pantry.

CUT OUT ADDED SUGAR AND SUGARY DRINKS

As discussed in Chapter 1, a single daily serving of a sweetened drink, such as a soft drink or fruit juice, can result in accelerated shrinking and aging of the brain, affecting memory. These changes are even more pronounced for someone taking two or more sugary drinks per day. Think thirteen years of brain aging affecting memory if you are drinking three or more servings per day, a great incentive to let go of these drinks. If you find it hard to give up these drinks all at once, cut down by one or two servings every couple of days until they are off your menu.

If you are adding sugar to your coffee or tea, or to anything else for that matter, consider cutting this out, a little at a time if necessary, and, if you must have something that tastes sweet, switch to a safe sugar substitute. Two sweeteners especially worth considering are stevia, a natural sweetener brewed from the leaves of a plant, and erythritol, a sugar alcohol that does not affect blood sugar or insulin levels or cause the intestinal side effects of diarrhea or gassiness, like some of the other sugar alcohols. Stevia comes in powder and liquid forms, including a concentrated extract; just a few drops may be all you need to take care of your sweet tooth, and it works well in coffee, tea, coconut milk, yogurt, baked foods, and many other types of foods. Products combining erythritol and stevia are also available and might provide just the right type of sweetness for your palate, if either of these sweeteners alone doesn't quite cut if for you. I have sometimes used a packet of sucralose (Splenda) or, rarely, saccharine or aspartame if I can't find anything else, but my brain thinks "poison" when I do this, so I have started carrying a resealable bag with Stevia packets in my purse. The best option would be to learn to do without the sweetener altogether.

DRINK PLENTY OF FLUIDS

When you begin a ketogenic diet, your muscles will tend to release water. The early weight loss may be largely from urinating larger volumes of water, and it is possible to become dehydrated. So it is important to drink plenty of fluids to avoid this problem, somewhere around eight to ten 8-ounce (240 ml) glasses per day. The best of all fluids is water, but coffee and tea, as well as clear fluids without added sugar, like sugar-free sparkling waters, are good alternatives as well.

CUT DOWN ON PORTIONS

If you are not quite ready to give up bread, pasta, cereal, rice, potatoes, pancakes, and dessert, you can start by cutting your portions in half and then in half again when you are ready. The first few bites of any food you might crave are the best bites—think of the rest of the portion as just filling your stomach and adding more sugar that you don't really need. If you are eating out, consider turning down the bread and substitute a vegetable for the potatoes, rice, or pasta. This might seem inconceivable at first, but it is quite easy to find menu items that will allow you to stay low-carb and enjoy the meal in most restaurants. For example, if you crave a hamburger, is it really the bun you want or everything else in between? Could you stack your deli sandwich like a Dagwood, between two half slices of whole grain bread? Or try a low-carb wrap? Restaurants want to please their customers, and most are more than willing to serve you the burger without the bun and substitute a vegetable for the pasta or fries. If they are not willing, you'll find plenty of other restaurants that are.

It is possible to include small portions of some of your favorite carbs and stay in ketosis if you eat enough fat at the same time. To figure out a good portion size, you might weigh out or measure a typical portion you are eating now and figure out how many carbs that portion would contain. Divide that number by two or four, and you'll soon learn how to fit that into your meal plan's total carb allotment for the day. This is discussed in more detail in Chapter 6.

Don't go to a party with a big appetite. Eat something keto before you go, and it will be easier to control the urge to binge. Spend more time with people and less at the food tables and avoid the dessert displays. Also avoid drinking too much alcohol, or you may find you just don't care what you eat after that.

START ADDING MORE HEALTHY FAT TO YOUR DIET

When I talk about fats, this includes oils, butters, creams, and the fat that is contained within foods such as meat, fish, cheese, other dairy products, nuts, and avocados.

One of the chief problems with the typical Western diet is that it is high in carbohydrates and low in fat. Transitioning to a higher-fat, lower-carbohydrate diet is the major factor that will make your new diet a ketogenic diet. Simply adding more fat to your diet will not be enough to get you into ketosis, whereas adding more healthy fats to your diet while cutting down on carbohydrates is the pathway that will take you there.

TAKE IT EASY

If you are not accustomed to eating much fat in your diet, adding too much fat too fast may result in intestinal distress (diarrhea, gassiness, bloating, possibly nausea and vomiting) for some people. People who have had their gall bladder removed may have more difficulty than the average person, however, the liver continues to make bile with the enzymes needed to digest most fats, so it is possible to slowly adjust to a higher fat diet. The type of fat or oil you add could also play a role in how well you tolerate it. Consider that this is a lifestyle change and does not need to happen overnight.

You can begin slowly and increase the amount of fat in your diet as tolerated, adding some to each meal and snack, one-half to one teaspoon (2.5 to 5 grams) at a time, or even less if you find you are overly sensitive. If this is tolerated without a problem, then increase by this same amount every two to three days as tolerated. If you experience some diarrhea, back off to the previous level, wait for several days and increase even more gradually. The total daily amount of fat to strive for will be determined by how much you can tolerate as well as by how deeply into ketosis you want to go. Coconut oil and medium-chain triglyceride (MCT) oil, alone or in combination with each other or with other oils, can help support ketosis. Coconut oil contains medium-chain triglycerides and can be ketogenic when taking at least two tablespoons (30 grams) per day. MCT oil is more ketogenic than coconut oil, so less is needed for the same results.

To give you an idea of how much fat to aim for eventually, let's say you decide to rework your diet so that roughly 50 percent of the calories come from fat. If your diet is around 2,000 calories per day, then the fat intake to aim for would be equivalent to about 7½ tablespoons (110 grams) of fat per day. Of course, the foods you eat will contain some naturally occurring fats, which must be considered in the total. In Chapter 6, we will discuss the "spectrum" of ketogenic diets and provide more practical information on how to plan your specific diet based on what percent fat you would like your diet to be.

CONSIDER "GOOD" FATS AND "BAD" FATS

All natural fats and oils contain a combination of saturated, monounsaturated, and polyunsaturated fatty acids. The ratios of these are different from fat to fat and the relative amounts affect certain properties of the fat such as color, taste, the temperature at which it melts, and the temperature at which it smokes when you are cooking with it. How the fat or oil is processed for packaging may affect its quality as well.

In reviewing suggestions from various experts on healthier, more whole food type diets, such as the Paleo and Mediterranean diets, the consensus for what constitutes a healthy fat appears to be one that is organic and is pressed or expeller-pressed without using excessive heat, called cold-pressed or cold expeller-pressed. These experts all agree that the fats to remove from your diet include all trans fats, hydrogenated fats, and partially hydrogenated fats (the latter two contain trans fats). The process of hydrogenation is a problem because it eliminates essential polyunsaturated omega-3 fatty acids from the fat. You can figure out which products contain these unhealthy fats by reading the nutrition facts and ingredients labels.

The fat and lard from animals raised in the traditional way, with exposure to pesticides, hormones, and antibiotics in the feed, tend to store these potentially harmful substances, something to consider when choosing your foods. The risk should be less with meat, dairy, and eggs from grass-fed or cage-free animals, and it is possible to purchase lard and tallow from grass-fed animals.

Exactly which fats are healthy is one of the biggest controversies in the world of nutrition, but based on everything I have read to this point, some healthy fats and high-fat foods include, but are not necessarily limited to, the organic, cold pressed, or cold expeller-pressed versions of:

- olive oil
- sunflower oil
- raw nuts, nut butters, nut milks, seeds, seed butters, and seed milks that do not have added sugar or chemicals, such as walnut, flaxseed, hemp, macadamia, sesame seed, almond, cashew, hazelnut and pecan
- avocados
- olives
- coconut, coconut oil, and coconut milk
- canola oil (controversial due to the ways it has been hybridized over time and how it is processed by some manufacturers—look for organic cold pressed)
- palm and palm kernel oil (RSPO or Roundtable on Sustainable Palm Oil certified)
- tallow or lard from free range, pasture fed animals (likely controversial for those who worry about animal saturated fats)

Consider limiting fats that are high in omega-6 polyunsaturated fatty acids. These include soybean, peanut, safflower, and corn oils, which are often used in larger quantities for cooking. Because they are polyunsaturated, they have sites on the fatty acid molecule that potentially can pick up reactive oxygen species and other harmful substances and easily spoil. The higher relative percentages of polyunsaturated fatty acids in these oils, compared to the healthier oils listed above, make them much more susceptible to becoming rancid. Also, much work has been done to determine the healthy ratio of omega-6 to omega-3 fats by Williams Lands and others, and the evidence suggest that a ratio of between 1:1 and 4:1 is worth aiming for. In the typical Western diet, which uses predominantly soybean and corn oils, the ratios may reach levels of 10:1 or even 20:1. An imbalance in these ratios in favor of omega-6 can result in increased inflammation, constriction of blood vessels and a tendency for blood to clot more easily (Lands, 2005).

IF YOU EAT DAIRY, CHOOSE FULL FAT

Whether to eat dairy or not is controversial as well in the world of keto and Paleo eating. Domestication of animals and use of their milk as a staple in the diet only occurred 4,000 to 9,000 years ago, so, technically, dairy is not considered "Paleo" (which emphasizes eating foods similar to those that our ancestor consumed before the advent of agriculture, i.e., 2.6 million to 10,000 years ago). The Paleo diet is discussed in more detail in Chapter 4. A mutation occurred somewhere along the way that allows some people to digest dairy, but many of us are mildly to severely lactose intolerant. Another consideration is that some people have allergies and sensitivities to the proteins contained in animal milks.

Dairy, including heavy cream and cheese, is used routinely in the classic ketogenic diet for epilepsy, which is explained in more detail in Chapter 6. If you do well with dairy and want to continue eating it, use the whole fat versions and look for organic products that do not contain added sugar. (You would be surprised to know that milk often contains added sugar.) Fresh raw milk is great if you can get it, but it is not widely available and not even allowed for human consumption in some states, mainly due to concerns about infection.

Goat's milk contains considerably more medium-chain triglycerides than cow's milk and even a little more than human milk, so this could be a good alternative for people who are sensitive to cow's milk.

SWITCH TO WHOLE GRAINS

Refined white flour and white rice may taste great but have been stripped of important fiber and other nutrients such as vitamins. For many people throughout the world, white flour or white rice is part of virtually every meal and snack. It is incredible to discover how many different foods are made from the combination of white flour and sugar held together with margarine or soybean oil and flavored with additives (natural or artificial). Even though they do not taste sweet, white flour and white rice are almost entirely made of non-fiber carbs, so you might start thinking and picturing "sugar" when you see white bread or white rice. While the whole-grain alternatives are better choices for nutritional value, keep in mind that they still contain considerable sugar, so adjusting to small portions is key if you wish to continue eating them. Whole grains can be an acquired taste for people used to the white alternatives, but they have more texture and flavor and you may soon find you prefer the whole grain versions. Some pastas are made of whole grains and/or with vegetables, even better.

CONSIDER WHOLE, GRASS FED, CAGE-FREE, NON-GMO, ORGANIC AND GLUTEN-FREE FOODS

Okay, you might not be quite ready for all of this, however, consider that packaged foods very often contain added sugar, trans fats, synthetic vitamins, and an abundance of artificial ingredients to prolong shelf life. Reading the ingredients on labels can help you learn what you are actually eating, and you might be very surprised. If you see sugar and/or chemicals you don't recognize on the list, consider passing up that food and looking at the whole foods options available in your market. By strict definition, a whole food is one that has been grown naturally, has not been processed, and contains no artificial ingredients. However, many whole foods are cleaned and packaged, and, in the case of oils, extracted from a nut, seed, or fruit, with debris and other substances removed to clean and purify the oil. Technically, this is considered processing. Also, some products, for example, organic ricotta, yogurt, mayonnaise, salad dressings, or an organic beet, walnut, and goat cheese salad with greens packaged before purchase, are combinations of just a few healthy whole foods, without added artificial chemicals. I see no reason not to buy these. Again, the ingredients label can help you decide if this is for you.

The animals we eat are often fed grains to fatten them up and may contain pesticides, hormones and antibiotics that could harm us. Grass-fed beef and eggs from cage-free chickens are healthier choices. Organic fruits and vegetables are grown using mulches, compost, manures, and other natural fertilizers rather than potentially harmful synthetic chemicals.

Genetically modified foods (GMOs) are quite prevalent and also controversial at this point; virtually no wheat or corn exists in the United States that has not been genetically engineered. Hopefully governments will require GMO labeling soon so that we can know whether we are eating genetically modified foods or not and decide for ourselves if we want to. Some manufacturers make a point of labeling their produce as "non-GMO."

Another consideration is whether to eat a gluten-free diet. Eliminating gluten could substantially reduce the amount of carbohydrate in the diet. There appears to be a strong gut-brain connection and, although the idea of eliminating gluten completely is controversial, there is evidence that diets high in gluten may contribute to development of insulin resistance and ultimately Alzheimer's or other neurologic diseases. This is discussed in detail in *Grain Brain* by David Perlmutter, MD, a Florida neurologist whose own neurosurgeon father suffered from Alzheimer's. Wheat is the most obvious source of gluten, but it turns up in many other grains and in unexpected places, for example, as an additive that provides a certain consistency to processed foods, such as cereals, ice cream and many condiments such as mayonnaise and ketchup. Dr. Perlmutter joins a growing number of experts who agree that the low-fat diet (which usually leads to high-carbohydrate intake) should be replaced with a diet higher in healthy fats and lower in carbohydrates.

Wheat has been greatly modified over the years and the effect of eating it is to substantially raise insulin levels, regardless of whether the wheat flour is refined or whole grain. According to Dr. William Davis in his book *Wheat Belly*, wheat contributes to accumulation of excessive fat around abdominal organs.

If gluten is contributing to brain fog or more serious symptoms, once you eliminate it, you will notice a difference in a matter of weeks, according to Perlmutter. Many available whole grains are not wheat and have no gluten, including rice, rolled or steel cut oats (if labeled gluten-free), corn, potato, buckwheat, tapioca, soy, quinoa, millet, chia, amaranth, arrowroot, sorghum, and teff. Coconut flour and flours made from some of these grains, or from almonds or other nuts, can be used to make breads, pancakes and other tasty gluten-free, lower carb foods.

ADD NEW VEGETABLES AND BERRIES TO YOUR FOOD REPERTOIRE

I didn't think I liked vegetables, except potatoes, lettuce, and corn, until 2006 when I became interested in healthier nutrition. The vegetables I ate as a child were mostly from cans and were salty and mushy. I was pleasantly surprised when I began to experiment with adding new vegetables to my diet, and now I am a big vegetable fan. Different colors and types of vegetables contain different vitamins, minerals, and other nutrients. It is a good idea to eat a variety of vegetables and choose from different categories of vegetables. Choose some leafy greens, like lettuces, chard, collards, kale, and spinach. Include sulfur-rich vegetables, such as asparagus, broccoli, cauliflower, cabbage, Brussels sprouts, garlic, onions, radishes, and turnips. Add dark green, red, purple, orange, and blue vegetables and fruits, such as sweet and bell peppers, tomatoes, beets, carrots, zucchini, and other squash, as well as berries, such as blueberries, strawberries, and raspberries, which are relatively low in sugar compared to many other fruits. I recently learned about a cool kitchen tool called the spiralizer that turns vegetables into noodles. This is a great way to eliminate pasta from the diet and have some fun with your vegetables. The veggie noodles could be attractive to children as well (See Figure 2.1).

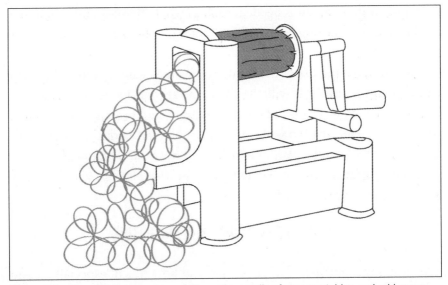

Figure 2.1. The spiralizer can be used to make noodles from vegetables and add some fun to your diet.

Seaweed, essentially algae plants, comes in three different color groups (green, red, and brown) and contains an abundance of nutrients, including vitamins, minerals, trace elements, amino acids, antioxidants, and about two grams of carbs in one-quarter cup. Like vegetables, each color has its own special nutrient composition. Some varieties of seaweed contain the important omega-3 fatty acids DHA and EPA, and fish ultimately acquire these omega-3s from algae through their food chain.

MAKE A LIST OF FOODS THAT WILL BE PART OF YOUR PLAN

Everyone has favorite foods, so it is very helpful to make a list of your own favorites and figure out how much fat, carbohydrate, and protein they contain for the serving size you would like to eat. Also write down the total number of calories in the serving to help you plan out a whole day of meals and snacks. If it is a packaged food, you can find this information directly on the label. For whole foods like vegetables, fruits, and meats, you can use a resource such as my favorite, *The Nutribase Complete Book of Food Counts* by Corrine T. Netzer (2017, 9th edition,), which contains more than nine hundred pages of complete nutrition information for thousands of whole foods and brand-name packaged and restaurant foods. The U.S. Department of Agriculture (USDA) Food Database website can also be helpful if more detail is needed, such as what vitamins and minerals a food contains or the breakdown of fatty acids (see https://ndb.nal.usda.gov /ndb/search/list).

As you make the list of the foods you usually eat and refer to the list while planning meals, it will soon become second nature to remember roughly how many grams of fat, carbohydrate, and protein are in each of them. Also, people tend to settle on a relatively small assortment of favorite meals, so, after a while, planning meals will not be too tedious.

There will be much more detail about how to plot out your keto day and plan meals in Chapter 6.

KEEP TRACK OF WHAT YOU ARE EATING

Start keeping a journal of what you eat and how much, especially if you hope to lose weight with the diet. A journal can keep you honest and can also help you analyze what you have been doing and make changes in the diet if you are not getting the desired results. If you are using the ketogenic to lose weight, as the pounds come off, your body may not need as many calories to carry out the basic functions. It takes quite a few more calories per day for the same person to maintain their weight at 200 pounds than at 150 pounds. A person weighing 300 pounds may be able to lose substantial weight while eating 3,000 calories per day in the beginning, for example, but with each 20- or 30-pound weight loss, may need to trim that number down to 2,800 and then 2,600 or more to keep losing weight. A person weighing 200 pounds may need to start out at 1,800 calories or less to lose weight. This can vary considerably from person to person. If your weight loss levels off, having your personal journal to refer to will help you figure out where you can make changes in your diet to reduce the overall calories.

If you are not using the ketogenic diet to lose weight, keeping a journal can also help you adjust the diet to figure out what percent of fat you need to eat and what ratio of fat, carbohydrate, and protein works best for you to achieve you desired ketone level.

DON'T GIVE UP IF YOU SLIP UP

Besides the advice to consult your doctor, the idea of not giving up if you slip up may be the most important pointer offered in this chapter. Making the transition to a low-carbohydrate ketogenic diet is a lifestyle change that could truly take you on a different path to a healthier future. It is natural for humans to crave sugar and, unless you are on the strictest ketogenic diet for a medical condition, such as cancer or epilepsy, a deviation here and there probably will not harm you. On the other hand, you need to be aware that one high-carb treat could blow you out of ketosis immediately and that it could take days to get back to the level of ketosis you were at before the deviation. Taking that into consideration, you might think twice before going that route. Also, if you aren't careful, old habits can sneak back in. As less-than-perfect human beings, we are bound to get off track here and there. Don't beat yourself up if that happens. Instead, applaud yourself for the great work you have done to this point. You have done this before, and you can do it again; your experience will give you the confidence to know that you will be back in ketosis in no time. This is a long-term plan, so if you walk off the path a little bit, you can just as easily get back on.

WHAT ABOUT ALCOHOL?

Two important points to address about alcohol are the carb content and the potential worsening of symptoms while adapting to a ketogenic diet.

Many alcoholic beverages contain small to large amounts of carbohydrates, including many beers, ales, lagers, wines, liquors, spirits, and especially sugary cocktails, so it is important to look closely for the sugar content on the label and factor these carb grams into your diet plan. A dark lager beer could have as much as 18 grams of carbs in a 12-ounce serving, and a nice rosé wine might have four or more grams of carbs. Consider switching to low-carb beers and wines. A company called Dry Farm Wines makes carb-free white and red wines.

Drinking alcohol has the potential to aggravate symptoms of the "keto flu" that many experience during the early weeks of adapting to the ketogenic lifestyle (see Chapter 10). It is wise to restrict or discontinue drinking alcoholic beverages if you feel woozier than usual while transitioning to a ketogenic diet. After you adapt, it may be quite possible to enjoy a beer or a glass of wine, so long as you factor in the carbs. Some people report that they feel the effects of alcohol much sooner with smaller amounts while on a ketogenic diet.

CHAPTER 3

KETONES AS A PRIMITIVE FUEL
Little Molecule, Big Effects

"Physicians have long been taught to fear ketosis . . .
This fear of ketosis may be exaggerated.
Mild ketosis can have therapeutic potential
in a variety of disparate disease states."
—**Richard L. Veech (Veech, 2001)**

If you are new to the world of ketones, ketogenic diets, and exogenous ketone supplements, you might have a very basic question: What are ketones, and where do they come from? Let's start with a lesson from Biochemistry 101 that I will try to make as simple as possible.

WHAT ARE KETONES? BIOCHEMISTRY 101

The English word *ketone* comes from the German word *keton* meaning "acetone," which is your basic fingernail polish remover. This is the very same acetone that is one of the three basic "ketone bodies" produced in the human body. (I will talk more about that later in this chapter.)

Atoms are the fundamental particles of matter. The basic atoms contained in living matter are oxygen, hydrogen, and carbon (See Figure 3.1). Atoms are connected

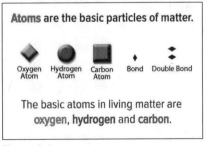

Atoms are the basic particles of matter.

Oxygen Atom   Hydrogen Atom   Carbon Atom   Bond   Double Bond

The basic atoms in living matter are oxygen, hydrogen and carbon.

Figure 3.1.

to each other by "bonds" that are much like magnetic attractions. When two or more atoms are connected, they are called "molecules." (See Figure 3.2.) Glucose (sugar), fats, and ketones are made of different combinations of oxygen, hydrogen, and carbon. The carbon atoms line up in a chain, and the hydrogen and

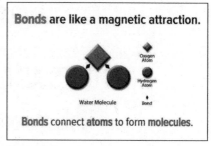

Figure 3.2.

oxygen atoms attach to the carbon atoms. The positions of the various atoms in a molecule determine what that molecule does in the body. Molecules become more complex by connecting with other molecules or with other atoms, such as nitrogen, sulfur, calcium, magnesium, phosphate, and many others. For example, amino acids, the building blocks of proteins, are made up of different combinations of carbon, hydrogen, and oxygen, with the addition of nitrogen (and sometimes also sulfur).

Remember that glucose is the main fuel for the cells in our body when we are on a higher carbohydrate diet. Chemically speaking, glucose starts with a chain of six carbons, each of which has hydrogen and oxygen atoms attached to it. (See Figure 3.3.) Betahydroxybutyrate, one of the three ketones made in the body, is a simpler molecule than glucose; it is composed of a chain of four carbons with hydrogens and oxygens attached. Betahydroxybutyrate becomes the predominant fuel for the brain during fasting or starvation—and while on a high-fat, low-carbohydrate diet that is otherwise known as a ketogenic diet. (See Figure 3.4.)

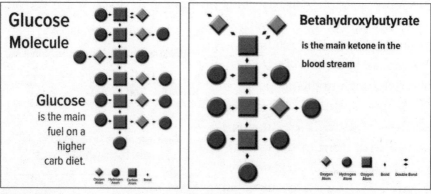

Figure 3.3.   Figure 3.4.

There are two forms of betahydroxybutyrate that are made up of the same atoms but have different shapes—sort of like mirror images, although it is more complicated than that. (See Figure 3.5.) D-betahydroxybutyrate is found mainly in the bloodstream, and L-betahydroxybutyrate is found mainly in mitochondria, the structures in our cells where the energy molecule ATP is produced. The "metabolic fates" of the D- and L- forms of betahydroxybutyrate are different, so each could potentially have different effects. (See Figure 3.6.) There are two other ketones produced by the human body: acetoacetate and acetone (fingernail polish remover!). Acetone evaporates easily and is mostly exhaled. It accounts for the fruity breath people may have when they are in ketosis. Acetoacetate converts easily to betahydroxybutyrate and vice versa. Acetoacetate also converts to acetone. (See Figure 3.7.)

Ketones are a primitive fuel, more efficient than glucose, since a chemically equivalent amount will produce more energy using less oxygen (Sato, 1995). These two fuels can drive our basic metabolism, an extraordinarily complex but organized intertwining of chemical reactions that are necessary to maintain life. How does this work? Stay with me while I get a bit technical. The tricarboxylic acid cycle (the TCA cycle, also known as the Krebs cycle or citric acid cycle, CAC) is a series of chain reactions (an

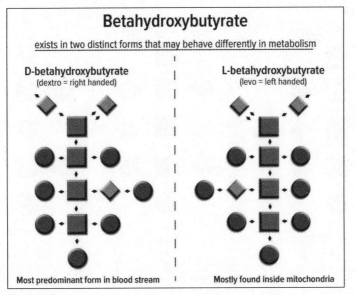

Figure 3.5.

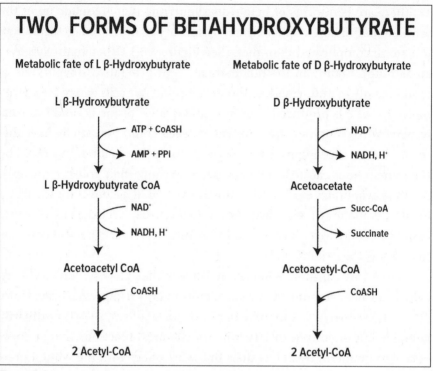

Figure 3.6.

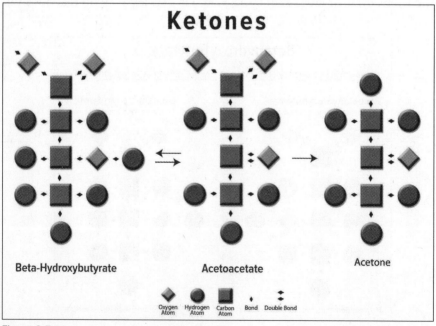

Figure 3.7.

eight-step process involving eighteen different enzymes and co-enzymes) that occurs within the hundreds to thousands of mitochondria in each cell. It is driven by a fuel—either glucose, ketones, fatty acids, or amino acids— that feeds into the electron transport chain (ETC) to yield the energy molecule known as adenosine triphosphate (ATP). ATP allows cells to carry out their vital functions. Throughout this whole process, an astonishing number of other substances are synthesized. Both glucose and ketones drive, and are part of, other biochemical processes besides the generation of energy. (See Figures 3.8 and 3.9.)

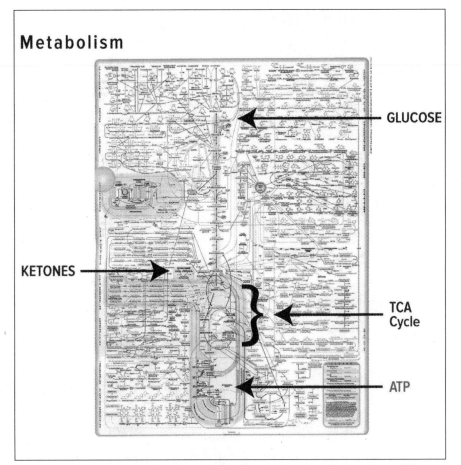

Figure 3.8. Metabolism consists of hundreds of intertwining chemical reactions. Glucose and ketones are fuels that can drive the TCA cycle leading to production of the energy molecule ATP. Ketones drive the TCA cycle more efficiently than glucose, requiring far fewer intermediary chemical reactions to take place before reaching the TCA cycle.

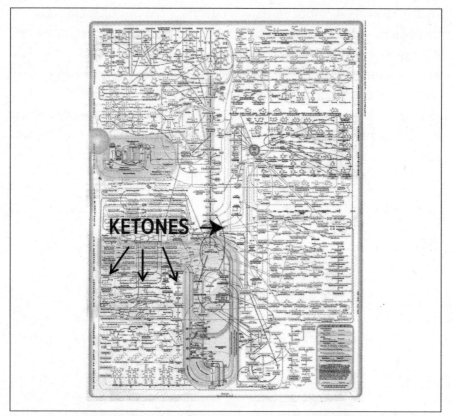

Figure 3.9. In addition to fueling the TCA cycle, ketones are involved in many other metabolic pathways as well.

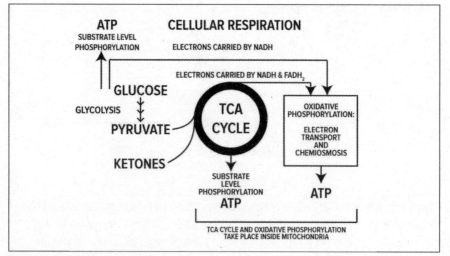

Figure 3.10. Aerobic cellular respiration.

The overall process of converting glucose to ATP under conditions in which oxygen is present is called "aerobic cellular respiration." (See Figure 3.10.) Though a lot happens in between, this process starts out with glucose and oxygen and ends up with carbon dioxide, water, and ATP. Here is the equation that describes the overall chemical reaction:

Aerobic cellular respiration:
1 glucose molecule + 6 oxygen molecules →
6 carbon dioxide molecules + 6 water molecules + 36 ATP molecules

Here, in a nutshell, is what makes ketones a more efficient energy source than glucose: when ketones are called on to provide energy, they feed into the TCA cycle more directly than glucose does, bypassing a number of chemical reactions required by glucose to enter the cycle. And they require less oxygen to produce more ATP than glucose. (See Figures 3.11.)

ENDOGENOUS AND EXOGENOUS KETONES

Endogenous ketones are ketones that originate inside our bodies; exogenous ketones originate outside of the body (See Figure 3.12).

The most common way that we generate endogenous ketones is when we do not eat for ten or more hours overnight; we will often be in mild ketosis in the morning until we eat something with carbohydrates (sugar) in it. Ketosis becomes much more pronounced over days to weeks in people

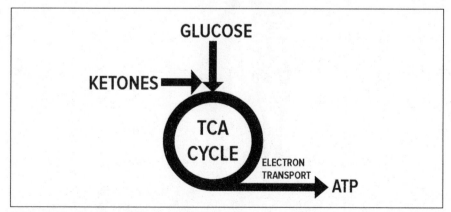

Figure 3.11. Greatly simplified version of the TCA cycle:—glucose or ketones enter the TCA cycle to ultimately produce ATP.

who are fasting intentionally, starving, or on a high-fat low-carbohydrate diet (Owen, 1967). In this situation, we begin to break down fat into fatty acids after the glucose stored in our body is used up, usually by forty-eight hours and often sooner. These relatively large fatty acids do not cross very

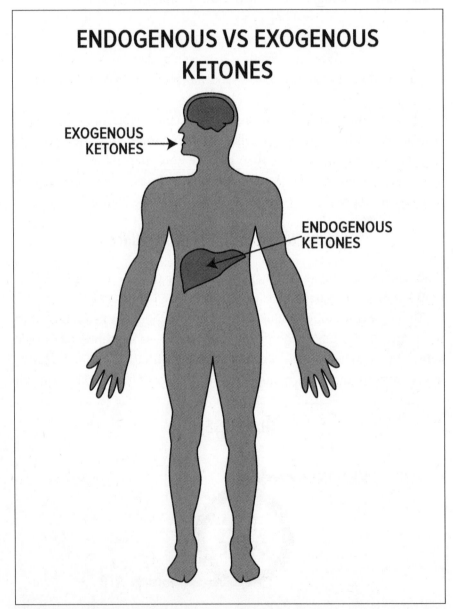

Figure 3.12. Endogenous ketones are ketones that originate inside our bodies, mainly in the liver, and exogenous ketones originate outside of the body.

well into the brain (meaning they don't provide fuel directly from the bloodstream to the brain), but they can be broken down in the liver to make ketones. (See Figure 3.13.) The cool thing about ketones is that they *do* cross the blood-brain barrier, providing fuel to the cells in our brain.

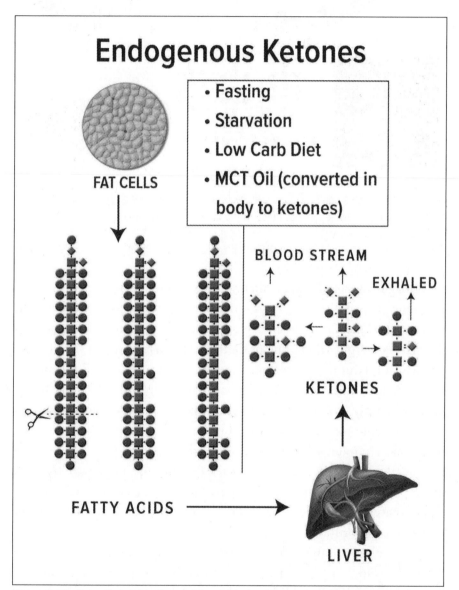

Figure 3.13. Fat cells release fatty acids, which are partly converted to ketones in the liver. The ketones betahydroxybutyrate and acetoacetate are carried in the bloodstream and acetone is carried to the lungs where it is mostly exhaled.

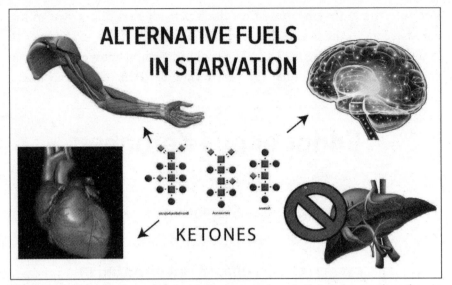

Figure 3.14. Ketones can provide fuel to the brain and most other organs, such as the heart and skeletal muscle, but not to the liver where ketones are made.

They can also provide fuel to our other organs (except the liver, where they are made). (See Figure 3.14.)

Both glucose and ketones enter the same chemical pathway—the TCA or Krebs cycle described above—that leads to the production of ATP. But, as mentioned, ketones enter this pathway several chemical reactions downstream from where glucose enters. Glucose requires insulin and the availability of insulin receptors on the surface of the cell membrane to enter most cells. It also requires substances known as glucose transporters, mainly GLUT 1 through GLUT 4, which ferry glucose through the cell membrane. Ketones instead use monocarboxylate transporters, which are channels that allow certain substances to pass through the cell membrane. Since ketones enter the cell and the TCA cycle through a completely different process than glucose, ketones can easily serve as an alternative fuel to the brain and other organs when there is a problem using glucose for fuel.

Dr. Stephen Cunnane and coauthors talk about the "push-pull" of brain-fuel supply in their article "Can Ketones Help Rescue Brain Fuel Supply in Later Life?" published in 2016 in *Frontiers in Molecular Neuroscience* (Cunnane, 2016). It explains that the amount of glucose taken up into the brain is driven by the demand for glucose in the brain, based on the activity of brain cells. Thus, glucose is pulled into the brain as needed. By contrast, ketone uptake into the brain is directly proportional to the level of ketones in the blood: the higher the level of ketones, the higher the percentage of energy that ketones supply to the brain, and so ketones are essentially "pushed" into the brain. The glucose level in the blood does not affect the amount of ketone entering the brain. Another point is that when ketones and glucose are both readily available, the brain will preferentially use ketones.

As mentioned, exogenous ketones originate from outside of the body. Consumers can purchase supplements that provide exogenous ketones. Generally speaking, the supplements fall into two categories: ketone salts and ketone esters. Ketone salts were the first products to be widely marketed to the public that contain the ketone betahydroxybutyrate. Beginning in early 2016, Pruvit Ventures became the first company to widely distribute ketone salts, which were developed and tested at University of South Florida in Dominic D'Agostino's lab. Ketone esters have been in development and tested in animal research labs for many years but just became available to the public at the beginning of 2018 from two companies, Ketoneaid (http://ketoneaid.com/) and Human (https://hvmn.com/). The ketone ester products are currently recognized by the FDA as safe for endurance athletes, but toxicity testing will soon be underway for use in the general public. Until then, caution should be exercised by anyone who plans to use ketone esters for any purpose other than athletic performance. More details about exogenous ketone supplements will be provided in Chapter 7 and other considerations related to age and health will be covered in Chapter 8.

WHAT DO KETONES DO?

Besides serving as fuel to make ATP in our cells, ketones enter a number of other pathways in metabolism as well and have an incredible array of effects. We will go into more detail about some of these effects after this summary and in later chapters, where I will provide the appropriate references. For now, here is a synopsis:

- Ketones provide alternative fuel for the brain and other organs and can benefit people with conditions that involve insulin resistance and decreased glucose uptake into the brain and other organs. This often translates into improved memory, better mental clarity and focus, better sleep, improved mood, and a feeling of having more energy. People with conditions such as Parkinson's and Alzheimer's diseases have reported improvement in physical symptoms and in day-to-day functioning as well. (See Figure 3.15.)

- Ketones provide super-efficient fuel to the heart and could potentially help improve heart function in congestive heart failure and after a heart attack.
- Ketones lower glucose and insulin levels, a great benefit to people with pre-diabetes and diabetes, while also stimulating fat loss.
- Ketones provide anti-inflammatory effects through several mechanisms; ketosis could improve conditions in which a key factor is inflammation. For example, ketones are antioxidants and neutralize the damaging effects of reactive oxygen species (ROS) by donating an electron (Figure 3.16). Numerous conditions share inflammation as a key factor, and reducing inflammation could improve symptoms and possibly slow down the progress of the disease. (See Figure 3.17.)

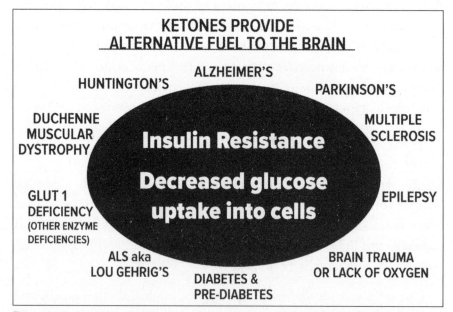

Figure 3.15. Ketosis could bring about improvement in many neurological and other disorders that are characterized by insulin resistance and/or poor glucose uptake into cells.

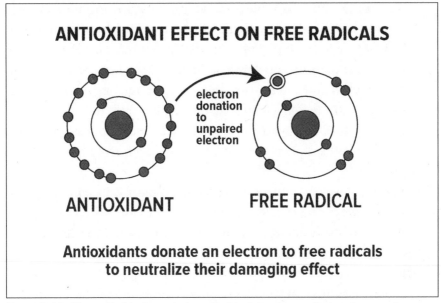

ANTIOXIDANT EFFECT ON FREE RADICALS

electron donation to unpaired electron

ANTIOXIDANT   **FREE RADICAL**

Antioxidants donate an electron to free radicals to neutralize their damaging effect

Figure 3.16. How antioxidants work. An antioxidant donates an electron to a reactive oxygen species molecule.

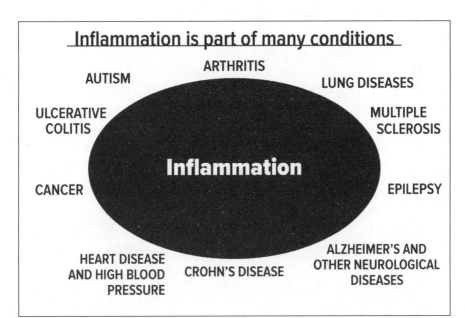

Inflammation is part of many conditions

ARTHRITIS

AUTISM   LUNG DISEASES

ULCERATIVE COLITIS   MULTIPLE SCLEROSIS

Inflammation

CANCER   EPILEPSY

HEART DISEASE AND HIGH BLOOD PRESSURE   CROHN'S DISEASE   ALZHEIMER'S AND OTHER NEUROLOGICAL DISEASES

Figure 3.17. Ketones are anti-inflammatory through several mechanisms and ketosis could improve conditions in which a key factor is inflammation. Many of these conditions are the same as those in Figure 3.15.

- Ketones help burn fat while preserving muscle. In the traditional diet, in which carbohydrates make up a high percent of the macronutrients and fat is reduced, it is almost inevitable that muscle loss will occur. Glucose remains the predominant fuel in this type of diet, and muscle is broken down to provide glucose when you burn more calories than you take in. On a ketogenic diet, fat becomes the predominant source of fuel, and muscle is not needed so much to make glucose.
- Ketones can suppress appetite, thereby supporting a weight loss program.
- Ketones have anti-cancer applications. Cancer cells love sugar, but most types of cancer cells cannot use ketones for fuel, so a ketogenic diet could lower blood sugar and starve cancer cells, while still supplying fuel for normal cells.
- Ketones have anti-aging properties, including many of those listed above that come together to improve quality of life and potentially extend life (Veech, 2017). Ketones have been shown to significantly extend life in a small roundworm called *Caenorhabditis elegans* (*C. elegans*), which is often used in studies to gauge the effects of substances on longevity. (See Figure 3.18.)

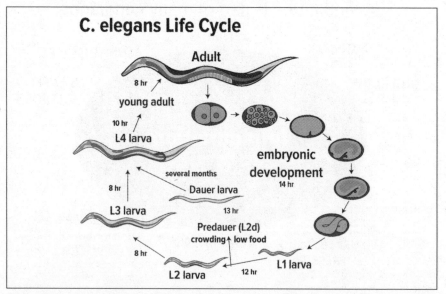

Figure 3.18. *Caenorhabditis elegans*, also known as *C. elegans*, has a relatively short life cycle that is modified by its surroundings, so it is often used in studies to gauge the effects of a particular substance on longevity.

Mark Mattson, PhD, of the National Institute on Aging (part of the NIH), and others have done extensive research on the effects of fasting and exercising on brain aging, and these studies are summarized in an excellent 2014 TEDxJohns Hopkins University talk, "Why Fasting Bolsters Brain Power," that can be viewed at https://www.youtube.com /watch?v=4UkZAwKoCP8, as well as on other longer recordings of his presentations. In the TEDx talk, Dr. Mattson reminds us that fasting was a way of life for humans until relatively recently (in terms of evolution), and our neural systems have evolved to be more active during fasting. Very literally we need to be able to go out and look for food. Ketones begin to increase quickly when we deplete the 900 or so calories of glucose stored as glycogen in our livers, which happens at about ten to fourteen hours of fasting if we do not exercise during that time, and sooner if we do. Thereafter we turn to the energy stored in our bodies as fat. He says fasting is a challenge to the brain, and the brain responds by activating stress response pathways that help the brain cope with this stress and resist disease.

Mattson and others have recently published an extensive review of the animal and human research in this area, detailing the many metabolic pathways affected by fasting (Mattson, 2018). He introduces the concept of "intermittent metabolic switching" and explains that different signaling pathways are enlisted when switching from glucose to ketones as the primary fuel, and again when switching back from ketones to glucose as the primary fuel. He explains that some cells, such as neurons and muscle, go into "cell-preservation mode" through activation of certain signaling pathways in response to switching from glucose to ketones as fuel; this effectively sets the stage for the recovery period when the fuel source is switched back from ketones to glucose, during which these cells adopt a "cell-growth mode." Muscle cells, for example, do not grow during exercise, but rather during the recovery period. How that happens is the result of the interaction between numerous biochemical pathways that are either activated or turned off depending on the prevailing level of ketones and glucose.

Mattson says that switching between short periods of negative energy balance (burning more calories than you consume due to either a short fast and/or exercise) and positive energy balance (eating and resting) can "optimize general health and brain health," resulting in improved insulin sensitivity, reduced abdominal fat, maintenance of muscle mass, reduced blood pressure, and a lower resting heart rate. *It is important to note that for some of the health outcomes, the best results may come not only from an increase in ketone levels but also from a significant reduction in blood glucose levels.* This appears to be the case for seizure reduction and for killing cancer cells and could apply to other conditions as well.

> It is important to note that for some of the health
> outcomes, the best results may come not only
> from an increase in ketone levels but also from a
> significant reduction in blood glucose levels.

The beneficial effects that occur from changes in signaling pathways during metabolic switching from glucose to ketones are many; if you want to delve into much greater detail on this topic, check out the 2018 Mattson article. The information in the review is based on results of numerous animal and human studies of intermittent fasting, alternate-day fasting, caloric restriction, vigorous and/or sustained exercise, and administration of exogenous ketone supplements, such as the betahydroxybutyrate ketone ester and betahydroxybutyrate salts, which are explained in more detail in Chapter 7.

If you don't want to dig that deeply, listed below are the highlights of some of the positive effects that can result when metabolism switches from burning glucose to burning ketones. (Bear in mind that this shift can be accomplished through regular intermittent fasting and/or through vigorous or sustained exercise.) The benefits of sustained nutritional ketosis—which involves achieving the state through dietary means rather than through deliberate fasting or a regimented exercise program—will be explored in later chapters:

- elevated ketone levels (and reduced glucose levels), which in turn
  - directly provide ketones as an alternative fuel to the brain and most other cells in the body, leading to increased production of ATP in mitochondria with improved cell function.
  - act as precursors to lipids that are prominent in brain cell membranes, including neurons and oligodendrocytes, and may also enhance myelination of axons.

- upregulate gene expression in numerous signaling pathways (discussed in the next bullet points).
- increased insulin sensitivity—that is, improved uptake and utilization of glucose in the brain and other organs.
- positive effects on the balance of neurotransmitters, leading to improvements in behavior and mood, reduction of anxiety and depression, and enhanced cognitive performance such as in learning and memory.
- setting the stage for increased neurogenesis (formation of new brain cells) and improved neuroplasticity (remodeling of the brain), thereby slowing brain aging and atrophy and enhancing cognitive and physical performance, strength, and coordination.
- increased mitochondrial biogenesis—that is, production of new mitochondria in cells to produce more of the energy molecule ATP
- promotion of autophagy (removal of damaged cells and recycling of usable substances from them) through the protein mTOR (mechanistic target of rapamycin), thereby preparing for cell growth during the subsequent recovery period and providing anti-aging effects as well as enhancement of physical and cognitive health.
- protection of neurons against metabolic and oxidative stress, through factors such as insulin-like growth factor (IGF1) and fibroblast growth factor 2 (FGF2), thereby enhancing anti-aging mechanisms by reducing and/or preventing damage to mitochondria, cells, tissues, and ultimately organs, while promoting DNA repair.
- reduction of inflammation by activating hydrocarboxylic acid receptor 2 and inhibiting the NRLP3 inflammasome—reduces damage from inflammation in many tissues, such as joints and walls of blood vessels, as well as inflammation in the brain that appears to contribute to neurologic and neurodegenerative diseases like Alzheimer's, Parkinson's, amyotrophic lateral sclerosis (ALS), autism, and many more
- an increase in cholinergic neurons that originate in the brainstem and provide the nerve supply for the heart, thereby lowering resting heart rate and blood pressure.
- burning of fat and activation of the thermogenic (heat producing) properties of brown fat, which include fat loss, increase in body temperature (thermogenesis), with greater utilization of energy.

- this is similar to the response from cold exposure—increase in cyclic adenosine monophosphate (cAMP) and transcription factor cAMP-responsive element-binding protein).
- an increase in levels of ghrelin and adiponectin and a reduction in levels of leptin, coupled with lower blood glucose and insulin and higher ketone levels, resulting in appetite suppression and promotion of fat burning.
- preservation of muscle mass by burning fat as fuel instead of breaking down muscle for amino acids to make glucose.
- several pathways come together to set the stage to make new muscle cells during recovery period by mitochondrial biogenesis, inhibition of mTOR and increase in autophagy during exercise and probably during fasting.
  - need to maintain daily protein intake at about 0.5 to 0.75 grams per pound of body weight (1.2 to 1.6 grams per kilogram of body weight).
  - long-term fasts may have detrimental effects on muscle mass.
- upregulation of these pathways to resist the development of chronic conditions, including obesity and its related chronic illnesses, such as diabetes and age-related mild cognitive impairment that may lead to dementia.

Another important and very thorough review of ketones—what they do and how they do it—was written by Patrycja Puchalska and Peter Crawford of the Metabolic Origins of Disease, at Sanford Burnham Prebys Medical Discovery Institute in Orlando, Florida. The paper is entitled "Multi-Dimensional Roles of Ketone Bodies in Fuel Metabolism, Signaling, and Therapeutics" and is published in *Cell Metabolism* (Puchalska, 2017). I recommend it to anyone who wants a serious review of the science.

How and why could a state of ketosis produce such a broad range of effects? World-renowned ketone expert Dr. Richard Veech has long spoken about this, but a flurry of new papers published in 2018 provide more proof that the marked increase in NAD (nicotinamide adenine dinucleotide) may be responsible. When NAD increases, the oxidized form of NAD, known as NAD+, also becomes elevated, resulting in a marked increase in the NAD+/NADH ratio. One of these recent papers describes NAD as "a pivotal molecule for redox reactions and the backbone of ATP generation". This relative increase in NAD+ "enhances mitochondrial function, protects against oxidative stress damage and decreases cell death". Enzymes related to metabolism, inflammation and DNA repair are dependent on NAD+ (Elamin, 2018). A study by Lijin Xin et al. demonstrates that ketones do, in fact, increase the redox NAD+/NADH ratio in the brains of healthy young adult humans when given a product containing 10 grams of 60% C8 and 40% C10 MCT oil. The total ketone levels increased to 0.4 mM/L and the NAD+/NADH ratio increased on average by 18% in these subjects (Xin, 2018).

Ketones are little molecules with big effects. As volumes of research now shows, ketones, once thought to be just harmful by-products of diabetic ketoacidosis, not only provide a wide range of potential benefits but are vital to our normal growth and development as individuals and to our survival as a species.

## CHAPTER 4

THE KETOGENIC LIFESTYLE
Evolution and Historical Perspectives

"Were it not for the betahydroxybutyrate
and acetoacetate providing brain fuel, we
Homo sapiens might not be here."
—George F. Cahill Jr. (Cahill, 2006)

The classic ketogenic diet, as we know it today, was first developed and named nearly a century ago, when it was discovered and reported by Rollin Woodyatt that either starvation or consuming a very low-carbohydrate, high-fat diet resulted in production of three ketone bodies—betahydroxybutyrate, acetoacetate, and acetone—in people who were otherwise healthy (Woodyatt, 1921). Shortly after, Russel Wilder of the Mayo Clinic coined the term "ketogenic diet" to describe a diet that resulted in high levels of ketones, a state known as ketonemia (Wilder, 1921). Wilder and C. E. Baker were the first to report on the use of the ketogenic diet for epilepsy (Baker, 1921), though fasting had been used well before then with some success. There is historical documentation of the use of fasting for seizures in the King James Version of the Bible, where Jesus stated that the "demon" causing a boy's convulsions could only be cured with prayer and fasting (Mark 9:14-29; not all translations include "fasting"). Likewise, in the fifth century BC, Hippocrates recognized that seizures were likely a medical and not a spiritual phenomenon and reported that fasting seemed to be the only effective treatment.

The story of ketones in evolution has much more to it than this. Relying on ketones for fuel goes all the way back to the beginnings of life itself, about 3.5 billion years ago. Oxygen levels in Earth's atmosphere have fluctuated considerably over the eons and ancient single-celled organisms called archaea, which still exist today, could use the ketone body betahydroxybutyrate (BHB) as one of three fuels, which may have been important to the survival of these tiniest creatures when atmospheric oxygen levels were low. Other fuels used by archaea include polysaccharides (complex sugars) and polyphosphates, both of which require considerable hydration, whereas BHB does not. BHB is stored in the form of poly-betahydroxybutyrate granules, which are made up of chains of BHB molecules connected end-to-end and are found in tiny quantities in our blood and in cell membranes, with many different functions in health and disease. Despite their presence in our bodies, humans do not appear to use poly-BHB granules as fuel. Most bacteria today (except coliforms) can use BHB as fuel, and some protozoa contain up to 90 percent of their dry weight as poly-BHB granules (Cahill, 2006).

> Relying on ketones for fuel
> goes all the way back to the beginnings
> of life itself, about 3.5 billion years ago.

It is very likely that the ability of our brains and other organs to use ketones as an alternative fuel to glucose factored heavily in the successful evolution of humans and in our survival as a species over millions of years. What separates humans so obviously from other primates and nearly all other critters on Earth is the size of our brains relative to our bodies. The adult human brain is so large and so active compared to the brains of other mammals that it requires 20 percent or more of the total calories we consume, even though it weighs only about three pounds (1,350 grams). By comparison, the chimpanzee brain weighs just 0.85 pounds (384 grams) and uses about 8 percent of the total calories eaten (Robson, 2008).

> The adult human brain is so large and so active
> compared to the brains of other mammals that it
> requires 20 percent or more of the total calories we
> consume, even though it weighs only about 3 pounds.

KETONES: CRITICAL TO THE NEWBORN BRAIN

Ketogenesis (production of ketones) in the newborn appears to be a normal adaptive process that helps the baby successfully transition from the womb to the outside world. The pathways for using ketones are well established before birth. The fetal brain just twelve weeks into the pregnancy (the earliest studied) is already quite capable of using ketones as an efficient fuel (Adam, 1974). Ketones cross the placenta from mother to the growing fetus, and a pregnant woman goes into ketosis more rapidly than a non-pregnant woman (Rudolph, 1983).

Babies are born fat and fat is the main energy source for the newborn, coming from their own fat stores as well as from breast milk, of which about 50 percent of the calories are fat. Women who have breastfed can confirm that there is very little milk—drops of colostrum—the first day or two. Newborns experience accelerated release of fatty acids from their fat stores during the first days of life at a rate of 4 to 5 grams per kilogram of body weight per day. This fat release allows for production of energy and, also, provides material for the production of ketone bodies. In the newborn, the blood sugar drops substantially shortly after birth, and ketone body levels increase within eight hours of fasting to levels of 2 to 3 mmol/L—a level that would require several days of total fasting by an adult. The turnover of ketones is directly proportional to the free fatty acid and ketone body concentrations in the blood. The uptake of ketones into the newborn brain is four times higher than the uptake in the adult brain and ketones account for as much as 25 percent of the total body energy requirement of the newborn during the first few days of life. At 0.8 pounds (360 grams), the human newborn brain at birth is already nearly the size of the full-grown chimp brain and uses a whopping 74 percent of caloric intake, of which nearly half is in the form of the ketone body betahydroxybutyrate (Bourgneres, 1986; Cahill, 2006; Robson, 2008; Holliday, 1971).

The baby who is breastfed and does not receive supplemental formula reaches higher ketone levels than formula-fed babies; ketone levels in breastfed infants increase steadily, from about 0.1 mmol/L at birth to 1 mmol/L or even higher by 48 hours of age. Small-for-age babies do not have much fat, and when they are strictly formula fed, they do not go into ketosis at all. These thin newborns are at risk for cognitive delays that may become more obvious during the first few years of life. We need to consider the possibility that the lack of availability of ketones to the brain in these tiny babies might contribute to the poor outcome and think about how they might be provided with this important fuel at this most critical time in their brain development. Large babies born to mothers who are not diabetic often have low blood sugar but this appears to be offset by the increase in ketone levels (Bourgneres, 1986; De Boissieu, 1995; De Rooy, 2002; Hawdon, 1992; Lucas, 1978).

Colostrum, the milk available to the baby during the first days of life, is very small in quantity and contains very little lactose sugar, but much triglyceride and protein, effectively "starting man's entry into society on an Atkins diet," according to George F. Cahill Jr., who studied human nutrition and wrote extensively about metabolic changes during fasting and starvation (Cahill, 2006). About 10 to 17 percent of the fats in breast milk are medium-chain triglycerides (MCTs), at the higher end of the range when the baby is premature, and this contributes to the increase in ketone levels in the infant's body, since MCTs are partly converted to ketones (De Rooy, 2002; Hamosh, 1985; Tantibhedhyangkul, 1971). MCT oil was added to the feedings of extremely premature newborns from the late 1970s to early 1980s, since these fats were well-tolerated and helped promote more rapid weight gain. In the mid-1980s, higher calorie formulas containing up to 50 percent of the fat as MCTs were developed for premature newborns along with formulas with about 25 percent MCTs for full-term infants (Wu, 1986). Most infant formulas around the world today contain coconut oil and/or palm kernel oil, which are rich sources of MCTs, and many also contain MCT oil, specifically, formulas for premature newborns and babies who have trouble digesting their feedings normally.

Stephen Cunnane, a star in the world of ketone research, has written extensively on this subject in his books *Survival of the Fattest: The Key to Human Brain Evolution* (2005, World Scientific) and in *Human Brain Evolution: The Influence of Freshwater and Marine Food Resources* (2010, Wiley-Blackwell) with co-editor Kathryn Stewart. He points out that humans are the only land mammals who give birth to fat babies and that our babies—completely dependent on their parents for every need— are born several months premature in their development compared to other mammals. The large brain provides a major disadvantage during childbirth, since the very large head does not pass easily through the pelvis, a potentially serious and often fatal complication for both mother and baby before the advent of modern medicine. The oxygen-dependent energy requirement of the massive brain is so great that just five to ten minutes without oxygen can result in brain damage, sometimes quite severe.

Cunnane believes that fatness in the newborn has played a crucial role in the evolution of the large human brain by providing a back-up source of fuel to glucose as ketones to meet the extraordinary demands imposed by that brain. He and his associates have learned that ketones also serve as the main building blocks for the lipid-rich brain. In 1999, they published the results of their studies in mice: using radioactive labels, they tracked the fate of carbon atoms from certain eighteen-carbon essential omega-3 and omega-6 fatty acids (alpha-linolenic acid and linoleic acid) and were surprised to learn that these fatty acids are quite ketogenic. They were largely beta-oxidized and therefore broken down into ketones, which picked up the labeled carbons in the brain, the gut, and the liver. The labeled carbons then appear in cholesterol and the other important saturated, monounsaturated, and polyunsaturated fats in the brain. Cholesterol, saturated and monounsaturated fats do not easily cross from the bloodstream into the brain and must be made "from scratch" *in situ* (inside) the brain. It appears from these studies then that fats in the bloodstream are broken down into ketones that do cross into the brain where they become the building blocks for cholesterol and these other vital fats (Cunnane, 1999; Cunnane, 2003).

> Fatness in the newborn has played a crucial role in
> the evolution of the large human brain by providing
> a backup source of fuel to glucose as ketones to meet
> the extraordinary demands imposed by that brain.

Cholesterol and saturated fats have been villainized for their alleged roles in heart disease and are often thought by the non-scientist to be harmful. However, cholesterol plays a vital role in the structure and normal functions of the brain and most other cells, and as a precursor to many hormones. Defects in the ability to make cholesterol lead to very severe abnormalities in the development of humans, such as Smith-Lemli-Opitz syndrome, which results in abnormal brain, face, and limb development. Saturated fats also serve many important and necessary functions in the lung, in white blood cells, and in many other tissues.

Another important point from Cunnane's research is that only min-iscule amounts of these eighteen-carbon essential omega-3 and omega-6 fatty acids end up as the vital DHA (docosahexaenoic acid) and ARA (ara-chidonic acid). For many years until about 2002, infant formula manufac-turers relied on soybean and corn oil, which contain the eighteen-carbon omega-3 and omega-6 fats, believing that this would result in adequate DHA and ARA for the newborn brain, however, in reality, they are not reliable sources. The fetus picks up DHA and ARA from the mother and stores them in its own fat, slowly releasing them as needed after birth. The mother's diet plays a very significant role in how much of these essential fats are available to the fetus. For this reason, these days, in the United States and in many other countries, pregnant women are advised to take a DHA supplement to ensure an adequate supply to the fetus and newborn. Studies performed in the 1990s showed improved visual acuity and IQ in newborns who were given a test formula with DHA and ARA and finally, in 2002, some manufacturers began to add them to their infant formulas.

Newborns are not capable of storing much glucose in their bodies, and the supply can be depleted in a matter of an hour or even less if the baby is premature or small for age with poor fat reserves. Hypoglycemia (low blood sugar) is a big problem in the first hours of life, sending many babies to the newborn intensive care unit (ICU) for the standard treatment with intravenous fluids. It is a particularly serious problem for infants of diabetic mothers. The fetus experiences chronically elevated blood-sugar levels along with the mother, and the fetus's pancreas will produce high levels of insulin—sometimes extremely high—in response to the high blood sugar. After birth, it takes time for the insulin level to come back down to normal, often days or even weeks. It is common for the blood sugar to plummet shortly after birth, which is a risk for seizures and brain damage if not treated immediately, since the brain requires more glucose than it is provided in this situation. The treatment often involves using a much-higher-than-usual concentration of dextrose (glucose), given intravenously, and then slowly weaning the baby, lowering the concentration while checking the blood glucose very frequently to ensure that it is not too high or too low.

Ketones can easily replace glucose for the energy needs of the brain at all ages, but this concept has been overlooked in the standard treatment of hypoglycemia in the newborn. It would be interesting to study what happens to the betahydroxybutyrate level in this situation and would take only a fraction of a drop of blood for testing at the same time as blood glucose testing. Intravenous solutions containing betahydroxybutyrate have been used in research in the past, and an intravenous emulsion containing 50 percent medium-chain triglycerides, which the liver partly converts to ketones, was used in the 1980s as part of routine intravenous nutrition in newborn ICUs in the United States but has not been available here for many years (though it is available in Europe). A study reported in 1993 used MCT oil given to thirteen babies through a tube into the stomach (a common feeding practice with newborns) to treat hypoglycemia in addition to the usual intravenous fluids with dextrose (sugar). They found that the MCT oil significantly increased both glucose and ketone levels in these babies (Bourgneres, 1989). Using ketones as an alternative fuel for the brain could be a useful additional treatment for newborn hypoglycemia and, therefore, giving MCT oil as an adjunct to feeding could potentially save a lot of babies a trip to the newborn ICU, which is a very disappointing experience for new parents.

The whole point in this discussion about the fetus and the newborn is to stress the critical importance of fat and ketones to the newborn human in the successful transition from the womb to the outside world, as well as to the normal growth and development of the infant's very large brain.

WHERE'S THE FAT?

The question then becomes, do fat and ketones abruptly become unimportant after the first year of life? Most babies are weaned from the breast by six to twelve months of age. Formula-fed babies are usually weaned to cow's milk by one year or sometimes a little later—around eighteen to twenty-four months of age—if the pediatrician recommends a junior formula to supplement cow's milk. The Women, Infants, and Children (WIC) Program is a federally-assisted program that provides nutritional help to low-income pregnant women (as well as breastfeeding and non-breastfeeding postpartum women), infants, and young children and follows USDA guidelines. Their current recommendations are summarized on a diagram called My Plate for Preschoolers (see Figure 4.1.) The plate is more than three-quarters carbohydrates as fruits, vegetables, and grains (carbs, carbs, and more carbs), less than one-quarter protein and a cup on the side showing dairy. It recommends making half of the grains whole grains (which means the rest can be nutrition-stripped refined grains), but even worse, there is no fat shown on My Plate, and it actually advises the parent to use skim or 1 percent milk and yogurt (https://www.choosemyplate.gov/MyPlate).

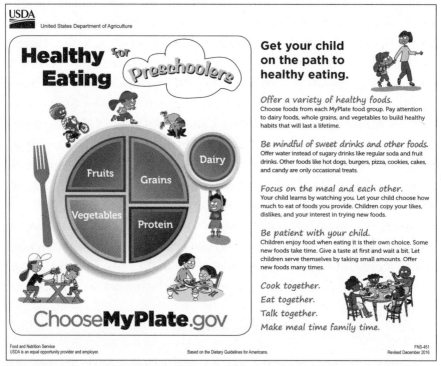

Figure 4.1. Where's the Fat? My Plate for Preschoolers is three-quarters carbohydrates and contains no fat; it recommends that up to half of grains can be refined and that milk should be skim or 1 percent fat. This sets up preschoolers for a very high-carb diet.

In the scenario typical in the United States, the one-year-old infant rather suddenly goes from consuming breast milk, which has about 50 percent of its calories as fat, or formula, which has a bit less fat, to eating a very-low-fat, high-carbohydrate diet. Is this really the right thing to do, given that the brain continues to grow rapidly at this point and needs cholesterol, fats, and ketones to do this well? In 2014, according to Centers for Disease Control and Prevention (CDC) surveys, 14.5 percent of children ages two to four who were on the WIC Program were obese, meaning that their weight was greater than the ninety-fifth percentile, and many more were considered overweight (CDC, 2016). In 1970, obesity rates in preschoolers were about a third of what they are now. Obese children are ten times more likely to grow up to be obese adults. Could the emphasis on eating large amounts of carbs, including refined flours and rice, at the expense of fat, have something to do with this?

Not only is obesity on the rise in children, but diabetes is as well. In a news release from the National Institutes of Health (NIH) on April 13, 2017, the first-ever study of trends in diabetes in children was published. Researchers found that between 2002 and 2012, rates of type 1 diabetes increased in children ages 0–19 by 1.8 percent per year, but even more significantly, type 2 diabetes increased by an astounding 4.8 percent per year. The news release remarked that development of diabetes at such a young age will "lessen [a person's] quality of life, shorten their life expectancy, and increase health-care costs." The release also noted that rates of diabetes are higher in certain ethnic groups that also have higher rates of low-income socioeconomic status and thus are more likely to participate in and receive nutrition counseling from the WIC Program. This study did not really attempt to identify the reasons for these trends but mentioned that other studies are in progress in this regard. (The report can be viewed at https://www.nih.gov/news-events/news-releases/rates-new-diagnosed-cases-type-1-type-2-diabetes-rise-among-children-teens.) Is it really possible that the current emphasis on the low-fat, high-carb diet would have nothing to do with these alarming trends? Most likely it has everything to do with it.

HUMAN EVOLUTION AND KETONES

So, what did people eat before the low-fat diet was promulgated and so many high sugar foods became readily available?

Humans have walked upright and eaten a larger proportion of meat than other primates have for more than 2.6 million years. According to Stephen C. Cunnane, eating meat would provide a higher quality diet—obviously more protein but also a specific micronutrient content that likely factored into the tripling of brain size compared to some of our closest upright pre-human relatives of two million years ago (Cunnane, 2010).

Our distant ancestors learned how to cook somewhere between 400,000 and 1.8 million years ago, which made the food more digestible and likely more palatable. There was an agricultural revolution about 10,000 to 12,000 years ago followed by domestication of animals for their milk and meat between 4,000 and 9,000 years ago at various places in the world. Before that, as far as we know, human life did not include plowed fields or rows of orchard trees from which to harvest grains, potatoes, or apples. Some of this information is detailed in an eye-opening article written by Ann Gibbons for National Geographic (www.nationalgeographic.com/foodfeatures/evolution-of-diet), who makes the point that, contrary to what the dicta of the current Paleo trend would have us believe, with rare exception, meat is not the whole story when it comes to how humans ate before agriculture became a way of life. (The rare exception is the Inuit population in the Arctic, who derive 99 percent of their calories from whales, seals, and other sea creatures.)

Most primitive humans were "hunter–gathers" who walked miles every day; the men hunted meat, fowl, and fish; the women foraged for enough vegetable and fruit matter, nuts, tubers, and bits of grain to keep themselves and their families alive. Some fortunate people managed to carve out a "garden" in the forests for themselves. A source of water was critical to survival and creeks, lakes, rivers, and oceans were, and still are, a great source of fish, shellfish, and other edible creatures. Some populations have even thrived on eating insects. Hunting was not a sport but a way of life for hunter–gatherers. We know this not only from fossil evidence and molecular genetics studies, but also from studying the very few remaining hunter–gatherer populations in our world today.

The 15,000 Tsimané Indians, who are spread out in about one hundred villages along the Amazon basin in Bolivia serve as just one example. Other groups in Africa, known as the Kung, Hadza and Aka and Baka Pygmies, as well as the Australian Aborigines, have been studied intensively as well. In some of these populations, the men are successful in bringing home game (meat and fish) only about half the time, and they rely heavily on what the women collect and make into porridge. While the wild gathered vegetable matter is mainly carbohydrate, it tends to be high in fiber (and many other nutrients) and would more likely than not have a low glycemic index and result in a low glycemic load (see Glycemic Index and Glycemic Load in Chapter 6) when combined with other foods. Tsimané women usually cook with rendered animal fat and rarely use vegetable oils, such as soy, corn, or safflower oil. Much of the fat intake is within the meat and fish they eat, and they do not eat dairy. The ability to tolerate dairy in humans is a fairly recent development in evolution. Very many people today have a problem with lactose (the main sugar in dairy) intolerance and therefore do not digest dairy well.

A study reported in *Lancet* in 2017 that the Tsimané people have the lowest rates of coronary atherosclerosis (hardening of the arteries) of any population yet studied, with 85 percent showing no accumulation of calcium (an indication of atherosclerosis) and only 8 percent of people older than seventy-five showing signs of an abnormal accumulation. They also have low blood pressure throughout their lives, low triglyceride levels, and low levels of LDL cholesterol. While the Tsimané do have to deal with high rates of infant and child mortality, parasites, and infections (the most common cause of death), and while they may not have ready access to the advances of modern day medicine, heart disease or high blood pressure are not problems they have to worry about. If they make it past infancy and childhood, the average lifespan is about seventy years (Kaplan, 2017; Cordain, 2002).

The Tsimané people say that their bodies "need meat," and they crave it. On average, meat and fish make up about 30 percent of their calorie intake, but they have periods of days to weeks when meat is scarce, so 70 percent of their calories overall come from plant matter. Other hunter–gatherer societies eat higher proportions of meat and fish, upward of 70 percent, with 30 percent from plant matter. Estimates of fat intake for most of these populations are between 36 and 45 percent of total calorie intake and, like the Tsimané, they tend to have very low rates of heart disease. But the types of fat they eat is much different from the types of fats eaten in modern societies. Most of their fat intake is animal fat, and their animals are wild and not fattened with grains. (The type of food an animal eats affects the composition of the fatty acids in their stored fat.) They use much less omega-6 fats and tend to have higher omega-3 DHA levels due to their fish intake, resulting in a much more favorable ratio of omega-6 to omega-3 fats in the 1:1 to 3:1 range, compared to people on a typical Western diet who may have a ratio of 10:1 or even 20:1. An imbalance in these ratios can result in increased inflammation, constriction of blood vessels, and a tendency for blood to clot more easily (Lands, 2005).

Many of the present-day hunter–gatherers are transitioning over to the modern-day way of eating, which may make life easier, but the downside, according to Gibbons's sources, is that they are acquiring modern-day diseases, such as diabetes and heart disease, in the process,.

THE SHIFT TO FARMING AND SHEPHERDING

The major shift in diet in most populations from hunter–gatherer to farming and shepherding had its advantages. The food supply became more dependable and predictable and women began to give birth more frequently, every 2.5 instead of 3.5 years on average, resulting in a population explosion. But a diet that consists of eating the same stored grain every day is less nutritionally diverse than a foraged diet, which may include upward of sixty or seventy different foods, and some of the trade-offs have been developmental delays related to iron and iodine deficiencies, periodontal disease, and cavities, rarely found in hunter–gatherers, along with harmful parasites, tuberculosis, and other infectious diseases contracted from the farm animals. Another trade-off was shorter stature, with the average height decreasing from 5 feet 10 inches to 5 feet 6 inches for men and from 5 feet 5 inches to 5 feet 1 inch for women. Average heights did not increase again until the twentieth century (Hermanussen, 2003).

On the other hand, the transition to agriculture and domestication of animals has been so successful to the propagation of humans that it is estimated by the turn of the next century there will be 4 billion more mouths to feed than the 7.5 billion people in the world today, according to the United Nations Population Fund. This compares with a population of about 370 million in the year 1350.

The daunting challenge of feeding such a huge mass of people has been met by major advances in agricultural science and the food industry. Keeping food cold or frozen in most parts of the world, except the iciest, has been possible only since the electric refrigerator was invented by General Electric less than a century ago in 1927. The trade-offs for all of this are that, as a group, we now tend to rely heavily on genetically modified foods that may be subjected to pesticides and other chemicals, created to make yields greater, food units larger, and shelf life longer, but resulting in foods that may have less nutritional value, might not be recognized and utilized the same way by our metabolic pathways, and may be contaminated with chemicals that are harmful to our health. Much has been written lately about the serious effects some of these dietary changes and chemical exposures have had on our microbiome (the universe of bacteria that live in our bowel and on our skin) and how this can affect our health profoundly. An excellent book to read on this topic and the gut-brain connection comes from David Perlmutter, the neurologist, in *Brain Maker* (Little, Brown and Company, 2015).

In her *National Geographic* article on "The Evolution of Diet," Ann Gibbons points out that "the real hallmark of being human isn't our taste for meat but our ability to adapt to many habitats—and to be able to combine many different foods to create many healthy diets. Unfortunately, the modern Western diet does not appear to be one of them."

> "The real hallmark of being human isn't our taste for meat but our ability to adapt to many habitats—and to be able to combine many different foods to create many healthy diets. Unfortunately, the modern Western diet does not appear to be one of them." Ann Gibbons.

DID OUR HUNTER-GATHERER ANCESTORS EXIST IN A STATE OF KETOSIS?

I have not been able to find any studies specifically looking at present day hunter–gatherer populations and whether they might exist mostly in a state of ketosis. There is little doubt that they eat part of what they find on their travels, but they bring the rest of their bounty and gatherings back home to share as a larger meal toward the end of the day. The infants and young children are breastfed until two to three years of age on average, until the next baby arrives, so they receive a high fat diet, including some medium-chain triglycerides (MCTs) in the mother's milk; on the other hand, toward the end of the first year they would also be fed some of what the older children and adults are eating. It is very likely that this dietary pattern was typical for our hunter–gatherer ancestors as well. The hunter–gatherer lifestyle would lend itself to going in and out of ketosis for several good reasons:

1. Periods of low food supply with inadequate intake of calories would result in ketosis, as the body turns to fat for fuel. "Intermittent fasting" is a technique deliberately used today to stimulate ketone production.

2. An overnight fast of just ten to twelve hours can mildly increase ketone levels, and it is likely that these people do not raid the kitchen pantry at night.

3. In contrast to sedentary Americans who may walk less than a kilometer per day, hunter–gatherers cruise for up to 10 miles per day, with men walking for about six to seven hours and women walking for four to six hours per day.

    a. Just thirty to forty minutes of vigorous exercise can result in an increase in ketones that lasts as long as nine hours, a phenomenon known as "post-exercise ketosis." (See Chapter 7 for details and references.)

    b. Cunnane, Castellano, and associates performed a study using ketone and glucose positron emission tomography (PET) scans, in which people with mild Alzheimer's participated in a twelve-week program of walking on a treadmill for forty minutes at 4 to 8 km/hour (2.5 to 5 mph) three times per week. By the end of the program, the participants had nearly triple the ketone uptake in the brain compared to ketone uptake before they started the program (Castellano, 2017).

    c. There are two types of muscle fibers, with type 1 using fatty acids and type 2 using glucose for fuel. During low intensity endurance type exercise (as opposed to high intensity bursts of exercise, like sprints), type 1 muscle fibers come into play and the fatty acids released over a period of hours per day may be partly converted to ketones.

Considering all of this, there is good reason to believe that, before the agricultural way of life took hold, our predecessors were in at least mild ketosis much, if not nearly all of the time.

There is good reason to believe that, before the agricultural
way of life took hold, our predecessors were in at least
mild ketosis much, if not nearly all of the time.

THE ROLE OF THE COCONUT IN HUMAN SURVIVAL

As a huge fan of coconut, because of what that food did for my husband, Steve, and because I just like it for many reasons, I cannot leave the subject of human survival throughout evolution without talking about the coconut palm and its role in human nutrition for eons. Another reason I want to touch on the topic is that some of the ketogenic strategies discussed in this book center around or can be enhanced with coconut oil and the medium-chain triglycerides it contains.

Fossil evidence places coconuts in Australia, India, Indonesia, and the Americas as far back as 37 to 55 million years—many millions of years before humans appeared on Earth, and the history of coconuts "is fundamentally intertwined with the history of humans in the tropics" (Gunn, 2011). The tree grows well in humid tropical regions, loves water, stands as high as 98 feet and can yield between thirty and seventy-five coconut fruits per year (See Photo 4.1.). Some genetic variations have been helpful in studying the migration patterns of the coconut palm, including a dwarf version that appears to be the result of human selection of specific traits.

The history of coconuts "is fundamentally intertwined
with the history of humans in the tropics."
Alistair Jan Gunn

The coconut can float on water for up to 3,000 miles (4,828 km) and still germinate more than 110 days later (Edmondson, 1941). Thus many experts believe that the coconut spread from India and Indonesia regions, eventually arriving at many other places in the world, by "float" distributing itself, riding on ocean currents and taking root wherever it landed.

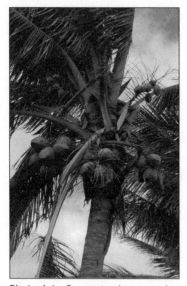

Photo 4.1. Coconut palms grow in tropical regions including southern Florida in the United States. One tree can produce thirty to seventy-five coconuts per year. Photo by Mary Newport.

Humans contributed to its spread by carrying the coconuts inland and planting them near good sources of water. Also, as a portable source of food and drink and a useful item for trade, the coconut was very often taken along for sea voyages on rafts and ships, turning up hundreds to thousands of miles away and planted at the end of the trip on islands and larger land masses, eventually arriving in the New World an estimated 2,250 years ago, brought first from Asia, most likely from the Philippines by way of Polynesia, to the Pacific coast of Latin America and later in the 1400s by European explorers to start plantations in the Caribbean islands (Edmondson, 1941).

Today, nearly 30 million acres (12 million hectares) of coconuts grow in eighty-nine-tropical countries (Batugal, 2005). Indonesia and the Philippines are the top exporters of coconuts and its products, while India is the largest producer and consumer of coconuts.

The coconut palm is called the "tree of life" in places like the Philippines because every bit of the tree and its fruit, the coconut, has a useful purpose. These days the coconut has hundreds of uses as whole food, an ingredient in other food products, drinks (coconut water found inside the nut, as well as coconut milk), fiber, charcoal, fertilizer for new trees, construction material and, of course, the oil, which is used in cooking, in skin and oral medications and supplements, soaps, industrial applications and even as biofuel (Gunn, 2011). Coconut oil is a great moisturizer for skin and hair, is a natural lubricant (suppositories and sex come to mind), and is even used for cleaning teeth by brushing (spit it into a garbage can or use hot water so you don't clog the sink) and a technique called oil pulling. With oil pulling, a teaspoon or two of the oil is worked around in the mouth for about twenty minutes to allow time for the oil to work its magic. With regular oil pulling, the teeth become quite clean and slick.

The use of coconut for oil pulling and in pharmaceuticals stems from the recognition that lauric acid, which composes about 50 percent of the coconut fats, is antimicrobial, as is capric acid, also contained in coconut, to a lesser extent. Chemist and coconut oil expert Fabian Dayrit of the Philippines cites numerous studies in his review of the properties of lauric acid, reporting that it kills viruses like herpes simplex and HIV, fungi such as Candida, protozoa, and dozens of bacteria, including the microorganisms that cause acne and dental caries (Dayrit, 2015).

Pure coconut water can be found inside the mature coconut and contains an abundance of vitamins and minerals. It was used in a pinch during World War II as an intravenous fluid due to its favorable electrolyte content and has become very popular in recent years as a sports rehydration drink and, medically, to treat dehydration orally. Immature green coconuts contain jelly instead of water at the center and have become popular for the potential health benefits. You can eat the jelly and then scoop out the delicious soft white meat with a spoon.

Pertinent to the ketogenic diet, the coconut is the richest natural source of medium-chain triglycerides (MCTs) at about 60 percent, which, when eaten, are partly converted to ketones in the liver. The next richest source of MCTs is the palm kernel at 54 percent from the oil palm tree. Historically, compared to the coconut palm, the oil palm is a latecomer in the world of commercial edible oils. The oil palm originated in the tropical forests of West Africa, and the oils in the palm fruits have been essential components of tasty food recipes for thousands of years. Somewhere between the fourteenth and seventeenth centuries, palm fruits arrived in the Americas, where they did not do particularly well. These palms were then taken to the Far East where they eventually became a major plantation crop in the twentieth century in some countries near the equator with high rainfall, such as Malaysia and Indonesia. The oil palm gives the highest yield of oil for the same land area for any crop and many MCT oil products are extracted from the palm kernel. The MCT oils extracted from coconut oil and palm kernel oil are identical in molecular composition, color, and taste.

The palm fruit is much smaller than the coconut, easily held in the palm of your hand, and unique in that two different kinds of oils can be extracted from it. The outer meat of the palm fruit, called the mesocarp, is orange and contains deep red and flavorful palm oil, which is extremely low in MCTs. The inner white kernel is separated from the mesocarp by a shell, is very rich in MCTs, including 47 percent lauric acid with a fatty acid composition quite similar to coconut oil. Both of the oils contain significant tocopherols (vitamin E) and some vitamin K (see Photo 4.2).

One issue that has plagued the oil palm industry (not involving the coconut palm) is the practice of slashing and burning the trees without replanting, often encroaching on protected forests, which affects the animal life as well. However, efforts have been made in recent years to educate the oil palm farmers in better, less-harmful practices, and a Roundtable on Sustainable Palm Oil (RSPO) certification has been put in place to designate companies that buy only from farmers who practice these sustainable techniques.

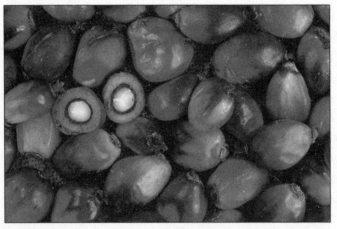

Photo 4.2. Red palm oil is extracted from the orange pulp of the palm; fruit and palm kernel oil comes from the white meat at the center of the fruit.

THE LOW-CARBOHYDRATE DIET FOR WEIGHT LOSS IN THE NINETEENTH CENTURY AND BEYOND

I have been on many different types of weight loss diets since I was eight years old, but I clearly remember that my pediatrician in the 1960s advised me to cut out sweets and starches, such as bread, potatoes, and desserts, to lose weight. Where did that idea come from?

David Diamond, PhD, a neuroscientist at University of South Florida, learned some interesting facts about this while on a quest to improve his own health. Dr. Diamond gives an outstanding presentation on low- versus high-fat diets, saturated fats, cholesterol, and statins that can be viewed at YouTube.com (David Diamond—An Update on Demonization and Deception in Research on Saturated Fat. https://www.youtube.com/watch?v=uc1XsO3mxX8). His presentation starts with a review of the historical perspective of diets, obesity, and health featuring a booklet published in London in 1863, written by sixty-five-year-old William Banting, who was considered to be very fat at 202 pounds and 5 feet 5 inches tall. The book is readily available and is a quick and interesting read for nutrition and history buffs.

As a retired Victorian undertaker to the royalty, Banting was relatively wealthy and lived a sedentary lifestyle compared to the average person at that time. He struggled immensely just to get up and down the stairs and could barely reach his feet to tie his shoes. Banting tried to lose weight by following suggestions from several physicians that only resulted in hunger and more health problems. He visited an ear, nose, and throat physician, Dr. William Harvey, who also gave him dietary advice that resulted in a weight loss of forty-six pounds over the following year; his sight and hearing improved substantially as well. He was easily able to negotiate the steps and tie his shoes. Banting was so excited that he decided to share Dr. Harvey's dietary advice so that others could be cured of the "disease of obesity." He wrote and published a booklet *Letter on Corpulence, Addressed to the Public* (Harrison, London, 1863). Banting writes that before receiving dietary advice from Dr. Harvey, he "partook of the simple aliments of bread, milk, butter, beer, sugar, and potatoes more freely than my aged nature required" and these foods were "the main elements of my existence." He believed that the lack of activity since his retirement contributed greatly to his obesity. So he tried rowing, but this gave him a "prodigious appetite." He tried other forms of exercise, like horseback riding and walking in the sea air, often prescribed by physicians for obesity, along with Turkish vapor baths and shampooing.

Eventually, from Dr. Harvey he received some very different advice: to eliminate the bread, milk, beer, sugar, and potatoes that he was so fond of because these foods "contain starch and saccharine matter, tending to create fat, and should be avoided altogether." Up to that point, Banting had eaten "bread and milk for breakfast, or a pint of tea with plenty of milk and sugar, buttered toast; meat, beer, much bread (of which [he] was always very fond) and pastry for dinner, the meal of tea similar to that of breakfast, and generally a fruit tart or bread and milk for supper"—in other words, a very high-carbohydrate diet. He "had little comfort and far less sound sleep." He wondered what he would eat instead but settled on three meals a day that consisted of meats, fish, and bacon (totaling about 12- to 15-ounces per day), any kind of vegetables but potatoes, two or three ounces of fruit, an ounce or less of bread, a glass or two of wine and a grog (hard liquor) without sugar before bed. He drank plenty of water and tea without sugar or milk. He steadily lost about 1 pound per week and soon found that he was sleeping well at night for six to eight hours.

Banting states in his book that, as a result of this diet, "I am very much better, bodily and mentally, and pleased to believe that I hold the reins of health and comfort in my own hands, and, though at sixty-five years of age, I cannot expect to remain free from some coming natural infirmity that all flesh is heir to, I cannot at the present time complain of one."

Banting also writes about a friend who decided to try out his diet and, after just eight weeks, stopped having frequent heart palpitations and "sensations of fainting," and was "a new man." In a later edition of the book, Banting reported that he was "restored in health, 'bodily and mentally,'" had more muscular power and "vigour," ate and drank "with a good appetite" and slept well. "All symptoms of acidity, indigestion, and heartburn (with which I was frequently tormented) have vanished."

Banting sold more than 63,000 copies of his pamphlet in England alone. It was translated into several other languages and even found its way to the United States. Though he received harsh criticism and resistance from doctors, he received letters from more than two thousand people thanking him for writing the booklet and received innumerable reports of successful weight loss and improvements in health using this dietary approach. Several times in the booklet he gave credit and thanks to Dr. Harvey. His only regret is that he did not have a photo taken before he started on the diet to compare with the more slender version of himself published in his booklet (Photo 4.3).

William Banting lived to age eighty-one, well beyond the average lifespan at that time. His book was so popular that a new verb came into the English language in the late 1800s—*bant*, which means "to diet"! Was William Banting on a ketogenic diet? The answer is very likely "Yes" since his meal plans included relatively

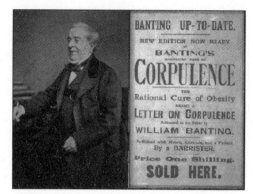

Photo 4.3.

small amounts of carbs, and Victorian meat, fish, and vegetable dishes were often cooked with butter and bacon. Sauces containing butter and cream were the norm. (See http://recipespastandpresent.org.uk/victoriancooking /fish.php.)

Another book, *How Nature Cures—Comprising a New System of Hygiene; Also The Natural Food of Man* was written in 1892 by English physician Emmet Densmore, MD (available on Amazon) and he explains that, "The central thought on which this book is written is the confident belief that sickness and acute attacks of illness bear the same relation to diet that drunkenness bears to drink." The subtitle of the book is, "A Statement of the Principal Arguments against the Use of Bread, Cereals, Pulses [peas or lentils], Potatoes, and Other Starch Foods."

Dr. Densmore tried various dietary approaches with his patients and for himself and his wife. He observed that when he advised the patient who was overweight with medical conditions to eat meat and non-starch foods, they would lose not only weight but their illnesses as well. When they improved, for a time he would then advise them to change back to a diet of "bread, fruit and pulse," and he was surprised to see many of them developed serious problems; the people who refused to change to the new diet retained their health. In 1889, Densmore himself was experiencing mental cloudiness and sleepiness in the afternoon and evening after eating and poor sleep at night and decided to try a "non-starch dietary." At about a week into the new diet, he found that he was "able to proceed at once to the transaction of business, or the writing of an essay, without any sense of having eaten, and without the slightest heaviness or drowsiness." He was alert and awake instead of dull and sleepy throughout the evening, and he began to sleep well. He was very likely following a ketogenic diet. Densmore came to the conclusions that that "the successful treatment, the world around, for obesity and diabetes, is the elimination of all starch foods from the dietary" and that "cereals, the universal food, are the primal source of universal disease." Thereafter, he recommended to his patients that they eat a non-starch diet and include eggs, milk and cheese, meat, nuts, and some fruit. His book is an interesting look back at the practice of medicine in that era, and his experience with diet is just part of it.

It is striking that both Banting and Densmore reported improved health benefits that go well beyond weight loss: sharper mental focus, increased energy, improved sleep, and the resolution of illnesses. That proved true both for themselves and others who tried their dietary plans and is consistent with what so many people report today when they make the transition from a high-carb to a low-carb ketogenic diet and/or take exogenous ketone supplements, such as ketone salts.

> It is striking that both Banting and Densmore reported improved health benefits for themselves and others who tried their dietary plans, that go well beyond just weight loss, such as sharper mental focus, increased energy, improved sleep and the resolution of illnesses.

BIRTH OF THE CLASSIC KETOGENIC DIET IN THE EARLY TWENTIETH CENTURY

In modern times, the successful use of fasting for epilepsy was first reported in the early twentieth century by two French physicians, G. Guelpa and A. Marie (Guelpa, 1911). Around that time, fitness expert and magazine publisher Bernarr MacFadden popularized the idea of using a three- to thirty-day fast to cure diseases, including epilepsy, and, not long after, Hugh W. Conklin, DO, an assistant to MacFadden, began to prescribe fasting for treatment of seizures.

In 1921, a pediatrician, Rawle Geyelin, MD, reported at an American Medical Association convention on Conklin's successful treatment of three patients with epilepsy. One of these patients was a ten-year-old boy with severe epilepsy who underwent two very long periods of fasting, after which he had no seizures for the next year. Dr. Geyelin also reported that eighteen of twenty-six patients he himself treated showed marked improvement, and two were seizure-free for more than a year. He found that a twenty-day fast appeared to have the best results. The working idea at the time was that fasting resulted in the release of toxins that were causing the seizures. Geyelin was the first to report that one could almost always clear a "clouded mentality" with fasting, an idea that did not appear again in the literature for decades.

On July 27, 1921, R. M. Wilder, MD, authored "The Effects of Ketonemia on the Course of Epilepsy," a brief article in *The Clinic Bulletin* of the Mayo Clinic, in which he reported that ketonemia (a state in which ketone levels are high) was produced during fasts. He wrote that ketones "are also formed from fat and protein whenever a disproportion exists between the amount of fatty acid and the amount of sugar actually burning in the tissues." He suggested that, in place of fasting, the ketogenic diet might also produce good results in treating epilepsy, since it was "long known" that it was possible to "provoke ketogenesis" by using a diet "very rich in fat and very low in carbohydrates." Another article, entitled "High-fat Diets in Epilepsy," ran in *The Clinic Bulletin* the very next day on July 28, 1921. In this article, C. E. Baker presents three brief case reports of patients, ages thirteen, thirty-one, and twenty-three, describing the successful use of the ketogenic diet initiated in the hospital to eliminate seizures. In the case report of the thirteen-year-old, Baker states that the diet consisted of 15 grams of carbohydrate, 57 grams of protein, and 231 grams of fat, putting fat at about 88 percent of total calories. This report was followed with a brief discussion written by Dr. Wilder in which he states, "It is impossible to draw conclusions from the results of these few patients treated with high-fat diets, but we have here a method of observing the effect of ketosis on the epileptic. If this is the mechanism responsible for the beneficial effects of fasting, it may be possible to substitute for that rather brutal procedure a dietary therapy which the patient can follow with little inconvenience and continue at home as long as seems necessary" (Wilder, 1921; Baker, 1921).

And so the classic ketogenic diet for epilepsy was born just less than one hundred years ago. The ratios of fat, protein, and carbohydrates used in the classic ketogenic diet today have not changed.

In the classic ketogenic diet, about 80 to 90 percent of calories come from fat, and the other 10 to 20 percent come from protein and carbohydrate combined. Protein is limited because it can be converted in the liver to carbohydrate, through a process called gluconeogenesis, which generates about ½ gram of glucose for each gram of protein eaten when carbohydrate stores have been used up. At the same time, it is necessary to provide enough protein to prevent the breakdown of muscle and other tissues in the body, the so-called lean body mass. For children with seizures who are on a ketogenic diet, protein is strictly calculated to allow for preservation of muscle and for adequate growth.

From the 1920s to the 1960s, there was considerable research on the ketogenic diet and epilepsy as well as the production of ketones during starvation. As lab techniques improved for measuring ketones, animal studies were performed and then confirmed by human studies to learn more about how ketones are made and metabolized. Two of these earliest pioneers in ketone research, George Cahill Jr. and Oliver Owen, MD, who though recently passed away, were still actively writing about ketones and the potential to treat disease through nutritional ketosis in the early twenty-first century. Physicians Sami Hashim and Richard Veech are still actively working on developing and testing exogenous ketone supplements. Dr. Theodore VanItallie, age ninety-eight at the time of this writing in 2018, studied medium-chain triglycerides with Dr. Hashim in the mid-twentieth century and discovered that MCTs are partly converted to ketones in the liver. Years later, VanItallie carried out an encouraging landmark study of the ketogenic diet in Parkinson's disease (VanItallie, 2005). He is still constantly researching and publishing on the potential therapeutic uses of ketones. Read more about these physicians and their important work in Chapter 5.

Unfortunately, for children with epilepsy, in the middle of the twentieth century, as various anti-seizure medications came into widespread use, the ketogenic diet as a treatment for epilepsy was forgotten by most pediatricians and neurologists for many years and, for that reason, fewer dieticians were trained to counsel people on it.

DR. ALFRED PENNINGTON IN THE MID-TWENTIETH CENTURY

Just as the ketogenic diet was moving toward the back burner for children with epilepsy, a low-carb diet came to the forefront for weight loss. In 1953, Alfred W. Pennington, MD, challenged the notion that obesity is simply the result of careless overeating (Pennington, 1953). Instead, he recognized from the evidence available at the time that appetite is "part of a complex mechanism for assuring an appropriate intake of food." He proposed that obesity could be the result of damage to the hypothalamus or due to abnormal neural or humoral influences, affecting the sensitivity of the hypothalamus, which controls appetite and hunger as one of its many hormonal functions, noting that people with hyperinsulinism (when the body produces too much insulin) are often obese. Another explanation is that there could be an "abnormally functioning fat storage mechanism." He quoted R. M. Wilder and G. M. Randall that, "In some individuals with obesity, fat stores are less available for oxidation while deposition of fat is accelerated" (Wilder, 1945). Pennington noted that some lab animals, and probably people too, seem to have a "retarded mobilization" of fat.

Obesity researchers at that time discovered that "pyruvic acid, which is formed as an intermediate product in the breakdown of carbohydrate, inhibits the oxidation of fat and stimulates the synthesis of fatty acids from smaller elements" (Pennington, 1953). Instead of simply restricting calories, Pennington suggested that severely restricting carbohydrate intake would result in less production of pyruvic acid and therefore decrease its effects of stimulating fat formation and inhibiting fat oxidation; at the same time, fatty acids in the bloodstream would be used instead of carbohydrate as fuel and would be replaced in the blood by fatty acids from the body's fat stores. He reported studies in which obese participants ate *ad libitum* (as much as they wanted), taking in 2,000 to 3,100 calories per day as lean and fat meat, and still lost weight; these people also experienced a 5 to 7 percent increase in their metabolic rates. Pennington proposed a diet in which a person could eat however much protein and fat they choose, while restricting only carbohydrate intake.

Later that year—1953—Pennington published an article discussing the use of this calorically unrestricted diet to treat obesity (Pennington, 1953).

He pointed out that the basal caloric expenditure (also called the basal metabolic rate—the minimum number of calories needed to keep the body functioning while at rest) does not decline when carbohydrate alone is restricted; however, there is a decline when total calories are restricted. Basically, in a typical low-calorie diet, which often includes significant carbohydrate, at some point, the body senses impending "starvation" and lowers the basal metabolic rate to conserve energy. This is a disadvantage when someone is trying to lose weight because far fewer calories will be burned and weight loss will slow down or even stop, resulting in the infamous and discouraging plateau. Also, very overweight people who lose weight will often find that they need to adjust to taking in significantly fewer calories to maintain their weight loss than people who are their age with similar height and weight.

Pennington also notes several studies showing that the use of "glucose, fatty acids and ketones by the tissues is influenced by the concentration of these substance in the blood." He then proposed that increasingthe mobilization and utilization of fat would allow adequate calories for the tissues to carry out their basic functions and therefore no decline in the basal metabolic rate. He goes on to say that a diet consisting of protein and fat is ketogenic and recognizes that ketogenesis appears to be the "normal mechanism by which the organism is enabled to utilize fat in much larger quantities than it normally would." The blood levels of ketones and fatty acids would increase, "causing the tissues to oxidize them in larger amounts" and, therefore, ketogenesis would be "the key to the possibility of weight reduction on calorically unrestricted diets." He said this would be especially applicable to the obese. He predicted that the appetite would decline on this type of diet based on such findings in animal experiments.

Pennington recommended eating eight ounces of meat for each of three meals per day, which would equal about 180 grams of protein in a day, give or take a little depending on the type of meat, fish, or poultry eaten. He emphasized that fat, as well as lean meat, should be eaten and that one part of fat should be eaten for every three parts of lean meat, which would equate to about 2 teaspoons of fat or oil for each 4-ounce serving of lean meat. He suggested buying extra beef kidney fat to fry along with the meat. Regarding carbohydrates, he notes studies showing that ketogenesis is reduced when more than 100 grams of carbohydrates are eaten per day, but ketogenesis is stimulated below 40, and possibly below 60 grams or less per day of carbohydrates, also mentioning that ketogenic diets seem to show "a very favorable protein-sparing action." This is important because our muscles use considerable calories, and muscle is often lost during a standard weight-loss diet. The basal metabolic rate will be lower with less muscle mass, making it more difficult to maintain the weight loss, along with less strength and power, a disadvantage to long-term health and survival.

Pennington suggested that the amount of carbohydrate restriction should be tailored to the individual and that some people may need even more-drastic restriction to result in ketogenesis. His diet proposed that the individual eat three big meals per day with meat and fat as above, suggesting various seasonings and condiments, each the same, including one "ordinary portion" of white or sweet potatoes, boiled rice, half grapefruit, grapes, slice of melon, a banana, a pear, raspberries, or blueberries. He also recommended consuming plenty of water and other fluids such as tea and coffee, a half lemon per day in water, and to limit salt and salty meats. He stated that "this diet contains no bread, flour, salt, sugar, alcohol, or anything else not mentioned." His references included the fourth edition of the book by our friend William Banting from 1863.

Pennington also recommended that people avoid oversleeping and that they consider taking a thirty-minute walk before breakfast, which would stimulate greater use of fat as fuel, especially after an overnight fast. He predicted that this type of diet would reduce appetite and, therefore, overall caloric intake and people would lose 7 pounds per month on average. Some very large patients were able to eat 3,000 calories per day on this diet and still lose weight. Worth noting: this diet contains virtually no vegetables, nuts, or dairy.

The Pennington diet stirred up some controversy. However, certain nutrition researchers found success for their highly motivated patients with the Pennington Diet, noting that those who stuck with the diet and lost weight were not hungry and found it much easier to maintain their weight two years later. Those who abandoned the diet did so because they found it to be monotonous and/or they missed eating sugary foods (Leith, 1961).

THE ATKINS DIET

Does the Pennington diet sound seem a lot like the Atkins diet? If the answer is "Yes," then you will not be surprised to learn that the Pennington diet inspired the Atkins diet. Robert C. Atkins, MD, a cardiologist, read an article by Alfred Pennington describing his low-carbohydrate ketogenic diet and developed his own diet plan outlined in his best seller book, *Dr. Atkins' New Diet Revolution,* published in 1992. The diet was wildly popular and stirred considerable controversy given that the USDA and American Heart Association were promoting the "low-fat diet," and this was quite the opposite, allowing a person to eat as much bacon and other foods as desired, a practice considered to be unhealthy by these establishment groups. The fact that Dr. Atkins was a cardiologist added fuel to the flames of the controversy. The fad subsided for a while but there was a resurgence of interest in the early 2000s that led to *Time* magazine naming Atkins as one of the ten most influential people of 2002.

The Atkins diet is considerably more structured than the Pennington diet but followed the same basic principles, allowing unrestricted consumption of protein and fat while greatly restricting carbohydrates. The diets differ in that Atkins allowed for other proteins such as eggs and cheese, as well as limited amounts of vegetables, fruits, nuts and dairy in the diet, so long as the carbohydrate content is counted. There is a two-week induction period during which carbohydrates are limited to 20 grams per day. Thereafter, carbohydrates are increased by 5 grams per week until weight loss stalls; then they are stepped back to the previous level and continued at that level until the weight loss goal is achieved. At that point, carbohydrates are increased in small increments to find the ideal maintenance amount of carbohydrates for that person. Considerable water is lost from muscle during the first week, which is very encouraging on the scale, and then the fat loss kicks in. Regarding the unrestricted protein allowed in both the Pennington and Atkins diets, it should be noted that excessive protein could be converted to glucose at a rate of about ½ gram for each gram of protein.

In his book, Dr. Atkins goes into detail about how insulin keeps us fat and how the low-carbohydrate ketogenic diet reduces blood sugar and insulin levels while increasing ketone levels, a sign of fat-burning. He discusses some of the problems associated with eating too much sugar and examines how the ketogenic diet makes you healthy. He also recommends a good vitamin supplement and suggests using lipolysis testing strips (one brand is Ketostix), which detect the ketone acetoacetate in the urine (but not the much more predominant ketone betahydroxybutyrate). I still have my original copy of *Dr. Atkins' New Diet Revolution* from the 1990s, heavily earmarked. Dr. Atkins died in 2003 after suffering a severe blunt head injury that put him into a coma. At the time, there was a rumor that he died from a heart attack, which set off a lot of "I told you so" comments in the media. Dr. Atkins did, in fact, suffer a cardiac arrest at one point before that, which is different from a heart attack. However, he suffered from a chronic viral infection involving his heart, called cardiomyopathy, and his doctor stated at that time that his angiogram (a test used to look for blockage of blood vessels in the heart) was pristine—the arteries were clean.

The Atkins diet, also called the Atkins Nutritional Approach, was redesigned and a new book was published in 2010 entitled *The New Atkins for a New You* written by Eric Westman, MD, Stephen Phinney, MD, and Jeff Volek, PhD, who have researched the low-carbohydrate diet extensively. The authors also have considerable practical experience using the diet with people with medical conditions, as well using it with healthy people and professional athletes. They have found that people with type 2 diabetes respond extremely well to this diet, particularly if they restrict carbohydrates to 20 grams or less per day, and they are often able to discontinue insulin and diabetic medications within weeks or even days. The main changes to the diet are a limitation on how much protein is eaten, recommending typically 13 to 22 ounces per day, and an emphasis on the importance of eating healthy fats and using amounts of fat that will allow the person to "savor" but not "smother" the food. Excessive calories from fat, the authors point out, could interfere with weight loss. They also stress the importance of including a marine source of the essential omega-3 fats. Finally, Colette Heimowitz has written an excellent resource for the diet called *The New Atkins Made Easy*.

As of early 2018, Dr. Volek has authored nearly three-hundred research studies, many of them in collaboration with Dr. Phinney, and they have co-authored in-depth books on low-carbohydrate diets, including *The Art* and *Science of Low Carbohydrate Living* and *The Art and Science of Low Carbohydrate Performance*. Some of their vast body of research will be discussed in later chapters.

THE SOUTH BEACH DIET

The South Beach Diet published in 2003, also a best seller launching another diet fad, had its roots in a diet plan that Arthur Agatson, MD, also a cardiologist, originally developed in the mid-1990s for patients coming to see him at his office in South Beach. It is often considered to be a low-carb diet, but it actually does not severely restrict carbohydrates. Instead, Agatson places more emphasis than the original Atkins diet did on eating healthy fats and "good" carbohydrates. He specifies avoiding white bread, potatoes and white rice and including foods with a low-glycemic impact that do not cause the sudden spike in glucose followed by a spike in insulin levels that are characteristic of "bad" carbohydrates, such as whole grains, nuts, legumes, and most vegetables. There is no fruit and higher-sugar vegetables are listed as "foods to avoid" during the initial phase of the diet. His book does not discuss ketosis or claim to be a ketogenic diet, but it could be, if small enough portions are eaten of the "carbs to enjoy," along with healthy fats and adequate but not too much protein. This book is a great resource for learning what a healthy whole-food diet should look like.

THE MEDITERRANEAN AND THE PALEO DIETS

Some other diets that should be mentioned here for completeness are the Paleo diet and the Mediterranean diet. Either of these diets could easily be adapted to become a ketogenic diet.

Loren Cordain, PhD spent two decades studying the natural human diet throughout evolution and is considered to be the world expert on the Paleolithic diet. Dr. Cordain is the founder of the very popular Paleo diet movement and author of the huge best-seller *The Paleo Diet*. According to his website, https://thepaleodiet.com, he has also authored more than one hundred scientific peer-reviewed articles that have appeared in major medical journals. He formulated the Paleo diet to bring to modern-day humans the health benefits that come from consuming the natural diet of our ancestors. The diet consists of meat from grass-fed animals, fish and other seafood, eggs, fresh fruits and vegetables, nuts and seeds, as well as healthful oils (including olive, walnut, flaxseed, macadamia, avocado and coconut oils). Foods to be avoided include cereal grains, legumes, dairy, refined sugar, potatoes, processed foods, refined vegetable oil, and salt. The Paleo diet could very easily provide a great foundation for a ketogenic diet, as long as dieters limit fruit, eat protein in reasonable amounts, and consume enough fat. (For more information see https://thepaleodiet.com /what-to-eat-on-the-paleo-diet-paul-vandyken/.)

The concept of the Mediterranean diet, which began to attract attention in the 1990s because of its potential health benefits, is based on the centuries-old eating habits of people who live in southern Europe and northern Africa. The roots of the diet may actually go back thousands of years or longer, to Hippocrates and other Greek physicians who wrote about the use of nutrition for their patients. Hippocrates is well-known for saying, "Let food be thy medicine and medicine be thy food."

The Mediterranean diet is mentioned repeatedly in a very interesting book by Dan Buettner entitled *The Blue Zones* (2nd edition 2012, National Geographic Society), which takes a close look at the diets and other habits of people living in locations around the world where there are heavy concentrations of centenarians. One of these spots is in Sardinia, a large island in the Mediterranean west of Italy, and another is on Ikaria, a Greek island in the Aegean Sea. In the course of writing his book, Buettner interviewed numerous centenarians to try to learn their secrets to longevity. The traditional Mediterranean diet varies from place to place, but the basic foods include plenty of olive oil, vegetables and fruits, legumes, fish, and some alcohol every day, but limited amounts of meat and dairy. Buettner interviewed a centenarian who lived on Ikaria and learned that, over the course of the seasons, the people in that area gather more than 150 different varieties of green to use in salads and that some of these greens contain more than ten times the amount of antioxidants found in red wine. The people in Ikaria also drink "mountain tea" every day from whatever herbs and greens are in season, and they start their day with a spoonful of honey, which they take like a medicine. Depending on how much olive oil one consumes, and if fruit is limited, the Mediterranean diet could easily provide the basis for a healthy ketogenic diet.

Steve and the Mediterranean Diet

In 2006, I began to consider the role that nutrition might play in Alzheimer's disease. I read every book I could find on healthy nutrition, and we made changes to our diet. Before then, we were eating the SAD (standard American diet), or, as I like the call it, the convenience-food diet. In 2007, I came across an article reporting that people with Alzheimer's who ate a diet most like the Mediterranean diet lived on average nearly four years longer than the people who followed an eating plan least like the Mediterranean diet: an average of 10.5 years following diagnosis compared to 6.59 years. This article sealed the deal. Steve and I both transitioned quickly from a relatively healthy to a more Mediterranean diet with plenty of olive oil, more fish than meat, different colors of vegetables and plenty of them, fruits, whole grain rice instead of bread, pasta, and potatoes, and considerably fewer carbohydrates than we had eaten in the past (Scarmeas, 2007).

VEGETARIAN AND VEGAN DIETS

The vegetarian and vegan diets have become more popular in recent years. Are these diets compatible with the ketogenic diet?

The vegetarian diet is a diet that eliminates the flesh of animals, including beef, poultry, pork, fish or any other animal. It also excludes the by-products of animal slaughter. On the other hand, unfertilized eggs, milk and milk products are permitted, although some vegetarians exclude dairy but eat eggs (ovo-vegetarians) and others eliminate eggs but use dairy (lacto-vegetarians). Since dairy and eggs are good sources of protein, and there are many vegetable oils to choose from, vegetarian diets can very easily be adapted to a ketogenic diet.

The vegan diet goes further than the vegetarian diet by eliminating any animal product from the diet, including eggs and dairy. Most of the protein in the diet comes from vegetables, grains, nuts, seeds, and legumes. To avoid nutritional deficiencies, the proteins need to be carefully balanced to include adequate amounts of each of the eight essential amino acids with each meal (a protein or combination of proteins that contain all eight essential amino acids is considered to be a "complete" protein). Soy (tofu, for example) is a rare food that contains all eight essential amino acids and is a mainstay for many vegans. Eating dishes with rice and beans is one example of combining two different sources of proteins to provide all eight essential amino acids. It is very possible to combine a vegan with a ketogenic diet. Research and good meal planning are paramount to successfully maintaining a healthy keto-vegan diet. Fortunately, there is a growing trend in the food industry to produce complete plant-based protein foods for the vegan market.

THE KETOGENIC DIET FOR EPILEPSY SIMMERS IN THE BACKGROUND

While utilization of the classic ketogenic diet for childhood epilepsy faded from the mainstream in the mid-twentieth century, Johns Hopkins Hospital in Baltimore, Maryland, continued using the ketogenic diet all along, thanks to the advocacy of John Freeman, MD (deceased) and dietician Millicent Kelly, who spent decades caring for hundreds of epileptic children. The ketogenic diet was a topic of discussion in the 1970s during my own medical school training and was used on occasion at the hospital where I did my pediatric residency for children with the most resistant forms of epilepsy. I could not have imagined at that time the role ketones would play in my own life and that of my husband several decades later.

Although physicians who used the ketogenic diet for epilepsy were few and far between, in 1971, a variation on the diet was introduced by Peter R. Huttenlocher, MD, as a more palatable alternative to the classic ketogenic diet. Like the original diet, Huttenlocher's plan showed good results in eliminating or reducing seizures. Instead of 80 to 90 percent of the calories coming from fat, as required in the classic ketogenic diet, this variation allowed 60 percent of total calories from MCT (medium-chain triglyceride) oil, more protein and carbohydrates, and more variety overall. A big drawback is that some people experience bloating, diarrhea, or other intestinal symptoms when taking this much MCT oil and, so, a further modification was later developed at John Radcliffe Hospital in Oxford, United Kingdom, by Ruby Schwartz, MD and her colleagues. This plan reduces the MCT in the diet from 60 to 30 percent of total calories in the beginning, allowing the other 30 percent of fat in the diet to come from longer-chain fats. If these proportions fail to raise ketone levels high enough or fail to control seizures, the quantity of MCT oil is then slowly increased as tolerated to 45 or 50 percent of calories (Huttenlocher, 1971).

In addition to the MCT oil diet, at least two other alternatives to the classic ketogenic diet exist: the low glycemic index diet and the modified Atkins diet. These two diets are easier to stay on for the long haul, and they show effective seizure control in many children and some adults. We will discuss these in more detail in Chapter 6, where you will find a chart from The Charlie Foundation with a comparison of the ratios of the three macronutrients—fat, protein, and carbohydrate—in these four diets compared to the typical Western diet.

Children with epilepsy who respond to ketogenic diets with cessation of seizures can sometimes be weaned successfully off the diet after two years or more without recurrence of their seizures, although there may be other good reasons to continue at least a modified form of the diet. In addition to seizure control, families often report improvement in cognition, behavior, and mood, and this is supported by at least one study of fifty children (twenty-eight on ketogenic diet and twenty-two controls not on the diet) conducted in the Netherlands. The study used extensive testing and showed reduction in anxiety and "mood-disturbed behavior," higher scores for "vigor" ("energy"), reaction time and word comprehension (Ijiff, 2016). As discovered by Banting and Densmore and their patients from the nineteenth century, there appear to be benefits for children and adults with epilepsy well beyond the problem they hoped to overcome by using the ketogenic diet.

THE KETOGENIC DIET FOR EPILEPSY MOVES TO THE FRONT BURNER ONCE AGAIN

The ketogenic diet for epilepsy experienced a major resurgence beginning in the early 1990s when Jim Abrahams came upon the diet in the course of his research as a potential treatment for his toddler son, who had severe epilepsy and was heavily sedated because of the multiple medications he took, all of which failed to control his frequent seizures. Abrahams is a Hollywood filmmaker. Born in 1944, he grew up near Milwaukee, Wisconsin, where he says he "killed four years" majoring in English at the

University of Wisconsin-Madison and
barely escaped with a bachelor's degree.
He and his longtime friends David and
Jerry Zucker began making funny vid-
eotapes to share with their friends and
family. This led to theater openings, first
in Madison and then in California where
they showed their films and even got on
stage themselves. They landed a gig on
the *Tonight Show*, and though Jim says
they were "terrible," they started writing
scripts in the same comedic vein and

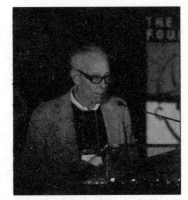

Photo 4.4. Jim Abrahams

soon found themselves making spoof movies in Hollywood as writers,
directors, and producers. Who could forget their biggest hit, *Airplane!*
from 1980? Some of their other hits included *Kentucky Fried Movie*, *Big
Business*, and *The Naked Gun* and *Hot Shots!* series. (See Photo 4.4.)

Jim's life took an unexpected turn in 1993 when his son Charlie began
to have numerous seizures at just eleven months of age. Jim, at a high point
in his career by this point, was well-connected and some of his associates
were big hospital donors who made it possible for Charlie to "skip to the
head of the line" to see prominent neurologists at major hospitals around
the country. The doctors were unanimous in their recommendations for
medications and surgery but no one mentioned the ketogenic diet. Jim
later learned that every one of them knew about the diet, about John Freeman's work with epileptic children and the ketogenic diet, and about the
research on it that had taken place at Johns Hopkins Hospital. He remains
mystified and upset that none of them thought it was important to offer the
diet as an alternative, even though Charlie's seizures were not controlled
even with a combination of four anti-convulsants or even after surgery.

At one and one-half years of age, Charlie underwent surgery to remove
a cyst that doctors thought might be causing the seizures; he suffered a
severe allergic reaction to morphine given during the procedure. When
his seizures resumed two days later, Charlie seemed doomed to living his
young life heavily sedated and wearing a helmet to protect his head.

When Charlie was twenty-one months old, Jim came across information about the ketogenic diet for epilepsy, and he learned that Johns

Hopkins had had a program in place for many years to start children on the diet under the direction of John Freeman, with counseling by dietician Millicent Kelly. Charlie was admitted to Johns Hopkins and, upon starting the diet, his seizures stopped completely within several days of starting the diet. Freeman was so certain that Charlie's seizures had stopped because of the ketogenic diet that he weaned the little boy off all four anti-convulsant medications over one month.

Charlie remained completely seizure free, but attempts to wean him off the diet after two years and then again after four years were unsuccessful. (He briefly resumed having seizures.) But the fifth year proved the charm: He was able to go off the diet without ever having another seizure. In 2018, as I write this, Charlie is twenty-six years old, plays piano, boxes, is a college graduate, and has a career as a schoolteacher. (See Photo 4.5.) He no longer adheres to the ketogenic diet, but, ironically, the rest of his family, including Jim, are on it! They never found the cause of Charlie's epilepsy, but he is well beyond two decades since his last seizure, which is considered cured in most people's book. Even so, doctors caution Jim to say Charlie's epilepsy is "controlled" not cured. Jim is bothered that the Epilepsy Foundation insists that epilepsy has no cure even in the face of cases like Charlie's: he stopped having seizures while on the diet and was eventually weaned off the diet and hasn't had another seizure. If that is not a cure, what is?

To increase awareness of the benefits of the ketogenic diet for people with epilepsy, Jim Abrahams filmed a made-for-TV movie called *First Do No Harm,* featuring his neighbor Meryl Streep (See Figure 4.2). It

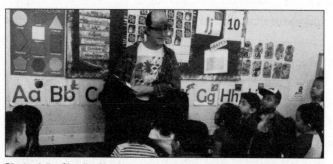

Photo 4.5. Charlie Abrahams, now a schoolteacher, is seizure-free from ketogenic diet for more than two decades. Permission from The Charlie Foundation.

was based on the true story of another boy who responded dramatically to the diet. (He lives a normal life and is now in his fifties.) Jim believed that millions would see the movie and that his fight to inform the world about the diet would be over. He says he was "dead wrong." He underestimated the opposition to the ketogenic diet—from drug companies and doctors who were not taught about the diet's therapeutic value; from the American Heart Association, which touts the low-fat diet; from the sugar industry, which does not take kindly to a low-carbohydrate diet; from hospitals that don't make a profit from the diet; from insurance companies that refuse to reimburse for counseling in the ketogenic diet therapy.

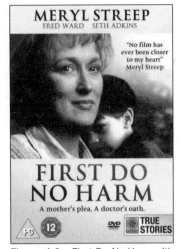

Figure 4.2. *First Do No Harm* with Meryl Streep, was filmed by Jim Abrahams to increase awareness of the ketogenic diet in treating epilepsy. With permission from Jim Abrahams.

With Dr. Freeman, Jim also made an informative video called *An Introduction to the Ketogenic Diet.* He took three hundred VHS tapes to distribute at the 1994 American Epilepsy Society meeting where there were thousands of participants; inexplicably, he couldn't give them away and left with 296 tapes. (See Figure 4.3.) Shortly thereafter, Jim founded The Charlie Foundation for Ketogenic Therapies to advocate for the diet. The foundation has organized and sponsored two dozen professional meetings to facilitate both medical awareness and scientific understanding (https://charliefoundation.org/). In 2006 it established an international committee of neurologists and dietitians with expertise in ketogenic diet therapies to come

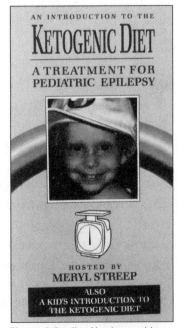

Figure 4.3. Jim Abrahams video, *An Introduction to the Ketogenic Diet* made with Dr. John Freeman.

up with practical recommendations for implementing it. The Consensus Guidelines were published in *Epilepsia* in 2008 and then updated in 2018 (Kossoff, 2009 , Kossoff, 2018). The Charlie Foundation has provided training under the guidance of dietician Beth Zupec-Kania to more than two hundred centers around the world and has helped tens of thousands of people globally learn about and benefit from the ketogenic diet. In April 2008, in Phoenix, Arizona, The Charlie Foundation sponsored the first ever Global Symposium on Ketogenic Therapies for Epilepsy and Other Disorders; related articles written by presenters were published in a special edition of the medical journal *Epilepsia* in October 2008.

In recent years, the foundation has taken turns organizing these biennial meetings with Matthew's Friends, a UK advocacy group that was founded in 2004 by Emma Williams, the mother of another child who experienced relief from severe seizures with the ketogenic diet. These days the symposia go well beyond the topic of epilepsy, with presentations on use of the ketogenic diet for cancer, Alzheimer's disease and other neurologic disorders, rare enzyme defects that respond to the diet, traumatic brain injury, and other conditions. In fall 2018, the sixth Global Symposium on Ketogenic Diet for Neurologic Conditions is scheduled to take place in Jeju, Korea.

Jim notes that neurology associations have not supported the ketogenic diet until recently. The American Epilepsy Society (AES) will finally hold its first-ever dietary symposium in the fall of 2018, more than thirty years after AES announced its "concerted effort to address issues on childhood onset epilepsy" and twenty-five years after Jim began his efforts to get the message out to the world that the ketogenic diet is a viable treatment—and maybe even a cure—for epilepsy. Jim feels a lot of unnecessary damage has been done in the meantime. He also says it is difficult for someone who is not a medical provider to be an advocate for a medical treatment. He senses that neurologists and others in the field may think he is just an uninformed, angry father spouting holistic ideas. However, Jim has had his own brush with a serious medical condition—leukemia—and went the traditional route to successfully treat the problem. He was cured with three months of chemotherapy and a stem cell transplant from his sister, so he is no stranger to the miracles of modern-day medicine.

Jim recognizes that there is a big gap in knowledge when it comes to epilepsy, and he hopes the science will catch up with the reality and that the medical world will soon recognize the value of the ketogenic nutritional approach to treating epilepsy and many other disorders. (From interview with Jim Abrahams on February 6, 2018.)

THE KETOGENIC DIET: NOT JUST FOR EPILEPSY

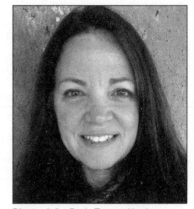

Photo 4.6. Beth Zupec-Kania

The work of Beth Zupec-Kania (see Photo 4.6) with The Charlie Foundation has been integral in the resurgence of the ketogenic diet for treating epilepsy and various other conditions. Beth was born in 1959 in Waukegan, Illinois, the fourth of ten children. Her father was diagnosed in his late forties with lung cancer, which rapidly metastasized to other organs. He was weakened by the debilitating effects of the intensive chemotherapy and radiation treatments typically used in the 1970s. It was clear to Beth that he suffered more from these archaic medical treatments then from the cancer itself. His interest in alternative nutrition-based options (such as laetrile) inspired her to pursue a degree in nutrition at the University of Wisconsin and become a registered dietician nutritionist.

While raising her two children and working part-time at Children's Hospital of Wisconsin, Beth became acquainted with the director of neurology. Together they resurrected a ketogenic program that had been active in the 1930s. She found records of a patient who had become seizure-free on the ketogenic diet. Beth contacted the patient and learned that she remained seizure-free, had children and grandchildren, and lived a healthy life. She told Beth that during her two years on the diet as a young child, she came to the hospital every Saturday to fast, playing all day with the nurses and with other children on the diet. Beth consulted with Millicent Kelly, the dietitian from Hopkins, about using the ketogenic diet in children. Beth has paid the help she received from Kelly forward by training nutritionists in ketogenic-diet therapies at more than two hundred medical centers, including ten in foreign countries. She has been involved with The Charlie Foundation since 2005 as a consultant, has written several guides on implementing the ketogenic diet, has mentored hundreds of nutritionists, and has helped to organize national and global ketogenic-diet meetings sponsored by the foundation. She also maintains a small private practice to assist people around the world who don't have local access to a ketogenic program.

Beth learned early on that working closely with each family, having a knack for math, and being extremely organized were key in implementing a ketogenic diet. But to spread use of the diet farther, she wanted to develop a computer program to help patients manage the diet themselves. With funding from a generous donor, the first ketogenic-diet calculator was created, eventually evolving into an online program, the Keto Diet Calculator (www.ketodietcalculator.com). The online program is a live database, updated daily and used by thousands of ketogenic professionals and their patients around the world.

Ketogenic-diet therapy for children with epilepsy experienced a surge in use after the first controlled study was published in the 2008 issue of *Epilepsia* that was dedicated to the ketogenic diet. Reports of benefit (both anecdotal and published) for other neurological disorders soon emerged including autism; rare genetic, mitochondrial and endocrine disorders; and brain cancer. Beth has seen many children with these disorders experience significant improvements in behavior and cognition after implementing the ketogenic diet. This led to her involvement with a parent-run initiative called TREND to test a modified ketogenic diet therapy in twelve children from around the world with Prader-Willi syndrome. Prader-Willi syndrome is a rare genetic disorder that results in behavioral and cognitive problems including a constant sense of hunger, often leading to obesity. The one-year collaboration involved providing online group and individual consultations, education, and collaborations with the children's physicians to monitor progress. Families were required to submit data throughout the year including laboratory studies, growth, behavior, and progress in school. All the children who completed the full year (ten of the twelve patients) of ketogenic-diet therapy reported improvements in quality of life that were significant. Beth published a white paper describing this informal study, hoping that it would lead to a larger study.

Another of Beth's special interests is working with people who have cancer, primarily brain cancer. One of her first patients was a teenager who had an inoperable brain tumor that also triggered seizures. Although the ketogenic diet was prescribed to control his seizures, he received other benefits from it as well. This occurred before the science was published showing efficacy of ketogenic diet therapy in thwarting tumor growth in mice with glioblastomas. His tumor was the size of a golf ball, which resulted in multiple issues including paralysis of his legs and the inability to speak, but he was alert and communicative through sign language, and his mother pursued every possible therapy to help him. After he started on a ketogenic diet he became more active and, to everyone's amazement, started wheeling himself in his wheelchair and even started playing wheelchair basketball. He lived much longer than predicted and with a better quality of life. Since then, Beth has worked with more than one hundred people with cancer.

Although only a few anecdotal cases have been reported in medical literature, migraine headaches are another condition that Beth has found to be responsive to ketogenic diet therapy. Eighteen percent of women experience migraine headaches. Most of these women are prescribed anti-seizure medications, which can have adverse effects. Beth has worked with more than a dozen women with migraines who have tried all available medications, and she has found that they experienced the best relief from using a modified ketogenic diet. Most of these women had such severe migraines that they needed to be hospitalized.

Another application of ketogenic diet therapy that hasn't been documented yet in medical literature is for perimenopausal hot flashes. During testing of a prototype breath acetone meter, Beth put herself on a ketogenic diet to achieve ketosis. She noticed that with each new batch of meters she tested, while she was in ketosis, her hot flashes vanished completely. When she came out of ketosis, they returned. She tested this theory several times by going in and out of ketosis, and the results were consistent. In addition to relief from debilitating hot flashes (including waking up in the middle of the night drenched in sweat), her complexion improved, and her energy level increased dramatically. Through a combination of a modified ketogenic diet and intermittent fasting, she has achieved a mild state of ketosis that she says makes her feel like she is in her twenties.

The impact of food on health has become a major point of conversation with anyone who comes to Beth for advice. She doesn't believe that everyone needs to be on a ketogenic diet but that everyone can benefit from improving their dietary habits including a practice of going without food for long periods, also known as intermittent fasting (although not for young children). Her advice usually starts out with a discussion of the universal human addiction to sugar. She explains that the first step is to recognize that it is a physical addiction. The next step is to relearn how to behave in our sugar-laden culture. Similar to how a recovering alcoholic relearns to manage their desire to consume alcohol, learning to avoid sugar (and most processed foods) is a process. Some recovering alcoholics choose to avoid situations where they would be exposed to alcohol; others learn tactics for coping or lean on a mentor for support during the temptation to drink. Similarly, it is easier to eat a sugar-free diet if you are doing it with someone else. She recommends to anyone who wants to try a ketogenic diet that they first try a whole-foods (no processed foods), sugar-free diet that includes healthy fat with each meal. Often, this alone can result in significant health benefit. Beth finds that those who try this strategy first are the ones who are willing and able to manage a ketogenic diet with success.

When asked what she sees on the horizon for the ketogenic diet, Beth points out that the ketogenic diet is highly underutilized for epilepsy as well as for other conditions. One of the most devastating epilepsy conditions in infancy, called infantile spasms (IS), is very responsive to ketogenic diet therapy. Infants and toddlers who have this particular type of epilepsy enjoy the highest success rate for eliminating seizures through adherence to the ketogenic diet, yet only a few hospitals use the diet for this condition. The standard treatment for IS is a steroid called ACTH that costs $250,000 dollars to treat one infant. The ketogenic diet has been shown in studies to be as effective as ACTH and with neither the adverse effects nor the extreme cost.

Beth has seen an evolution in the use of the ketogenic diet therapy in her twenty-six years of working with it but is disappointed by the lack in advances in making it more available to people who can benefit. Funding of both animal and human studies is a major roadblock in advancing use of ketogenic diet therapies since no pharmaceutical company benefits. Still, she has seen gradual advances, including recognition by several leading organizations that appeared in two Cochrane Reports, from 2012 and 2016, prepared by the American Academy of Nutrition, American College of Nutrition, Child Neurology Society, American Epilepsy Society, and the International League Against Epilepsy.

Beth has dedicated her career to designing resources for health professionals and patients to make it easier for them to access and implement ketogenic diets including the Ketodietcalculator.com, a help line, and webinar library for professionals. She recently mentored a group of Ketogenic Specialists called Charlie's Angels (unofficial title) who are available to consult for individuals worldwide (accessible through The Charlie Foundation's website). (From Interview with Beth Zupec-Kania on January 27, 2018.)

GROWING AWARENESS OF THE KETOGENIC DIET

The growing awareness of the ketogenic diet for epilepsy has been accompanied by an explosion of research—more than 2,000 results come up with a simple search of the text words "ketogenic diet" on PubMed.Gov, with more than 1,800 of these published after 1999. A search for the word *ketosis* yields more than 9,100 results.

It is important to note that children with epilepsy who are on a strict ketogenic diet can greatly reduce the frequency of seizures and even become seizure-free over time, but it requires rigid adherence to the diet, with precise calculation of the ratios of fat to carbohydrate and protein, as well as weighing and measuring every meal and snack. For this reason, it is vital that the family work closely with a dietician qualified and experienced in the use of the ketogenic diet. Other families are a great source of support as well, sharing recipes and providing encouragement. Recently, the diet has been tried by older people, and some adults with epilepsy benefit significantly from the ketogenic diet as well. Not everyone with epilepsy responds dramatically to the diet, but some do completely stop having seizures, and many more experience a 50 to 90 percent reduction in their seizures.

A ketogenic diet is not easy for most people to follow as a long-term strategy, due to the very small amount of carbohydrate allowed and the requirement to accurately measure every bite of food eaten. On the other hand, adhering to the classic ketogenic diet has a distinct advantage: It produces levels of ketone bodies five to ten times higher than levels produced by ingesting medium-chain-triglyceride (MCT) oils, while substantially lowering blood sugar—more than would be expected from MCTs. It is still not known exactly why the classic ketogenic diet stops or reduces the number of seizures, and it is quite possible that achieving a very low blood sugar is as important as obtaining high levels of ketones. The elevation of ketones will provide fuel to the cells and protect brain and other tissues from the effects of low blood sugar.

The use of the classic ketogenic diet and its modifications are not limited to children and adults with epilepsy, and nearly everyone, healthy or otherwise, could benefit from adopting some form of the ketogenic diet. People with Alzheimer's disease, Parkinson's, and other neurodegenerative diseases who do not see improvement by adding oils with medium-chain triglycerides to their diet might consider going all the way with a ketogenic diet. Modifications of the ketogenic diet to include medium-chain triglycerides may allow for a slightly less-restrictive diet and assurance that some ketone production will occur, even if there is a slip-up in how much carbohydrate is consumed.

A strict ketogenic diet is very challenging to maintain; for this reason, a modified ketogenic diet is often suggested first to treat epilepsy and other conditions. If the various alternative diets fail to produce satisfactory results, the classic ketogenic diet may be a viable alternative, since it would, on average, result in higher levels of ketones and lower blood sugar levels than any of the modifications that are typically recommended. The Charlie Foundation, Matthew's Friends, Ketogenic.com, and many other organizations have done considerable work to create a variety of palatable recipes that are compatible with both the classic and the modified ketogenic diets.

Ketogenic diets have shown promising results in studies of people with a variety of medical conditions as well as in athletes seeking improved performance and in people who are relatively healthy but want to feel and look better. As we see from the books and articles I've discussed so far, people who follow a ketogenic diet report improvements in weight loss and diabetes, as well as in memory and focus, energy level, mood, behavior, sleep, alertness, endurance and relief from some physical symptoms, such as aches, pains, and tremors.

Use of exogenous ketone supplements to support the ketogenic diet could be considered as well and will be discussed at length in Chapter 7. As of early 2018, only a handful of human studies on the use of exogenous ketones for athletic performance and for specific medical conditions have been published. Over the next few years, we can expect an increase in animal and human studies that look at the effects of ketone salts, ketone esters, and other exogenous ketone supplements.

If a person is healthy but wants to make the most of the ketogenic diet, the help of a qualified dietician or nutritionist who has experience with the classic ketogenic diet could be invaluable. For someone with epilepsy, cancer, Alzheimer's, Parkinson's, diabetes, or other medical condition, such help is vital, along with support and monitoring by the person's medical provider.

Ketogenic diets have a very long history, as long as humans have been around on Earth and throughout our evolution. We have deviated so far off course in recent decades that we are seeing historically unparalleled increases in rates of obesity, diabetes, chronic illnesses, cancer, neurologic diseases like Alzheimer's, as well as diseases related to inflammation and accelerated aging. As the typical high-carbohydrate, low-fat Western diet has spread throughout the world, these diseases have traveled with it. The only credible explanation for this phenomenon is what we put in our mouths. Sugar is highly addictive, and we are not designed to eat as much of it as most of us now do. Ketones are a primitive, effective, and powerful fuel for the brain and most other organs, and they participate in pathways that reduce inflammation and slow the aging process. Steering ourselves away from sugar and toward a ketogenic lifestyle could undo much of the damage and lead us along a path to a better quality of life as we grow older.

CHAPTER 5

PIONEERS AND RISING STARS IN KETONE RESEARCH AND PRACTICE
A Historical Review

"The mind is like a parachute—
it only works if it is open."
—Anonymous

Beginning around 1921, ketone research focused mainly on the use of the classic ketogenic diet for drug-resistant epilepsy in children. This simmered on the back burner for decades followed by a resurgence beginning in the 1990s that has contributed greatly to awareness of ketones and ketogenic diets today. This story is discussed at length in Chapter 4. In the meantime, other developments were unfolding, as various researchers became interested in studying ketones, what they do, and how ketones might be therapeutic for many other medical conditions. Many of the people involved in this story were kind enough to allow me to interview them so I could present this information from their perspective and describe what motivated them to pursue careers in science or medicine. For some, a family tragedy spurred them to do what they are doing today. I believe their stories will serve as inspiration for the next generation of ketone researchers and physicians.

Each researcher's story is like a puzzle piece that contributes to the larger picture of where we are today. Ultimately, they are all interconnected. Scientists are often secretive and protective of their niche of research and this interferes with real progress in helping mankind. Open mindedness, curiosity, creativity, sharing of ideas, advocacy, support for one another's ideas, and collaboration are qualities that separate the individuals featured here from many others. Recognition that nutrition is fundamental to health and to disease is an idea embraced by all of them. Thanks to these people and their cooperation with each other, we have a real chance at finding preventive and therapeutic treatments for a wide range of disorders.

Many individuals have been involved in ketone research; whether from the past or the present, from the United States or from other parts of the world—I apologize that I couldn't mention each of them here.

THE EARLY TWENTIETH CENTURY

The earliest ketone research I uncovered began just a few years before the introduction of the idea of using the ketogenic diet for epilepsy. It was concerned with postexercise ketosis.

In 1909, G. Forssner noticed that the levels of ketones always increased in his urine after a brisk four-kilometer walk lasting over thirty-six minutes, and in 1911, L. Preti reported the same phenomenon in a patient who had a minor stomach complaint after climbing up and down stairs until exhausted. In 1936, F. C. Courtice and C. G. Douglas reported that following moderate early morning exercise after fasting overnight, ketones begin to rise upon completion of exercise and continue and remain elevated for at least nine hours. They hypothesized that the muscles, which were glucose-deprived due to lack of food overnight, use the circulating ketones while the exercise occurs. When the exercise ceases, the liver continues to make ketones for a short period, which then accumulate in the circulation. This phenomenon was thereafter called the "Courtice Douglas effect" and is also known as "post-exercise ketosis." In all three of these studies, the subjects were on restricted diets, either low-carbohydrate or high-protein diets, for a period of time before the experiments. Later, researchers noted that if a high-carbohydrate meal was taken before the exercise, ketones did not increase; one group found that typically inactive people tended to have higher ketone levels following exercise than trained athletes (Forssner, 1909; Preti, 1911; Courtice, 1936; Passmore, 1958; Johnson, 1974; Koeslag, 1979).

More recent research on post-exercise ketosis continues to confirm these very early findings. Dr. Stephen Cunnane and his associates have learned through ketone PET scans that exercise nearly triples ketone uptake in the brain, suggesting that post exercise ketosis may play a role in the benefits to physical and cognitive performance conferred by exercise (Castellano, 2017). You will find more details about this in Chapter 7. Could there be a connection between post-exercise ketosis and other metabolic changes that occur with exercise that explain the benefits of exercise? A substance known as brain-derived neurotrophic factor (BDNF) has widespread functions throughout the brain, such as promoting the growth and survival of neurons and strengthening of synapses; it is important to normal cognitive function and is reduced in the brain in Alzheimer's disease (Blurton-Jones, 2009). Like ketones, BDNF also increases with exercise and it is conceivable that there is a connection between BDNF and ketosis, but this is still unknown as of early 2018.

One of the major scientific discoveries of the mid-twentieth century will impact millions now living in the twenty-first century: Ketones are an alternative fuel for the brain. How this idea and application of this idea has unfolded can be told through the stories of the pioneers of ketone research.

THEODORE VANITALLIE, MD:
THE OLDEST LIVING PIONEER IN KETONE RESEARCH

At ninety-eight and going strong in early 2018, Dr. Theodore VanItallie, a pioneer in nutrition research, believes so strongly in the concept of ketones as an alternative fuel for the brain and the application of that idea as a therapeutic to help others that he continues to research, write, and publish on the subject, when most people would have long since handed over this mission to others.

Theodore ("Ted") VanItallie was born in the Hackensack Hospital (New Jersey) in 1919, not long after the end

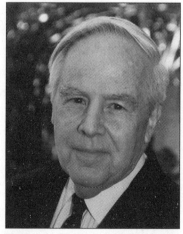

Photo 5.1. Theodore B. VanItallie, MD.

of World War I. Following his birth, his parents moved to a permanent home in Ridgewood, New Jersey, a friendly and prosperous suburb within commuting distance from New York City. At that time the George Washington Bridge and the river tunnels had not yet been constructed. Every working day, Ted's father, a hard-driving manufacturer of core-drilling equipment and abrasive tools, had to take a steam-powered Erie Railroad train from Ridgewood to Hoboken, New Jersey. From there, he boarded a ferry to get across the Hudson to his small factory and offices in downtown Manhattan.

At a very early age, VanItallie became involved with Presbyterian Church activities and with some of the YMCA's outreach programs. From these experiences, he learned firsthand how important it is to be concerned about and help other people—particularly those in financial and/or social difficulty. VanItallie attended Deerfield Academy, where he grew interested in science and medicine. His chemistry teacher, Helen Boyden (also the headmaster's wife), exerted a powerful influence on his choice of career, as did a novel by Sinclair Lewis called *Arrowsmith*, about an idealistic young physician who selflessly served humanity. The book further stimulated VanItallie's long-term interest in pursuing medical training.

As an undergraduate at Harvard College, VanItallie took the required premedical courses but chose to focus on philosophy and comparative literature. He believes that this broadening of his education enhanced his understanding of humans and helped make him a better physician and a more humane person. He attended medical school at Columbia University and did his internship and residency at St. Luke's Hospital in New York. In 1950, after finishing two years of active duty as a U.S. Navy medical officer and having completed his residency in internal medicine, he accepted an offer from Dr. Frederick J. Stare, chairman of the Department of Nutrition at Harvard's School of Public Health, to serve as a research fellow at Harvard. This appointment encompassed activities in the departments of nutrition, surgery, and medicine at the Peter Bent Brigham Hospital, a major teaching arm of the Harvard Medical School. His principal mentors at the Brigham were Francis D. Moore, MD, chairman of the department of surgery, and George W. Thorn, MD, chairman of the department of medicine.

After completing two years of research training at Harvard and three more years of independent research as director of the Clinical Nutrition

Laboratory at St. Luke's, VanItallie returned to Boston as an assistant professor of clinical nutrition and medicine at Harvard's Schools of Medicine and Public Health. As a member of the associate medical staff at the Brigham, he also taught medical residents and medical students. In 1957 he was invited to return to St. Luke's Hospital as its first full-time physician-in-chief. He served as director of medicine there from 1957 to 1975. He also became a full professor of medicine at Columbia in 1971.

VanItallie's long-time research partner, Sami A. Hashim, MD, who completed clinical training as an intern and resident at the Peter Bent Brigham Hospital, joined the medical staff at St. Luke's in 1959. At about the same time, VanItallie became a Columbia University faculty member, working closely with Dr. W. H. ("Henry") Sebrell, founding director of Columbia's Institute of Human Nutrition. The St. Luke's metabolic research unit also acted as the institute's clinical investigation facility. It is noteworthy that Henry Sebrell had served as an early director of the National Institutes of Health (1950–1955).

Most of VanItallie's research work after 1959 was conducted in partnership with Hashim. Together they founded the internationally recognized program in metabolism research at St. Luke's, with an early focus on obesity and body composition. They also conducted a wide range of laboratory and clinical studies, including their pioneering research in the physiology and clinical uses of a (then) novel nutritional entity, medium-chain triglycerides (MCTs). The MCT work grew in part from their friendship and collaborative activities with the noted industrial chemist Vigen Babayan, a national leader in the development of the classic distillation method used to extract medium-chain triglycerides from coconut oil. For a number of years "Vig" Babayan worked closely with Hashim and other members of the metabolic program.

Dr. F. Xavier ("Xave") Pi-Sunyer, a Columbia Medical School graduate, completed a medical residency at St. Luke's and then joined the metabolic research program, becoming an internationally recognized expert in the field of diabetes. He played a leading role in many of the Endocrine-Nutrition Division's metabolic studies. Pi-Sunyer was the son of parents who migrated from Barcelona to the United States as refugees from the Spanish Civil War to escape the dominance of the oppressive and cruel Franco dictatorship. The Pi-Sunyers were part of a distinguished Barcelona family who, for many generations, were academic medical leaders in Spain's Catalonia province.

For a time, part of the Nutrition/Metabolism/Diabetes Division's work centered on the study of odd-chain medium length triglycerides, C7, C9, and C11, which occur naturally only under rare conditions. (The shorthand C7, C9, etc., indicates how many carbons the fat molecule contains—that is, how long it is. For more detail, see the section titled "The Unique Properties of Medium-Chain Triglycerides," in Chapter 7.) The terminal three carbons of these molecules are converted to glucose in the liver, and these are the only class of fatty acids that are partly "carbohydrate." Researchers fed rats odd-chain fatty acids, some of which ended up being stored in the rats' adipose tissue. The researchers learned that these unusual fatty acids were partly converted to glucose, especially when the laboratory animals were subjected to fasting. They found that this nutritional strategy helped to conserve liver and muscle glycogen during starvation. The results of one of the studies of odd-carbon triglycerides was published in *Science* in 1969 (VanItallie, 1969).

One of the most important findings from this research group's work occurred in the 1960s. It was discovered that after ingestion and absorption, medium-chain triglycerides (MCTs) are partly converted to ketones in the liver (Bergen, 1966; Pi-Sunyer, 1969). These observations were the basis for a seminal idea, which, forty years later, occurred to Samuel Henderson, the University of Chicago molecular biologist. Henderson predicted that the mild state of ketosis achieved through ingestion of medium-chain triglycerides could potentially bring about cognitive improvement in people with early or mild Alzheimer's disease. Based on this principle, Henderson went on to develop and test the "medical food" now called Axona.

VanItallie considers Dr. Hashim to be one of the world's experts on the use of MCTs for treatment of various types of intestinal malabsorption. Hashim was also leader of a group at St. Luke's who were responsible for the use of MCTs for micropreemies (babies born weighing less than 1 pound 4 ounces [1,000 g]) to help them gain weight (Tantibhedhyangkul, 1971). This was a common practice in the newborn intensive care unit when I was doing my pediatric residency and fellowship training in the late 1970s and early 1980s. When I first read about MCT oil as a possible treatment for Alzheimer's disease (AD) in 2008, I was familiar with the substances because of this experience so many years earlier.

VanItallie also worked on developing lipid emulsions at Harvard University and wrote several papers on lipid emulsions for intravenous administration before they became generally available. These intravenous fat preparations have saved the lives of many patients with gluten enteropathy (celiac disease), surgical patients, and untold numbers of tiny premature newborns around the world.

At Harvard, VanItallie connected with Dr. George Cahill Jr., who with Owen and other colleagues, discovered that ketone bodies provide alternative fuel to the brain during prolonged fasting (Owen, 1967). This was the first demonstration that the brain can subsist on ketone bodies when glucose is unavailable. VanItallie first met Cahill during a lecture on glucagon that VanItallie was delivering to the Peter Bent Brigham staff, of which Cahill was a member. The two young medical scientists became friends.

In 2001, Cahill told VanItallie about Dr. Richard Veech's work with ketone bodies. Veech was director of the Laboratory of Metabolic Control at NIH's NIAAA division. VanItallie began to read papers by Cahill and Veech on the subject of ketone bodies as an alternative energy source for the brain, and on the therapeutic possibilities of this remarkable fuel—particularly its potential for the treatment of neurodegenerative diseases like Alzheimer's disease and Parkinson's disease. Veech's pioneering work and his vision of the potential clinical benefits of ketone bodies in treatment of a variety of major medical disorders stimulated VanItallie 's own intense interest in ketones. He wrote his first article on ketone bodies in 2003, with coauthor Thomas Nufert, who also recognized the enormous scientific and medical potential of ketone bodies. Their article was appropriately entitled *Ketones: Metabolism's Ugly Duckling* (VanItallie, 2003).

Veech's ketone research stimulated VanItallie to perform and publish a landmark study demonstrating that people with Parkinson's who maintained a strict ketogenic diet for a month responded with a marked improvement in the signs and symptoms of the disease (VanItallie, 2005). These were just the first of a number of scientific papers VanItallie published on the subject of ketone bodies. He gave me great encouragement and guidance in helping Steve use medium-chain triglycerides to treat his Alzheimer's. Together, we and others, including Dr. Veech, coauthored a case report on my husband's very positive experience with medium-chain triglycerides and Veech's ketone ester (Newport, 2015).

Ted VanItallie continues reading and writing scientific articles on the subject of ketone bodies. He believes that ketone bodies for the prevention and/or treatment of dreadful disorders like dementia, Alzheimer's disease, Parkinson's disease, and traumatic brain injury could potentially help millions. As someone once told him, "The mind is like a parachute—it only works if it is open." He says he hopes that physicians will open their minds and examine with care the concept of ketone bodies as a potentially effective therapeutic modality. (From interview with Theodore VanItallie on February 8, 2018.)

SAMI HASHIM, MD: WORLD EXPERT ON MEDIUM-CHAIN TRIGLYCERIDE OIL

Now eighty-eight years old, Sami Hashim was born in Lebanon in 1929, though his grandparents had lived in the United States for years before he was born. He attended an American high school in Lebanon, where he became interested in science, and then went to the American University in Beirut for college, leading to a master's degree in biochemistry. He originally wanted to pursue a PhD but instead came to the United States to attend the University of Buffalo for medical school. After completing his internship and residency at

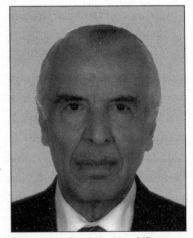

Photo 5.2. Sami Hashim, MD.

the Peter Bent Brigham Hospital at Harvard University, the dean of Harvard recommended that he do a research fellowship in nutrition at the Harvard School of Nutrition. During this period, he met Dr. Theodore VanItallie, who was chief of medicine at St. Luke's Hospital. VanItallie lured Hashim to New York for work, and the two began a lifelong relationship as friends and research collaborators. Part of their work together involves the invention of MCT oil and the discovery that medium-chain triglycerides are ketogenic.

While Hashim was doing his fellowship at Peter Bent Brigham Hospital, he also got to know another pioneer in ketone research, George F. Cahill Jr., who was chief resident. Hashim later worked on an experiment with Cahill in which a very obese nurse fasted under supervision for forty days. (He says that Cahill chose forty days because Christ and Moses had each fasted for forty days.) At the end of the experiment, they inserted lines to draw blood into the arteries and veins around her brain and liver and found that ketones had supplied the majority of the fuel to keep her brain alive. He recalls that her ketone levels were up to at least 7 mmol/L and her blood sugar was very low, about 40 mg/dL. They calculated that she was producing about 150 grams of ketones per day (Owen, 1967). They followed this up with other experiments in dogs and humans. They were aware of the use of ketogenic diets to treat childhood epilepsy, as described in articles by Dr. Russell Wilder from the early 1920s, and that awareness sowed the seeds of an idea that came later for the use of ketones as therapy for other conditions.

In the mid-1950s, Dr. Ancel Keys and other researchers published reports of small-animal and human studies showing that certain dietary fats, such as coconut oil, increased cholesterol levels. They hypothesized that this effect had something to do with the iodine value or the linoleic acid content of the fat. Dr. Hashim and his associates published their own study in 1959 with conflicting results, showing that coconut oil alone, as well as a combination of safflower and coconut oil, decreased cholesterol levels in the ten patients they studied (Hashim, 1959).

Two PhD students who worked in Hashim's lab noted that coconut oil sales were dropping due to the news that coconut oil appeared to increase cholesterol levels. He and Vigan Babayan, an industrial chemist, decided to analyze coconut oil. They learned that 8 to 10 percent of the fats in coconut oil were the medium-chain fatty acids C8 and C10. (Recall from earlier in the book that the abbreviations C8, C10, etc., indicate the number of carbon atoms contained in the fatty acid molecule and thus how long it is. See the section titled "The Unique Properties of Medium-Chain Triglycerides," in Chapter 7, for more information about the significance of these numbers.) They used a distillation process to separate these fatty acids from the other fats in coconut oil, a process that also brought along with it very small amounts of C6 and C12. This signaled the invention of

MCT oil in the United States and took Hashim and his associates on the path along which they discovered the unique properties and therapeutic uses of this class of fatty acids. They found that MCT oil is easily absorbed and is beneficial when used in people with malabsorption syndromes and following bowel surgery.

In association with Dr. Phienvit Tantibhedhyangkul, from Thailand (where coconut oil is both a staple in the diet and a major export), they studied the use of MCT oil in premature newborns and found that it was well-tolerated and could help them gain weight more quickly (Tantib-hedhyangkul, 1971). These studies directly led to the use of MCT oil in the newborn intensive care units where I did my pediatric residency and neonatology fellowship. They also discovered that MCTs are absorbed from the bowel directly into the portal vein and carried to the liver where they are partly converted to ketones, resulting in an increase in ketones in the blood (Bergen, 1966).

During the ten years after Hashim, VanItallie, and their associates first began studying MCT oil, other researchers joined in, leading to an abundance of new information. Their work was thoroughly documented in a 1968 book entitled *Medium Chain Triglycerides*, which is available on Amazon as an anniversary edition. In 1970, a review article was published by Michael Gracey and others on the use of medium-chain triglycerides in pediatric practice, including for children with cystic fibrosis who have serious problems absorbing fat, children who have had bowel surgery or other bowel conditions leading to malabsorption, and children with liver disease and biliary atresia as well as those with other rare conditions affecting fat absorption from the bowel (Gracey, 1970). In just ten short years, the discovery of medium-chain triglycerides as a therapy provided help for countless newborns, children, and adults affected by these diseases. Another important use for MCT oil came as the result of an animal study Hashim and his associates published in 1983, strongly suggesting that MCT oil could be used for prevention of human obesity, since it is completely oxidized and not stored as fat (Geliebter, 1983).

Awareness increased that medium-chain triglycerides are converted to ketones in the liver. In 1971 Dr. Peter Huttenlocher from Yale University published his idea of supplementing the ketogenic diet with 60 percent medium-chain triglycerides, which would allow for the inclusion of more protein and carbohydrates in the diet, making it more palatable (Hutten-locher, 1971). After Hashim gave a lecture in Germany, researchers there began to make and study MCT oil.

In the early 2000s, Dr. Veech published his landmark study demonstrating the neuroprotective effects of ketones in neurons exposed to toxins that cause Alzheimer's and Parkinson's disease. This inspired Hashim to think it might be worthwhile to try MCT oil in the treatment of Parkinson's disease. This idea instead evolved into a feasibility study using a strict ketogenic diet (without MCT oil) for twenty-eight days with the help of a knowledgeable dietician, referred to in the paper as a "hyperketogenic" diet. Five people with Parkinson's disease completed the study, most reaching ketone levels in the 6 to 7 mmol/L range, with an average decrease of 43.4 percent in their Unified Parkinson's Disease Rating Scale (UPDRS) scores, a very significant improvement (VanItallie, 2005). They postulated that this worked because the condition of hyperketonemia would bypass the complex I defect that interferes with glucose uptake in Parkinson's and, thereby, boost mitochondrial function and ATP production.

Recognizing that a strict ketogenic diet of this nature is very difficult for most people to follow, it occurred to Hashim that using betahydroxy-butyrate directly to increase ketone levels could potentially have results similar to those created by the diet for people with Parkinson's disease. To begin testing this idea, he drank a 5 percent solution of betahydroxybu-tyrate and, after he became quite ill because it was so acidic, quickly realized that something needed to be done to make it drinkable. He decided to make a product with D-betahydroxybutyrate as a triglyceride, which he now refers to as the glyceride ester, and he applied for a patent in 2010 for use of this ester in Alzheimer's disease, Parkinson's disease, ALS, Huntington's disease, epilepsy, and other disorders characterized by impaired glucose metabolism.

Hashim obtained a grant from DARPA to study his glyceride ester—on the condition that he would cooperate with Dr. Serge Przedborski of Columbia University, an expert on Parkinson's disease models of mice and rats. The two designed an experiment in which they fed Hashim's betahy-droxybutyrate glyceride ester to mice that had been injected with MPTP (1-methyl-4-phenyl-1,2,3,6-tetrahydropyridine), a toxin that induces Parkinson's disease. This substance was discovered in the 1976 when a chemistry graduate student accidentally made MPTP while trying to make another compound and developed Parkinson's symptoms several days after injecting himself with it. To their delight, the glyceride ester preserved the dopamine producing neurons in the mice that were injected with MPTP. The study was presented to the Society of Neuroscience meeting in New Orleans in 2012 with Hashim listed as one of the authors (Blesa, 2012).

Still going strong in early 2018, Dr. Hashim has been one of the world's leading authorities on medium-chain triglycerides for more than five decades. He has published more than 240 papers on the topic, as well as a number of books and book chapters. He has written more than thirty papers on medium-chain triglycerides alone. The extraction and invention of medium-chain triglycerides, and the recognition of their therapeutic benefits, have improved the lives of countless people of all ages, from the tiniest preemies to elderly adults. The discovery of the conversion of medium-chain triglycerides to ketones in 1966 by Hashim and his associates, Theodore VanItallie and Stanley Bergen, laid a foundation for other ideas to build on, ultimately leading to the therapeutic use of ketones to prevent and treat a whole host of conditions, which will ultimately benefit many more millions of people around the world. Like VanItallie, Hashim continues to write and publish to increase awareness of ketones as an alternative fuel for the brain. In 2014 they co-wrote an article on the subject (Hashim, 2014) (Hashim, 2018).

GEORGE F. CAHILL JR., MD: DISCOVERER OF KETONES AS AN ALTERNATIVE FUEL FOR THE BRAIN

I had the great pleasure of speaking with Dr. George Cahill in mid-2008, not long after my husband Steve's Alzheimer's disease improved when he simply started taking coconut oil. Steve was screened for clinical trials for two different potential Alzheimer's drugs two days in a row in two different locations. I had chanced on a press release that reported that nearly half of the people with Alzheimer's showed improvement in their cognitive scores when they consumed a medical food, Axona, that was not yet available. Axona was composed of the medium-chain triglyceride tricaprylic acid (C8), which is extracted from coconut oil or palm kernel oil. Steve had a four-point improvement in his score on the mini-mental status exam

(MMSE) within one day of starting to consume coconut oil, and he continued to steadily improve thereafter. The day he started taking coconut oil, Steve said it was as if the light switch came on in his head. As part of his testing, he was asked to draw a clock, and the image he drew showed a few small disorganized circles and some numbers. A doctor told me then that Steve was on the verge of severe Alzheimer's, which prompted me that very day to buy coconut oil, learn its fatty acid composition, and figure out

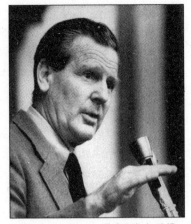

Photo 5.3. George F. Cahill Jr., MD.

what dosage to give Steve to equal the MCTs in the medical food. Two weeks after he started taking coconut oil, Steve drew another clock; although the drawing was still messy, it was much more organized with all the numbers in the right order around the clock. It was a huge improvement.

Within a few days of Steve's improvement, I started communicating with Dr. Richard Veech of the National Institutes of Health, a world expert on ketones, at first not revealing Steve's response to coconut oil but asking Veech's opinion of whether the MCTs in coconut oil could help someone with Alzheimer's. He did not believe the levels of ketones from taking coconut oil could be high enough to help, but he was taken aback when I later faxed him Steve's two clocks from the day before and two weeks after starting the coconut oil regimen. (See Introduction Figures Intro.1 and Intro.2.) He sent me several hypothesis papers that he and several of his long-time associates had written, and within the next twenty-four hours, I received phone calls from Dr. Theodore VanItallie, Dr. Sami Hashim, and Dr. George Cahill Jr., all of whom were thrilled to learn that a man with Alzheimer's apparently responded to ketones as an alternative fuel to the brain. Each of them believed and had written about the idea that increasing ketone levels could provide a therapy for and possibly prevention of Alzheimer's disease; Steve was the first person they were aware of who had tested the idea, showing them that their idea had merit.

The first time I spoke with Dr. Cahill, I did not yet know of his studies from forty years earlier that focused on the energy used by the brain during starvation. It was this study that laid the foundation for the idea that ultimately helped Steve, but it did not take long for me to make the connection. In February 2009, Cahill, Veech, and I met in Washington, D.C., with Rep. Ginnie Brown-Waite the Congressional representative from my district. Cahill came prepared with slides on paper, which he used to tell Brown-Waite the story of ketones as an alternative fuel for the brain and the possibility that ketones could help people like my husband who suffered from Alzheimer's disease and other progressive neurologic disorders. Cahill was a tall, handsome, principled but humble man with a pleasant demeanor. I spoke with him several times after that, mostly regarding his wife who suffered from a neurologic disorder and responded well to C8 but could not tolerate it. He told me that he was writing a book on ketones in evolution and explained that the first one-celled organisms used (and still use) ketones as one of their fuels. (There is more on this in Chapter 4.) To my knowledge, the book was never finished. Due to his passing in 2012, I did not have the opportunity to interview him for this book, so the details of his life come from public sources and from a chapter he wrote entitled "Fuel Metabolism in Starvation" for *Annual Reviews in Nutrition* published in 2006 (Cahill, 2006).

George Cahill was born in 1927 in Manhattan. His father, George Sr., was a urologic surgeon at Columbia. George attended the private prep school the Hotchkiss School, in Lakeville, Connecticut, where he fell in love with biology, chemistry, and mathematics. He began college at Yale at age sixteen. He enlisted in the navy near the end of World War II and was scheduled to be part of an invasion of Japan, but the war ended with the atomic bombings before that happened. Instead George served in the Naval Hospital in Oakland, California, taking care of wounded soldiers from Okinawa. He returned to Yale as a pre-med student and then attended Columbia for medical school. He married Sarah duPont (of the famous duPont family); they had six children and fifteen grandchildren.

Cahill completed his internship and residency at the Peter Bent Brigham Hospital in Boston, where he met Dr. Sami Hashim and Dr. Theodore VanItallie, both of whom became his lifelong friends and associates. He described the hospital as an "exciting hotbed of medical research" and told the story of a young patient who presented to the emergency room in a diabetic coma with the classic sweet smell of acetone in his urine. As

Cahill and his senior resident successfully treated the patient, they spent the night discussing "the how and the why of ketosis." This experience set him off on a research path, and he studied nutrition and metabolism, obesity, adipose tissue, diabetes, glucose and insulin, fasting and starvation, which ultimately led to his discovery that ketones are an alternative fuel for the brain.

Cahill joined the Hastings lab for two years, where he performed research on glucose and insulin. He returned to Brigham for another clinical year and then moved on to do research at the Baker labs, which later became the Joslin Diabetes Center, where he stayed from 1958 until 1978. Throughout his career, he was professor of medicine at Harvard, until retiring in 1990, and served from 1962 until 1990 as researcher and administrator for the Howard Hughes Medical Institute, which supports medical research. A PubMed.gov search for author George F. Cahill Jr. yields 171 articles, the first in 1956 on carbohydrate metabolism in the liver (Ashmore, 1956). He also wrote books and book chapters.

Of his many accomplishments in the field of nutrition and metabolism research, one that clearly stands out is his discovery of ketones as an alternative fuel for the brain. In the "Fuel Metabolism in Starvation" chapter of *Annual Reviews in Nutrition* (Cahill, 2006), he states that fasting was "in vogue" in the 1950s and 1960s. He and his associates wanted to learn more about the role of insulin in fasting; in 1965 they conducted an experiment with six divinity students they recruited to fast for eight days while they studied the levels of "every metabolic substrate and hormone we could measure" (Cahill, 1966). He noted that better methods to measure ketones had just become available from the lab of Hans Krebs. Among the many interesting findings, they observed that by day eight of the fast, levels of free fatty acids had nearly doubled, and total ketone levels had greatly increased from virtually nil to an average of 5.83 mmol/L with acetoacetate up to 1.11 mmol/L and betahydroxybutyrate at 4.72 mmol/L. Simultaneously, glucose levels gradually drifted down from 98 to 59 mg/dL.

During an informal conversation with a researcher who knew of his work on fasting, it occurred to Cahill that glucose could not provide all the fuel for the brain during prolonged starvation since too much muscle would need to be broken down to provide enough substrate to produce glucose from gluconeogenesis. So what was fueling the brain during fasting?

Around that time a Johns Hopkins medical resident, Oliver Owen, MD (who passed away in 2010), joined his team, and they launched a series of studies to find the answers to that question. Their first patient was an obese nurse who fasted for forty days, receiving only water, vitamins, and salt tablets. They placed catheters to draw blood from the arteries and veins around her brain and liver and were able to determine that ketones provided about two-thirds of the fuel to her brain, which greatly reduced the need to break down muscle to produce glucose. They confirmed these findings with two other patients, a man and a woman who fasted for thirty-eight and forty days respectively (Owen, 1967; Owen 2005). (See Figure 5.1 and Figure 5.2.)

In a series of experiments that followed, and in collaboration with many other researchers, Cahill, Owen, and their colleagues learned that

- about two-fifths of fatty acid metabolism in the whole body is by way of ketone production in the liver.
- about 100 to 150 grams of ketones are produced daily by the liver.
- During starvation, about 80 grams of glucose is produced daily by the internal organs, of which about 10–11 grams come from ketones, 35–40 grams from recycled lactate and pyruvate, 20 grams from the glycerol backbone of fatty acids, and the remaining 15–20 grams from amino acids, mainly alanine but also glutamine (See Figure 5.3).

Ultimately, it appears that long-term survival depends on how much muscle nitrogen is available. The use of fat as a fuel and ketones as an alternative fuel for the brain and other organs (except the liver, where ketones are made) greatly reduces how quickly muscle is used up and allows people to survive sixty days or longer, depending on how large the fat stores are and the availability of water.

In one bold experiment, three obese college-age men fasted for several days until their betahydroxybutyrate levels increased. They were then given a dose of insulin to drive down blood sugar into the severely hypoglycemic range. Normally, without the availability of ketones, such low levels of glucose would be expected to cause serious symptoms, including confusion, difficulty thinking and speaking, weakness, poor coordination, paleness, sweating, rapid heartbeat, and even seizures, loss of consciousness, or coma. In this study, the high level of ketones protected the subjects from experiencing symptoms typical of hypoglycemia (Cahill, 1980).

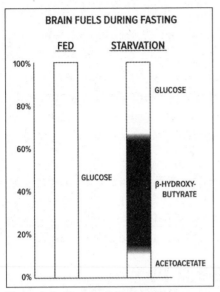

Figure 5.1. During an overnight fast, virtually 100 percent of fuel is from glucose, whereas with prolonged fasting, ketones supply two-thirds of the fuel to the brain.

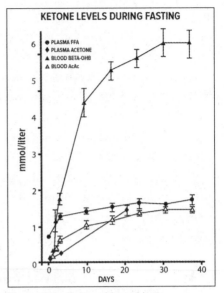

Figure 5.2. Fatty acids and ketones increase during a prolonged fast. Betahydroxybutyrate increases dramatically over seven to ten days.

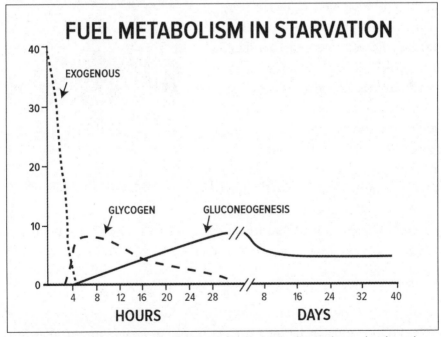

Figure 5.3. During starvation, as exogenous glucose intake drops, glucose is released from glycogen in muscle and liver, and gluconeogenesis increases.

In 2000, about thirty-three years after Cahill, Owen, and their associates discovered that ketones are an alternative fuel for the brain and that they protect the brain from the effects of low blood sugar and from starvation, Richard Veech made another important discovery: that ketones could protect brain cells from the processes that result in Alzheimer's, Parkinson's, and possibly other serious neurologic disorders. In 2003, they joined forces and wrote one of the several hypothesis papers on the subject: "Ketoacids? Good Medicine?" (Cahill, 2003).

George F. Cahill Jr. died of pneumonia at eighty-five years of age in 2012, comforted by the beautiful strains of the "Hallelujah" chorus from George Handel's *Messiah*; for someone who helped and will continue to help humankind, it was a particularly befitting way to exit this world.

RUSSELL SWERDLOW, MD: DISCOVERER OF THE KETONE-ALZHEIMER CONNECTION

When Russell Swerdlow was young, his grandmother told him that he could be anything he wanted to be, so long as he became a physician. With that and the fact that his other grandmother had Alzheimer's disease, his interest in the brain was stimulated at an early age.

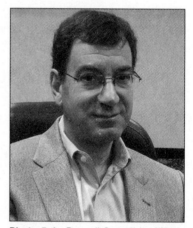

Swerdlow was born in New York City, grew up in the suburbs of northern New Jersey, and completed pre-medicine and medical school at New York University (NYU), where his father taught graphic communications and teacher education.

Photo 5.4. Russell Swerdlow, MD.

He considered the various ways he might combine his love of the brain and biochemistry with the practice of medicine and decided on the specialty of neurology.

By 1987, the evidence for decreased uptake of glucose into the brain in Alzheimer's cases was beginning to accumulate with the availability of FDG-PET imaging, including work performed by Drs. Mony de Leon, Steven Ferris, and Barry Reisberg at NYU. The idea of studying brain energy metabolism struck a chord with Swerdlow, and the summer before starting medical school at NYU, he landed a job in the lab of David Marcus, who was doing this type of research. Marcus and his associates, including Swerdlow, began to study glucose transport cross the blood-brain barrier as a possible explanation for the poor glucose uptake in the areas of the brain affected by Alzheimer's. One day during Swerdlow's first semester of medical school and the standard lecture on fatty acids in biochemistry class, the professor instructed the students that ketones can be produced by fatty acid oxidation and mentioned the decades-old use of ketogenic diet as a treatment for childhood epilepsy. In a lightbulb moment, it occurred to Swerdlow that, if their working hypothesis was correct about a problem with glucose transport into the brain, perhaps ketones could bypass this problem in Alzheimer's. The idea became the subject of his thesis, "Brain Glucose and Ketone Body Metabolism in Alzheimer's Disease."

Swerdlow spent several years after hours during medical school working on the ketone concept in a lab at old Bellevue Hospital in New York City. He and his associates used homogenates (tissues removed and liquefied) from the brains of people who had died with and without Alzheimer's and performed experiments in which the ketone body betahydroxybutyrate was radiolabeled and added to the homogenate in a closed container. As the ketone body was taken up and metabolized by brain cells, the radiolabeled carbon was released as carbon dioxide (CO_2) into the atmosphere of the closed container and taken up by hyamine hydroxide in a hanging bowl, which made it possible to measure the amount of CO_2 produced. The more betahydroxybutyrate that was used by the brain matter, the more CO_2 was released. The team found that the brains from the Alzheimer's patients and the non-Alzheimer's patients generated the same amount of CO_2 and, therefore, were equally capable of using the ketone body betahydroxybutyrate. However, when they performed the same study, but substituted radiolabeled glucose in place of the ketone bodies, they learned that there was more glucose used in the brains of non-Alzheimer's patients compared to those of the Alzheimer's patients. Whatever defect affected the glucose pathway in the brain did not affect the ketone pathway. They also showed with their experiments that decreased uptake of glucose in the Alzheimer's brain is not fully explained by the problem of transport across the blood-brain barrier.

Swerdlow reported these results along with the abstract of his thesis (mentioned above) at the 1989 meeting of the American Geriatric Society in Washington, D.C. (Swerdlow, 1989). Soon thereafter, he and his associates decided to try the ketogenic diet in treatment of Alzheimer's. They were awarded funding for a clinical trial, which, unfortunately was never completed after Swerdlow moved to University of Virginia (UVA) to begin his residency training in neurology. He continued his research in the lab of Davis Parker at UVA on energy metabolism and the contribution of mitochondrial DNA to mitochondrial changes in people with Alzheimer's and Parkinson's diseases. He completed a fellowship in cognitive disorders and a post-doctorate fellowship in the lab.

In 2004, Swerdlow proposed the "mitochondrial cascade hypothesis" for Alzheimer's disease. Around the same time, the first promising results were published of a pilot study of the medical food Axona in Alzheimer's disease (Reger, 2004). Remember that medium-chain triglycerides, the components of Axona, are partly converted to ketones in the liver and can provide alternative fuel to the brain. Based on this research, it occurred to Swerdlow that there might be a way to manipulate brain energy that would not require adhering to the strictest form of the ketogenic diet. In July 2017, at the Alzheimer's Association International Conference in London, he presented promising results in a trial of the ketogenic diet supported with medium-chain triglyceride (MCT) oil in people with Alzheimer's (Taylor, 2017). Back in the lab, he continues to study brain energy metabolism and mitochondria and is developing biomarker approaches for use in clinical trials to look at the targeting of mitochondria by specific interventions. He still sees patients and learns from them, knowledge that informs his lab work—an extraordinary career that started with a young boy who became interested in the brain because his grandmother had Alzheimer's disease (Swerdlow, 2017).

For the Scientist: Swerdlow's Study Shows Normal Ketone Uptake in Alzheimer's Brain

Brain Glucose and Ketone Body Metabolism In Alzheimer's Disease

R. Swerdlow, D. L. Marcus, J. Landman, M. Harooni, and M. L. Freedman. Dept. of Medicine, NYU Medical Center, NY, NY.
(Adapted from the original abstract with permission of Russell Swerdlow, MD.)

In vitro assays of Alzheimer's brain glucose metabolism were performed using autopic temporal cortex preincubated with 2.5 Mm ATP/NAD^+ mixture followed by an 18.5 hour incubation in the presence of 5uCi of D- $[^{14}C-[U]]$-Glucose. Three unique periods of differing metabolic rates were observed: (1) An initial period of low linear glucose metabolism; (2) a period of exponential rise; (3) a final period of elevated linear glucose metabolism. During the initial period (0–4 hrs), AD brain metabolism was 24 percent of control levels; during the final period (14.5–18.5 hrs) all metabolism was essentially equal between the AD and control brains.

GLUCOSE METABOLIC RATE (p Moles CO_2/minute)

	(0–4 hrs)	(14.5–18.5 hrs)
AD	11.2± 8.2 (n=7)	930± 83.0 (n=3)
Control	46.1± 33.2 (n=6)	960± 81.0 (n=3)

We also examined the metabolism of D-3-hydroxy $[3-^{14}C]$ butyrate and found no significant difference in rate between either AD/control or ketone body/glucose

BETA-OH BUTYRATE METABOLISM (n Moles CO_2/minute)

	(14.5–18.5 hrs)
AD	1.13 ± .363 (n=3)
Control	1.10 ± .687 (n=3)

These patterns suggest that decreased metabolism in AD is related to vascular mediated glucose deprivation rather than to intrinsic cortical pathology, and that ketone bodies may serve as a potential alternate metabolic substrate in AD.

RICHARD L. VEECH, MD, D. PHIL.–INVENTOR OF BETAHYDROXYBUTYRATE–BUTANEDIOL ESTER

Richard L. Veech was born in 1935 and grew up in Illinois where his parents were both school teachers. Because Veech was unaware of Harvard University's reputation, his biology teacher, taking note of his promise as a science student as well as his interest in history and literature, personally filled out Veech's application to the Harvard pre-medicine program. He was accepted. He stayed at Harvard for medical school and then went to Cornell University to complete a research fellowship. As his interest in metabolic diseases increased, he wanted to work with physician and biochemist Hans Krebs, a pioneer in the study of cellular respiration and namesake of the Krebs cycle. Through a mutual friend, Veech was able to get a position in Krebs's lab at Oxford to work on his doctor of philosophy degree.

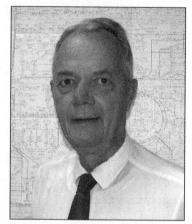

Photo 5.5. Richard L. Veech, MD, DPhil.

In 1968, Veech was a passenger in an airplane that crashed into Moose Mountain near Lebanon, New Hampshire. Thirty-five people died; Veech was one of only eight fortunate survivors. He and another man returned to the plane and managed to rescue two more people, in spite of sustaining a fractured vertebra in his lower back. Veech was hospitalized for the next three months, which he spent in a Stryker frame, a large contraption that encloses the patient like a sandwich and can be rotated. He returned to Oxford to finish his studies of cellular energy metabolism, spending a total of three years in Krebs's lab and completing his PhD.

Veech joined the National Institutes of Health in Bethesda, Maryland, where he works to this day, though there was a five-year hiatus in the early 1990s when his lab was shut down. He thought a lot about ketones during that time. From his medical school studies, he was somewhat aware of the use of the ketogenic diet for drug-resistant childhood epilepsy. When his lab was up and running again, Veech and his associates began to study ketone bodies intensively. The first article about their study of ketones, "Control of Glucose Utilization in Working Perfused Rat Heart," appeared in the October 14, 1994, issue of the *Journal of Biological Chemistry*. The study examined how the enzymes involved in glucose metabolism in the rat heart were affected by various substrates, one of which was the addition of ketones (Kashiwaya, 1994).

The second study, entitled "Insulin, Ketone Bodies, and Mitochondrial Energy Transduction," involved perfusing working rat hearts with a solution containing glucose. To this solution the researchers added either insulin or the ketone bodies betahydroxybutyrate and acetoacetate, or a combination of insulin and the ketone-body mixture. The amount of ketones added was equivalent to ketone levels that occur during starvation. They found that the addition of either insulin or ketone bodies increased the efficiency of the heart by about 25 percent, and the combination of insulin and ketone bodies increased the efficiency by about 36 percent. In other words, the hearts pumped harder using less oxygen. They also learned that ketone bodies were able to duplicate nearly all the acute effects of insulin (Sato, 1995).

Ketones Are Neuroprotective–A Landmark Study

The results of their second study with the heart were so encouraging that Veech decided to focus his research efforts on ketones. He was awarded a multimillion dollar grant from the U.S. Department of Defense to study whether a ketone ester could support and enhance the physical and cognitive performance of troops, who are often sent out on extended and grueling missions. The results also suggested to Veech that insulin resistance could be overcome with ketones and that therapeutic ketones could be used to overcome the problem of glucose uptake in the brain in Alzheimer's disease. While developing the ketone ester, Veech decided to test this hypothesis. Neurons collected from different areas of the brain— from the hippocampus to study Alzheimer's and from the mesencephalon to study Parkinson's—were grown separately in cultures. The cells were then subjected to a toxin known to cause these diseases: $A\beta_{1\text{-}42}$ for Alzheimer's, and 1-methyl-4-phenylpyridinium for Parkinson's. The ketone body betahydroxybutyrate was added to some of the cell cultures at levels found during starvation, but not to other cultures that were serving as controls. The researchers found that addition of the ketones significantly increased the survival of the neurons compared to those of the control cultures. They also found that the size of the neurons was larger and had a greater outgrowth of neurites (axons and dendrites that connect neurons with other cells), suggesting that ketones can act as growth factors to neurons in culture (Kashiwaya, 2000).

The results of this landmark study were so significant that a series of hypothesis papers followed to increase awareness for the potential use of ketones in preventing and treating Alzheimer's, Parkinson's and many other conditions.

- The first paper, entitled "Ketone Bodies, Potential Therapeutic Uses," appeared in the *International Union of Biochemistry and Molecular Biology (IUBMB) Life* in 2001 and was co-authored with Britton Chance, Yoshihiro Kashiwaya, Henry A. Lardy, and George F. Cahill Jr., the physician who discovered that neurons can use ketones as an alternative fuel to glucose.
- A second paper entitled "Ketoacids? Good Medicine?" was published in 2003 following a presentation by Cahill for the American Clinical and Climatological Association; it was co-written by Veech. This paper emphasized the importance of ketones in the evolution of humans with our large brain relative to other creatures.
- A third paper published in 2004, "The Therapeutic Implications of Ketone Bodies: The Effects of Ketone Bodies in Pathological Conditions," written solely by Veech for *Prostaglandins, Leukotrienes and Essential Fatty Acids,* explains the metabolic effects of ketones in exquisite detail: how ketones function as a fuel in the cell and in mitochondria and how they actually provide a more potent fuel than glucose; how ketones replace insulin during starvation, carrying out the same effects but in a more primitive way; and how ketones reduce oxygen-free radical damage.
- Another important paper, "Ketones: Metabolism's Ugly Duckling," written by Dr. Theodore VanItallie and Thomas H. Nufert (and mentioned earlier this chapter) appeared in the October 2003 *Nutrition Reviews.* The article provides an elegant discussion of how ketones

work along with the basis for treatment with ketones of certain neurodegenerative diseases.

Developing the Betahydroxybutyrate-Butanediol Ketone Ester

Ketones cannot be consumed as free molecules because the acidity would burn a hole in the stomach. The ketone molecule needs to be combined with another molecule to be taken orally. Veech considered many different formulations and looked to other researchers for ideas. Myron Mehlman, chief toxicologist at Mobil Oil at that time, suggested that he consider butanediol, which was used in Mehlman's native Ukraine as a by-product to feed pigs and was known to increase betahydroxybutyrate when consumed. The beauty of combining betahydroxybutyrate with butanediol is that the betahydroxybutyrate level increases directly and rapidly after consuming the ketone ester. Further, when the ketone and butanediol separate after consumption, there is a second increase in the betahydroxybutyrate level from metabolism of the butanediol. Betahydroxybutyrate exists in two forms that are mirror images. D-betahydroxybutyrate (also called R-betahydroxybutyrate to indicate the "right handed" form NOT the racemic form) is the circulating form, according to Veech and therefore more likely to produce the beneficial effects for people with Alzheimer's and other conditions that might respond to this treatment. It is possible to make a much less expensive product that is racemic, meaning that it is an equal mixture of D- and L-betahydroxybutyrate, but Veech believes it would not be as effective.

Chemist Todd King has spent countless hours making the betahydroxybutyrate-butanediol ester in Veech's lab at the NIH, one drop at a time. They have developed a process that could greatly reduce the cost by using fermentation technology, and Veech has been trying to convince the powers that be at the NIH to mass produce the ketone ester and perform clinical trials for Alzheimer's, Parkinson's, ALS, traumatic brain injury, and other conditions that might benefit from its use. He believes taking the ketone ester could be a prevention strategy and even a cure for Alzheimer's disease if taken early enough, since the problem of insulin resistance in the brain begins decades before symptoms of the disease appear (Veech, 2017).

How Ketones Work

The intensive work of Dr. Richard Veech and his associates at the NIH has revealed much about what ketones do in our metabolism and how this comes about.

The effects of insulin or ketones on the ability of the heart to work more efficiently is the result of increased production within the mitochondria of acetyl-CoA, the coenzyme from which the energy molecule ATP is made. This increased production of acetyl-CoA results in the generation of more ATP. The researchers were able to work out the biochemical details of exactly how this occurs. Ketones cause a sixteen-fold increase in the production of acetyl-CoA, similar to the effect of insulin. These findings indicate that during starvation, when glucose is not readily available and insulin levels are low, ketones can substitute for both glucose and insulin to ensure that cells continue to survive and function normally.

Ketones do not require insulin to enter the cell. Instead ketones use a monocarboxylate transporter to cross the cell membrane. Ketones bypass several steps in the process normally used by glucose to enter the mitochondria and start the process of making acetyl-CoA and eventually ATP. This is particularly important in the brain, since insulin cannot cross the blood-brain barrier. For example, in the brains of people with Alzheimer's, which have become both deficient in insulin and resistant to insulin, ketones can provide an alternative source of fuel. Ketones can also carry out many of the effects that are carried out by insulin in the normal healthy brain. Ketones can even stimulate the production of glycogen, the stored form of glucose, a function normally provided by insulin.

Veech learned that by increasing the efficiency of ATP, ketones have the added benefit of increasing the efficiency of how cells use sodium, potassium, and calcium, the three major electrolytes in our bodies. These electrolytes are very important to the transport of substances into and out of the cell. Sodium, potassium, and calcium must be maintained within very specific ranges both inside and outside the cell, or there will be dire consequences. For example, when a brain cell is injured, let's say by trauma to the head, potassium leaks out of the cell and too much sodium and calcium enter the cell. This causes the cell to swell and lose its ability to function normally. Ketones prevent or correct this problem of electrolyte imbalance by increasing ATP. Thus, injuries to the brain by direct trauma or lack of oxygen could be treated by administering ketones.

Studies of the use of ketones in traumatic brain injury are a major area of interest for the armed forces and everyday people who are injured in accidents. It is conceivable that an intravenous solution containing ketones could be given immediately to an injured soldier, an accident victim, or a newborn who has suffered a lack of oxygen during delivery to reduce damage to the brain and other organs. Veech has proposed in one of his ketone hypothesis papers from 2003 that the ketogenic diet might reduce seizures in people with epilepsy through the effect of ketones on ATP and the major electrolytes.

Veech has also found that ketones are able to reduce the amount of damage from free radicals within the tiny energy-generating mitochondria by their action on coenzyme Q_{10} (also called CoQ_{10}). Coenzyme Q_{10} is another important coenzyme required for making ATP, and it also acts as an antioxidant. Ketones can decrease damage to the cell by reducing the amount of hydrogen peroxide in the cytoplasm (the fluid within the cell).

In the discussion section of the team's 1995 paper, Veech states: "Provision of acetyl moieties within mitochondria has been suggested to reverse many age-related defects in mitochondrial ATP synthesis. Use of ketones may therefore provide unexpected benefits in the treatment of elderly patients or others suffering from oxidative damage to mitochondria." He also states in the abstract summary: ". . . the moderate ketosis characteristic of prolonged fasting or type 2 diabetes appears to be an elegant compensation for the defects in mitochondrial energy transduction associated with acute insulin deficiency or mitochondrial senescence." Simply put, raising the levels of ketones could be beneficial to people with diseases that involve a problem with damaged or aging mitochondria (Sato, 1995).

Some other important ketone studies that have come out of Veech's lab at the NIH follow hereafter.

Ketone Ester and Brown Fat - A Treatment for Obesity?

In a study published in 2012, Veech reported some unexpected findings. Two groups of mice received the same diet containing equal amounts of fat, protein, and micronutrients, but for one group part of the carbohydrate was replaced with an equal number of calories as the ketone ester. The mice were allowed to eat the amount they wanted (*ad libitum*). Compared to the control group, in the mice fed the ketone ester:

- D-betahydroxybutyrate levels were three to five times higher.
- The mice eating the diet with the ketone ester ate less.
- After one month, in the interscapular (between the shoulder blades) brown fat, the number of mitochondria increased, and there were double the number of electron chain proteins, uncoupling protein 1, and mitochondrial biogenesis-regulating proteins.
- Plasma leptin (a hormone that inhibits hunger) levels were more than double.
- Measurement of glucose uptake was double, and the quantitative insulin-sensitivity check index was 73 percent higher.
- There was increased sympathetic nervous system activity to the brown fat.
- The number of calories used while at rest was 14 percent higher.

They concluded from these very interesting results that the ketone ester could be a potential antiobesity supplement (Srivastava, 2012).

The Ketone Ester Improves an Alzheimer's Mouse Model

In their study published in print in 2013 (online in 2012), Veech's group studied a "triple transgenic" (3xTGAD) mouse model of Alzheimer's disease. In this mouse model, both the beta-amyloid plaques and tau tangles accumulate abnormally over time, and their cognition worsens as they age. Two groups of these mice were fed the same diet except that the control group received a diet enriched with carbohydrate and the other with a calorically equivalent amount of the ketone ester. In this study, Veech's group found that, compared to the control group, the mice consuming the ketone ester

- weighed 10 to 12 percent less on average after fifty days on the diet
- showed signs of less anxiety on two standard tests
- had superior cognitive performance on a test of memory
- showed significantly less accumulation of beta-amyloid and tau pathology.

They concluded that their "preclinical findings suggest that a ketone ester-containing diet has the potential to retard the disease process and improve cognitive function of patients with Alzheimer's disease" (Kashiwaya, 2013).

Case Report–Ketone Ester Helps Man with Early-onset Alzheimer's Disease

In 2015, I was deeply honored to appear as first author with Dr. Richard Veech, Dr. Theodore VanItallie, and others, on the case report of my husband Steve with early-onset Alzheimer's disease detailing his response, first to medium-chain triglycerides, and then to Dr. Veech's ketone ester as a pilot study of one person (Newport, 2015). Steve improved substantially during his first year of consuming large amounts of coconut and MCT oil, then leveled off for another year before his first setback, which I believe was related to the drug, semagacestat, that he received while participating in a clinical trial. We eventually learned that Steve was on the placebo for the first twelve to fourteen months and then crossed over to taking the drug for about five to seven months before we decided to withdraw from the study due to adverse effects. A few months later, we were notified that the trial was stopped because semagacestat was found to accelerate Alzheimer's destructive path. This was April 2010, nearly two years after Steve began taking coconut and MCT oil and his relatively sudden setback coincided with taking the drug.

Veech came to the rescue by suggesting that Steve receive the ketone ester as a pilot study of one person. Steve and I eagerly accepted his proposal, and one can only imagine how grateful we were (and still are) to have Steve chosen as the first Alzheimer's patient in the world to receive Dr. Veech's ketone ester. To Veech's way of thinking, it helped that I was a physician and would be able to monitor Steve closely, recognize adverse effects and obtain lab work as needed. Steve experienced a remarkable turnaround of his memory and a renewed ability to "do things" beginning within two hours after the first dose. He continued to improve over six to eight weeks and stabilized for about twenty months before another serious setback, unrelated to the ketone ester, changed things. You'll find more details about Steve's setback and recovery while on the ketone ester in the introduction under "Dr. Veech's Ketone Ester to the Rescue."

At age eighty-two, Dr. Veech refuses to retire from the NIH. He is determined to finish the work he started on ketones more than twenty years ago and to see that his ketone ester gets mass produced and studied in clinical trials so that people like my husband Steve and others with Alzheimer's, Parkinson's, and many other neurologic and other types of conditions can benefit from ketone as an alternative fuel for the brain and its many other life-improving and life-extending benefits.

STEPHEN CUNNANE, PHD—KETONES ARE IMPORTANT TO THE NEWBORN AND THE ELDERLY BRAIN

Since the early 1970s, considerable research has looked at the fuels used by the brain of the developing fetus and how they change in newborn life with the introduction of breast milk and formula. (See Chapter 4.) Dr. Stephen Cunnane was one of the researchers who contributed to this understanding, learning that ketones not only provide fuel but also provide the building blocks for lipids in the newborn brain. He has written about the importance of ketones in human evolution (Cunnane, 1999).

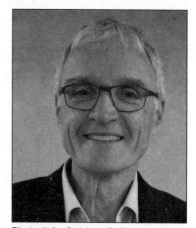

Photo 5.6. Stephen C. Cunnane, PhD.

His work shifted to the opposite end of the life spectrum when access to ketone and glucose PET scan technology became available.

Stephen C. Cunnane was born in London in 1952; his family emigrated to Canada when he was one and a half years old. He majored in biology at Bishop's University, a very small university east of Montreal, after which, pursuing his interest in research, he completed his PhD in physiology at McGill University in 1980. Cunnane's thesis focused on nutritional cofactors needed to convert the omega-6 fatty acid linoleic acid (LA) to arachidonic acid (ARA). His post-doctoral studies took him to Nova Scotia and Aberdeen, London, where he worked with renowned lipid researcher and Imperial College of London professor Michael Crawford, PhD.

Dr. Cunnane landed a faculty position at University of Toronto, where he taught a course on controversies in nutrition and continued his research. The university had a nuclear magnetic resonance (NMR) spectrometer, which permits one to visualize in real time the processes involved in fatty acid metabolism—for example, the conversion of omega-3 alpha-linolenic acid (ALA) labeled with carbon-13 to docosahexanoic acid (DHA). Using live rats as subjects, they were able to see that the tracer found its way into many other lipids in the brain besides DHA, including cholesterol and other saturated fatty acids. Indeed, the tracer accumulated in lipids by a factor of fifty to one-hundred times more than it was going into DHA. This unexpected finding was occurring by way of ketones. Hence they determined that ALA was actually moderately ketogenic (Cunnane, 1999; Cunnane 2004). Cunnane was aware of the use of ketogenic diet for epilepsy and focused some of his work on whether ALA might help with the ketogenic diet. These results also revealed that even relatively large amounts of dietary ALA do not result in adequate production of the essential omega-3 fat DHA and, therefore, this work strongly suggests that it is important to get DHA directly from a marine source and not rely on soybean and other vegetable oils to get adequate DHA from the diet (Plourde, 2007).

It turns out that ALA is about 80 percent beta-oxidized and is the most ketogenic of the common dietary long-chain fatty acids. The breastfed, full-term newborn goes into ketosis shortly after birth, supported by the fat accumulated during the last third of the pregnancy, as well as by the medium-chain fats in breast milk, which are partly converted to ketones. Cunnane's work has shown that ketones are vital to the development of the newborn brain, which represents roughly 10 percent of the baby's weight but uses about 70 percent of the total energy requirement. Premature and underweight newborns lack fat and often suffer from cognitive deficits that become apparent as they grow older. Cunnane's work points to ALA as a moderately good way for the infant to get ketones after being weaned from breast milk. ALA is ketogenic as well, but less so. Some of the resulting ketones are converted to new fatty acids and cholesterol in the brain. His book, *Survival of the Fattest: The Key to Human Brain Evolution* (World Scientific, 2005), details these ideas and the supporting research.

Cunnane-accepted a research chair position at Sherbrooke University, in Montreal, where he would have access to state-of-the-art brain imaging. An important focus for him became whether ketones could fill the energy deficit in the aging brain and also bypass the problem of glucose uptake in the Alzheimer's brain. There was a precedent for this idea in a report published in 1981 by Ulla Lying-Tunell and others of Karolinska Institute in Sweden (Lying-Tunell, 1981). Using a technique called arteriovenous difference expressed as a cerebral metabolic rate (CMR), they showed that glucose uptake in the brain is decreased but ketone uptake is the same for people with mild to moderate pre-senile dementia compared to normal healthy adults. An important question was whether the problem with glucose uptake in the Alzheimer's brain, well-documented by FDG PET imaging by that time, is a result of the death of the neurons in those areas, or simply due to the neurons being starved from a lack of fuel (glucose). The 1981 Lying-Tunell results suggest that the neurons might not be dead because they could still take up ketones normally. In 2003, with newer imaging techniques, Cunnane and his associates confirmed the earlier results and answered their own questions about ketones, brain aging, and Alzheimer's. They are the first in the world to study Alzheimer's using ketone PET imaging to achieve this end.

Another idea Cunnane was interested in was the role of brain inflammation in Alzheimer's. Specialized brain cells called microglia become activated when there is brain inflammation, and these cells might require more energy once activated. If so, then they would use more glucose as they attacked the beta-amyloid that makes up the well-known plaques that have been considered a hallmark of Alzheimer's disease for decades. These microglia might be competing for glucose coming into the brain, possibly contributing to the decreased glucose uptake into the areas of the brain affected by Alzheimer's. Cunnane and his associates wondered: If brain inflammation could be reduced, would more glucose be available for brain function?

Using a combination of the FDG PET scan to look at glucose uptake and ketone PET scan using the ketone acetoacetate labeled with carbon-11, they completed animal studies and human studies in healthy young adults (n=20) and older adults (n=24) (Nugent, 2014A, Nugent 2014B), followed by studies of cognitively healthy older adults compared to people with mild cognitive impairment and Alzheimer's disease (Croteau, 2018A). They learned that ketones provide about 3 percent of the brain's energy requirement in young healthy and cognitively older adults, with glucose supplying the remainder of the energy requirement; however, there is an energy deficit overall of about 7 percent in the older brain that grows to 8–9 percent with the development of mild cognitive impairment (MCI) and even higher in Alzheimer's. One of the group's profound findings regarding Alzheimer's disease is that ketone uptake is the same as in cognitively healthy older adults, supporting the idea that ketones could provide alternative fuel to the Alzheimer's brain (Cunnane 2016).

Cunnane and the team then attacked the next logical question of whether the brain of someone with Alzheimer's disease would use ketones from medium-chain triglycerides, which are partly converted to ketones in the liver. If so, how much would be needed to bridge the gap in the energy deficit in the brain for healthy aging people as well as those with MCI and Alzheimer's? So far, they have learned that the higher the plasma level of ketones, the greater their contribution for brain energy, just like in healthy adults. They also determined that MCT oil could help to bridge that gap by increasing plasma levels of ketones (Courchesne-Loyer, 2013; Courchesne-Loyer, 2016): 30 grams of MCT oil per day could reduce the energy gap 3–5 percent and 45 grams could increase the contribution of ketones from 3 percent to 10–12 percent of the energy required by the brain and bridge the gap in people with MCI. These results were reported at the Alzheimer's Association International Conference in London in July 2017.

At the time of this writing, Dr. Cunnane and his associates are engaged in the BENEFIC clinical trial looking at a key question: Can MCT oil delay progression of MCI to Alzheimer's disease? Their studies are producing preliminary promising results. A shorter proof-of-concept trial was recently completed showing that a 30-grams-per-day MCT supplement does increase ketone uptake in the brain showing mild to moderate Alzheimer's disease and the results will be published in 2018 (Croteau, 2018 B). In the meantime, they have completed a study of an individualized exercise program for people with mild Alzheimer's, which showed that walking on a treadmill at moderate intensity three times a week can nearly triple ketone uptake in the brain (Castellano, 2017). Could combining MCT with exercise double the impact of either alone? Another interesting finding is that caffeine increases breakdown of fat and transiently increases ketone levels to roughly double the levels seen following an overnight fast (Vandenverghe, 2016). It is still too early to know whether, if used together, these different approaches to raising ketones in the blood would really delay Alzheimer's. At the 2017 Alzheimer's conference in London, Cunnane headed up the first-ever session on the role of brain ketone metabolism and ketogenic interventions in Alzheimer's disease. On October 10, 2017, at the Lipids and Brain 4: Lipids in Alzheimer's Disease conference in Nancy, France, he was awarded the prestigious Chevreul Medal for his important body of research (Cunnane, 2018).

KETONES IMPACT BETA-AMYLOID IN ALZHEIMER'S MODEL

Dr. Marwan Maalouf of Scottsdale, Arizona, a promising young researcher in the area of ketones as an alternative fuel for treating Alzheimer's, was tragically killed in an accident while riding his bicycle. He spoke at the 2012 Charlie Foundation Global Symposium on Ketogenic Diets for Epilepsy and Other Disorders in Chicago just two weeks before he died. He was one of several authors on a paper published in *Neurobiology of Aging* in 2016 that reported on an important collection of studies looking at the direct effects of ketones on beta-amyloid, the substance that makes up the infamous plaques in the Alzheimer's disease brain. Some of the various studies were performed *in vitro* (outside of a living organism) and others in living mice (Yin, 2016). In summary, they found that a mixture of the ketones betahydroxybutyrate and acetoacetate protected neurons from the toxic effects of beta-amyloid by several different mechanisms. They also found that treatment with the ketone mixture from an early age drastically improved cognitive performance in a mouse model of Alzheimer's.

For the Scientist: Details of 2016 Study by Yin and Others on Effects of Ketones on Beta-Amyloid

In the preface, the authors note that:

- Beta-amyloid (Aβ) is absorbed into and is transported through distal axons.
- Aβ accumulates in mitochondria of cell bodies.
- Aβ is further transferred to nearby neurons.
- Accumulation of Aβ 1-42 causes mitochondrial dysfunction and failure by binding to mitochondrial proteins and increasing formation of reactive oxygen species (ROS).
- Alzheimer's is associated with mitochondrial dysfunction and oxidative stress.

In vitro experiments on primary cortical neurons of newborn rat or mouse pups showed that ketones (a roughly 4:1 mixture of BOHB and AcAc)

- prevented oligo Aβ42-induced membrane dysfunction, neuronal injury, mitochondrial dysfunction, and ROS formation.
- reduced intracellular levels of Aβ42 by preventing perforation of cell membrane by Aβ42.
- protected synaptic plasticity against oligo Aβ42 toxicity.

They also performed a study with APP mice, an Alzheimer's mouse model, which shows synapse loss and learning deficits at three to four months and increased Aβ plaques at six months. The *in vivo* experiments were performed on wild type and APP mice with daily subcutaneous injections of 0.9 percent saline or betahydroxybutyrate (600 mg/kg) and acetoacetate (150 mg/kg) for two months beginning at three to four months of age. This study showed that ketones:

- improved mitochondrial dysfunction by restoring complex 1 activity and reducing soluble Aβ42 level.
- ketones did not affect wild type mice but drastically improved memory performance in APP mice on Morris water maze and novel object recognition tests.

This is all good news for people with Alzheimer's and indicates that ketones could come to the rescue.

CASE STUDIES: HOW KETOGENIC THERAPIES HAVE HELPED TWO PEOPLE

William Curtis (Parkinson's)

William "Bill" Curtis, sixty-two years old at the time of this writing, describes himself as a nerd. He and his father, an aeronautic engineer, once tried to design and build the world's fastest bike, but it didn't quite make the cut. Bill acquired an undergraduate degree in agriculture but also studied chemistry and math and then spent many years taking graduate-level courses in physics, math, and other sciences without ever completing a master's degree. Eventually he found his niche in computer programming and creating software, working for a large financial institution.

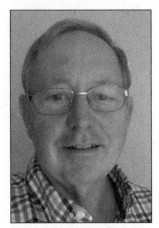

Photo 5.7. William Curtis

At about age forty-five, Bill began to have trouble remembering phone numbers and showed other symptoms of cognitive impairment. His right arm stopped swinging normally when he walked, and he had trouble doing things that he could easily do before. He developed a "pill-rolling" movement, a tremor in which the thumb rolls back and forth over the index finger. His ability to organize and carry out daily activities, as well as manage administrative and executive type work, deteriorated—a problem known as executive dysfunction. In 2004, at just forty-nine years old, he was diagnosed with Parkinson's disease, and that was just the beginning. The prescribed medications made him drowsy, and he could no longer drive without serious risk. If he stopped the medications, his memory was much worse. He tried to compensate for his disability by working more hours, but this seemed to make the problem worse and left little time for his wife, a nurse, and their three sons.

Curtis and his neurologist kept their eyes open for new treatments. He switched from the Mirapex, which made him drowsy, to Sinemet. He contemplated retiring early. However, it seemed that every few years there was another drug that came along that made a great difference. Azilect, Comptan, and the Neupro-patch were particularly effective. With the help of his neurologist, Curtis was able to keep functioning at work until 2012.

The tremor, which started on his right side, progressed to affecting his whole body. He developed dystonia (abnormal movements), had to give up driving, and recalls an episode at work when a coworker said, "Bill, I noticed you have been looking at the computer screen for several minutes and looking at that empty document. Are you okay?"

In 2006, his father told him about a scientific article written by Dr. Theodore VanItallie, reporting a pilot study of the positive results of ketogenic diet in five people with Parkinson's disease (VanItallie, 2005). He also looked at hypothesis papers written by Dr. Richard Veech on ketones as alternative fuel for the brain in Alzheimer's, Parkinson's and other diseases (Veech, 2001). Bill was in the early stages of the disease, and his symptoms were not severe, so he didn't try the ketogenic approach. Instead, he participated in a Michael J. Fox Foundation exercise study and found he could walk a little further but saw no other obvious improvement. He suffered from fatigue, and he would struggle to complete a simple task such as washing the car windows. About half of the people who struggle with Parkinson's list fatigue as the major cause of disability. Bill's condition continued to deteriorate, and he became completely disabled, sat in a chair having tremors most of day, and couldn't finish writing a sentence without reading and re-reading to recall what he wanted to say.

Bill began to correspond with Dr. Veech. Starting with a phone call he made to Veech in 2013, and with Veech's guidance and encouragement, Bill decided to try various ketogenic strategies. He has found that what works for him are an overnight fast, broken by coffee charged with coconut or MCT oil and butter, exercise, and, more recently, a strict ketogenic diet with low-carbohydrates and limited protein intake. At one point, Bill completed a ten-day trial of Veech's betahydroxybutyrate-butanediol ketone ester, which brought about remarkable improvement in his tremors, his ability to get around, and his mental clarity and even gave him better control of his bladder. He found that the ketone ester gave him the best results when combined with restriction of carbohydrates. He is waiting to resume taking the ketone ester until toxicity/safety testing is completed and it is recognized by the FDA for use in the general public.

Bill's philosophy is that the body "makes ketones for free," and so he continues to adhere to a strict ketogenic diet, which has allowed him to get up out of the chair and become more involved in life again, though he still considers his condition fragile. He continues to use the standard medications to treat his symptoms but has had a marginal reduction in how much he takes. Bill helps other people with Parkinson's get started on the ketogenic lifestyle by telling them what he has learned. He notes that, while the ketogenic lifestyle has not helped all of them, it does seem to work for most people with severe symptoms. He suggests that people with Parkinson's try one of the following three strategies:

1. Fast overnight and drink coffee with coconut and/or MCT oil in morning. Limit eating to about a six-hour window each day.
2. Reduce carbs and avoid excessive protein in addition to the overnight fast and morning coffee with fat.
3. Eat a more ketogenic diet by adding healthy fats as snacks and completely avoid high glycemic index foods.

Bill recognizes how difficult a ketogenic diet can be and advises people that there is "no rush" with this type of diet as there would be during starvation—there are "plenty of days to get it right." He works with nutritionist Miriam Kalamian, who is certified in the ketogenic diet, and encourages others to do so as well.

Bill says that the fateful telephone call he made to Dr. Veech in 2013 took him on a new pathway toward a ketogenic lifestyle and a new lease on life. Veech often says that Parkinson's is easy to study compared to Alzheimer's disease—"You either have a tremor, or you don't"—and the effect of a treatment on symptoms can easily be observed. To increase awareness, Bill posted videos on YouTube.com showing his symptoms while off and on ketones (https://www.youtube.com/watch?v=riGYq5iD2SM and https://www.youtube.com/watch?v=oYaFv-8dv58). The difference is obvious and truly remarkable (Curtis, 2017).

Joe Prata (Alzheimer's)

On the day I interviewed Carol Henry Prata, she and her husband, Joe, had just returned from the office of his neurologist with some good news. He had been previously diagnosed by four different neurologists with different opinions: two thought he had beginning dementia, most likely Alzheimer's; one said definitely Alzheimer's; and another said he probably had the beginnings of dementia with a vascular component. On this day, six years after Joe's symptoms first became noticeable, his tests related to speech were normal and, putting all the results of his tests together, the doctor had arrived at a diagnosis of amnestic mild cognitive impairment (MCI)—welcome news by compari-

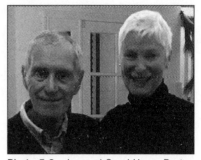

Photo 5.8. Joe and Carol Henry Prata

son, since MCI does not always progress to full-blown dementia. MCI mainly affects memory and executive functioning, which translates into "trouble doing things."

Joe Prata is eighty-nine years old and not someone you would ever expect to develop dementia. He was a world-class swimmer, narrowly missing a slot on the U.S. team during the trials for the 1952 Helsinki Olympics. He swims laps continuously for 30 to 35 minutes four to six days per weeks, surfs once a week, walks, and uses an exercise bike. He came from a family who liked to laugh and believed you should do something you enjoy every day. As a first-generation Italian-American, he has eaten a Mediterranean diet his entire life, has never smoked or used recreational drugs, and doesn't drink. He sleeps well and never lost consciousness from a head injury. But his family history is worrisome, with personality changes in his mother at the end of her life, dementia in his maternal grandmother, who also had diabetes, and hints of problems with both of his grandfathers. Joe obtained a bachelor's degree in speech/public speaking with a minor in social studies at Ohio State University, and a master's degree in theater from San Francisco State University. He worked as an English teacher and also coached swimming and water polo until he retired.

Carol Henry Prata prefers to be known as a citizen scientist and activist. At age seventy, she considers herself Joe's advocate-in-chief. Carol and Joe met when she was nineteen and he was thirty-seven. Early on, she was a working actress, but she eventually shifted to television and film production. She went back to school at age fifty-four and became a financial planner with her own business, which, as it turned out, made it easier to take care of Joe when he began having problems. In early 2012, when Joe was eighty-three, Carol began seeing signs of dementia in him. Having lived with her mother's Lewy body dementia, Carol knew that something was wrong. At first, they thought it might be the statin drug he was taking, and he did seem to improve five weeks after stopping the drug. However, he began to have periods of confusion and trouble doing things he had been able to do routinely, such as opening or closing up a package. He was often non-verbal in the morning and would sometimes stand in the middle of the room staring as if he were in another world. Looking back, Carol realized that, over the previous five to ten years, Joe had become quieter and more withdrawn, less optimistic, and more somber, with changes in his personality and levels of alertness and engagement. For about three years, he had slowly developed a problem with remembering nouns and would describe objects as, "The thing! You know—the thing!" By 2012, his love of relaying humorous memories and anecdotes had given way to aphasia and complaints about health issues, often with agitation and frustration. He experienced physical changes as well, such as difficulty with walking and balance, with navigating on land while carrying his surfboard, and with swimming freestyle with his head completely under water, which is uncharacteristic of a former elite swimmer.

Carol quickly adapted to the new reality. She attended caregiver classes and workshops and made a list of doctors and other people who could help Joe if something happened to her. After Joe first became symptomatic, a friend told Carol about Steve's story of improvement in his Alzheimer's symptoms while taking coconut and MCT oil. A few months later, Joe began a similar protocol. Carol noticed obvious changes each time she increased the amount of coconut and MCT oil he received, with dramatic improvements in his comprehension, memory, alertness, word recall, and personality. Carol wasn't the only one who noticed the changes; friends, neighbors, and the medical professionals who saw Joe regularly saw them, too.

In August 2012, Carol started giving Joe a coconut oil/MCT smoothie once a day and increased it to three servings daily in April 2013. In June 2014, she began to substitute Fuel for Thought® (no longer available) in a glass of coconut milk twice a day while continuing the mid-day smoothie, and, in October 2016, she began to substitute one-half serving twice per day of Keto//OS Orange Dream caffeine-free, a ketone salts product from Pruvit, in place of Fuel for Thought®, keeping his mid-day smoothie. In April 2017, she switched to Pruvit Keto//OS Max Swiss Cacao.

While Joe has done remarkably well over six years with ketone therapy, he has experienced some setbacks, mainly when he has had surgery or an illness that interferes with getting his full daily rations of ketogenic drinks. He has had setbacks during periods of stress and some that could be explained by episodes of atrial fibrillation. Carol says he declines just as dramatically as he improves when he misses his ketogenic drinks versus when he is taking them. When these setbacks are behind him and he gets back on track, he sometimes returns to his baseline quickly, and other times it has taken a couple of months.

She and Joe both eat a Mediterranean-type low glycemic index diet, and they aim for mild ketosis. They take coconut oil, MCT oil, and olive oil; drink coconut milk; and use butter as a treat. She and Joe both take ketone salts, but he takes more, consuming one packet total per day in two servings.

These days, Carol reports that, although Joe still has trouble with word retrieval and understanding concepts, his conversations and vocabulary are much more complex, and he is far more focused and engaged. Friends and family are amazed by the difference. His long- and short-term memory have improved exponentially since she started giving Joe the ketone salts in 2016. She reports that Joe is sometimes quick to come up with creative solutions that astonish her. His remaining cognitive problems are largely related to comprehension and task performance (e.g., he is vexed by packaging, the television remote control, unlocking the gas cap on the car, and putting in his hearing aids).

Carol has turned her personal challenges into advocacy. She has worked hard to let others know about ketones as an alternative fuel for the brain and their anti-inflammatory properties. She has been relentless in trying to get this information to doctors at University of California Los Angeles and University of Southern California, and other universities. She has found that Dr. Helena Chiu of University of Southern California and Dr. Rudolph Tanzi of Harvard University and Massachusetts General Hospital are receptive but, as a group, she finds most doctors do not seem open to the idea at all.

Carol describes Joe as a confident person with a positive attitude and enthusiasm for life. He never seems depressed but will lament on occasion when he is discouraged by physical ailments by saying, "I've passed my expiration date!" Carol states, "Since beginning this dietary intervention in September 2012, Joe has re-emerged from his private, silent world to rejoin me as a friend and partner. Our conversations about the news, politics, weather, and the observations of daily life are very much as they have been during our forty-nine years together. . . . Now his sense of humor is returning—the greatest gift of all." Carol says Joe looked out for her when she was young, and now she looks out for him (Prata, 2018).

DOMINIC D'AGOSTINO, PHD: TAKING KETONE RESEARCH TO A WHOLE NEW LEVEL

In July 2008, just two months after Steve began to improve due to the use of coconut and MCT oil, we traveled to Chicago for the Alzheimer's Association International Conference where five thousand researchers and physicians from all around the world would convene to share and learn the latest information on the disease. I wrote up a self-published case report about Steve's dramatic improvement after he began taking coconut oil to illustrate the need

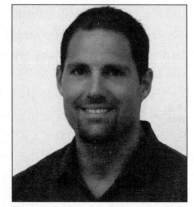

Photo 5.9. Dominic D'Agostino, PhD.

to increase awareness of the idea that ketones are an alternative fuel for the brain and could help people with Alzheimer's and other neurodegenerative diseases (Newport, 2008). I wanted to let people know that this treatment was already available on the shelf as coconut oil and MCT oil, and that a ketone ester had been developed in Dr. Richard Veech's lab at the NIH that could produce even greater results but that he lacked funding for mass production and testing. I hoped to inspire some of these researchers to take an interest in studying ketones.

At the last minute, the Alzheimer's Association reversed their decision to allow me to distribute my article in the exhibit hall at their conference, but I attended the presentations, looked at hundreds of posters on nutrition, glucose, insulin, and fatty acids, and spoke with as many of the participants as I could. I left with at least 1,400 copies of my case report, disappointed that I had not been able to get the message about ketones out in a big way. Little did I know that a researcher lived right in my own backyard at University of South Florida in Tampa and that he would step up, take the lead, and take ketone research to a whole new level.

Dominic D'Agostino was born in 1975 in a rural area of New Jersey and grew up working on a farm. He loved being outdoors and thought he might become a farmer or park ranger. He describes himself as a mediocre student until junior high school when he became super curious to figure out his own biology and physiology and to learn everything he could to maximize his athletic performance in sports and cognitive performance in school. Strength training became a big part of his life (and still is), but during his senior year in high school, he came to the realization that good nutrition was the key to overall health and to maximizing his efforts in the gym. This motivated him to major in nutrition science in college at Rutgers/The State University of New Jersey. He finished with a double major in biological science and gained valuable experience in a neurobiology research lab. His project was to identify the neurotransmitter phenotype (genetic characteristics) of specialized neurons that control cardiovascular and respiratory functions in the brainstem. This undergraduate project was the gateway for him toward getting accepted into a neuroscience and physiology PhD program at University of Medicine and Dentistry of New Jersey–Robert Wood Johnson Medical School. During the course of his PhD research, among other studies, D'Agostino further delineated how specialized neurons sense oxygen levels in the brain and how they affect cardiovascular and respiratory functions under conditions of low oxygen. He also discovered a previously unknown oxygen sensing mechanism in the brainstem. The American Physiology Society presented him with an award for his discoveries.

D'Agostino completed two years of post-doctoral fellowship at Wright State University Boonshoft School of Medicine before moving, in 2006, to the University of South Florida College of Medicine, where he did two more years of fellowship before becoming an assistant professor. Now a tenured associate professor, D'Agostino teaches molecular pharmacology, neuroscience, metabolism and physiology at the USF College of Medicine, and his research program at USF is funded in part by the Office of Navy Research (ONR). His primary focus is on the problem of seizures caused by central nervous system oxygen toxicity, a limitation for Navy SEAL divers, who breathe 100 percent oxygen using a closed-circuit system to eliminate bubbles, which could cause them to be detected under water.

In 2007, D'Agostino discovered that the ketogenic diet was not just a passing fad but is a powerful metabolic therapy for epilepsy and seizures of all kinds that do not respond to drugs, including seizures that occur during continuous exposure to 100 percent oxygen. At that time D'Agostino was charged with developing a countermeasure to prevent these seizures, and the ketogenic diet was one potential option. However, his ONR program officer was not enthusiastic about putting elite warfighters on a high-fat diet, so D'Agostino looked for alternative methods to induce nutritional ketosis. He connected with Mike Dancer, a man in his late thirties who suffered three to five severe seizures every week. Dancer's condition did not respond to multiple drug therapies and resulted in post-ictal (after seizure) periods, often lasting more than twenty-four hours during which he was nonfunctional and barely conscious. Mike Dancer believed he was dying and was on the verge of undergoing brain surgery to remove the defective area near his hippocampus. D'Agostino told him about the ketogenic diet and referred him to The Charlie Foundation (www.charliefoundation.org), explaining that the organization was dedicated to helping families use the ketogenic diet mainly for epilepsy but for some other disorders as well. Dancer followed a modified ketogenic diet approach (popularized by Dr. Eric Kossoff at Johns Hopkins), which quickly put a stop to nearly all of his seizures. Dancer has maintained this diet and remained nearly seizure-free status for almost ten years and, because of this turnaround, he has become a messenger for ketones as well. These days, when Dancer does have seizures, they are less severe and the recovery phase is shortened to the point that he becomes lucid in minutes instead of hours. It was Dancer's experience with the ketogenic diet that convinced D'Agostino that nutritional ketosis was a very powerful neuroprotective and anti-convulsant strategy.

Continuing his research, D'Agostino read an article by Jong Rho, MD, and Raman Sankar, MD. asking the question of whether the ketogenic diet might be packaged in a pill. At the time, the answer was "likely no" (Rho, 2008). He also read about Steve's dramatic improvement while using coconut and MCT oil in his early-onset Alzheimer's symptoms in an article that appeared in the *St. Petersburg Times* (Hosley-Moore, 2008). This article included an interview with Richard Veech about the ketone ester—an "Aha!" moment for D'Agostino that took him in new directions in his search for an anti-seizure strategy for Navy SEALs.

D'Agostino was able to acquire funding for research into the idea of using an exogenous ketone substance to prevent seizures and to develop a "deliverable"—a tangible product that could be used by Navy SEALs and the special operations community to prevent oxygen toxicity seizures. D'Agostino and his colleagues developed technologies to study this problem using atmospheric chambers that allowed for telemetry measurement of brain activity under these extreme conditions. They put rats on the equivalent of human fasting for one week (ketone levels of ~5mM), which significantly delayed the onset of the seizures. It is important to note that these rats were allowed to eat as much as they wanted of standard high-carbohydrate rat chow before being given the dose of ketone ester (in this case: 1,3-butanediol - acetoacetate diester) through a feeding tube (to give precise dose) thirty minutes prior to being given high pressure oxygen (5 ATA O_2), which would normally produce a seizure within five minutes. They started with one rat; sixty minutes later, the rat was grooming itself and appeared to be under little stress. D'Agostino says that they stared into the chamber in astonishment. The experiment was repeated, and tests with dozens more rats confirmed the results. While the rats each eventually had a seizure, they were 600 percent more resilient to seizures than rats who did not receive this ketone ester. In addition, the seizures that the ketone ester rats endured were not as strong and the rats recovered faster. This particular ketone ester raises betahydroxybutyrate and acetoacetate levels in a 1:1 ratio (D'Agostino, 2013).

Shortly after this, one of D'Agostino's PhD students, now Dr. Angela Poff, undertook a cancer research project for her dissertation. By this time, it was known that caloric restriction and the ketogenic diet could potentially suppress cancer-cell growth and prolong life in cases of glioblastoma, an aggressive brain cancer (Zuccoli, 2010). In Poff's project, her results found that raising ketones by adding a ketone ester to standard high-carb rat chow also had a remarkable cancer-suppressing effect in rats that had aggressive brain cancer cells implanted in their abdomens (Poff, 2014). This line of research has evolved into looking at the effects of various combinations of diet, exogenous ketones, glucose-lowering substances, and hyperbaric oxygen therapy on cancer. Other projects have studied the effects of ketogenic strategies on neurodegenerative diseases, rare enzyme deficiencies that cause seizures, status epilepticus (prolonged continuous seizures), muscle wasting (cachexia), wound healing, inflammation, exercise performance and resilience, and improvement of health biomarkers related to obesity, metabolic syndrome, and type 2 diabetes. These studies focus on effectiveness, safety, and the pharmacokinetics and the goal is to move these therapies from animal studies to human clinical trials, which have just started at the time of this writing. The ketone salts, an exciting product combining ketone molecules with minerals (or amino acids) to produce instant ketosis, were developed and studied extensively in D'Agostino's lab and widely available to the public since early 2016. D'Agostino currently has numerous pre-medical students, PhD students, and post-docs working with him on no fewer than ten projects to study various therapeutic possibilities for ketones in treating disease.

Dr. D'Agostino is most excited about the emerging treatments involving the ketogenic diet and/or exogenous ketone supplementation and has found that a combination of these two strategies appears to be most effective. He foresees limitless possibilities of engineering a wide variety of exogenous ketone molecules and formulations of those molecules to treat many different types of diseases and conditions and to enhance physical and cognitive performance in healthy people. His high school focus on maximizing his own performance and his recognition of the power of good nutrition has taken him on a path that will potentially help millions of people (D'Agostino, 2017).

THOMAS SEYFRIED, PHD: CANCER AND THE KETOGENIC DIET

I first heard of Dr. Thomas Seyfried's work with the ketogenic diet and cancer in March 2009 when Steve and I were asked by Dr. Veech to bring one of Seyfried's scientific articles to our meeting in the office of Senator Ted Kennedy, who was suffering from glioblastoma, an aggressive brain cancer that most do not survive for more than six months from diagnosis. In 2010 in Edinburgh, Scotland, we heard Seyfried speak at the Global Symposium on the Ketogenic Diet for Epilepsy and Other Disorders and witnessed the fateful first encounter between Seyfried and Dominic D'Agostino during the poster presentations that directly led to their first collaboration and now long-time partnership in the study of the ketogenic diet for cancer.

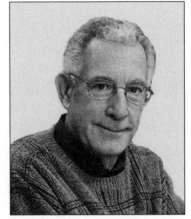

Photo 5.10. Thomas N. Seyfried, PhD.

Thomas N. Seyfried, was born in 1946 and raised in Queens, New York, where he had a traditional public-school upbringing. During his senior year of high school, his family moved to Brockton, Massachusetts, where he worked in the shoe industry to make money for college. He majored in biology at St. Francis College in Maine (now called University of New England) and recently received their alumni achievement award.

Seyfried finished his bachelor's degree during the height of the Vietnam War, when the draft was about to go into effect. He decided to join the army and attend officer candidate school, figuring this would give him the best odds of working behind the scenes rather than on the frontlines in Vietnam. He describes the training as brutal, recalling he was initially sent to Germany and then to Vietnam, where he found himself in the much lauded First Cavalry Division of the infantry. The soldiers patrolled the jungle, fighting off not only the enemy but also rats and other animals of all kinds, including ants, wasps, and snakes. Of Vietnam he said that if the enemy didn't kill you, the animals might. One of the division's many dangerous jobs was to move aboriginal people to safer locations. Although Seyfried achieved the rank of captain during his military career, ultimately the life wasn't for him. Years earlier, his high school biology teacher had encouraged him to go to graduate school at Illinois State University; Seyfried recalls filling out his application while sitting in the Vietnam jungle and getting mud on it.

After surviving Vietnam and army life, Seyfried pursued his master's degree in genetics at Illinois State University. For his thesis, he studied the mechanisms of mutagenesis, specifically the influence of oxygen on two chemical carcinogens. He attended the University of Illinois for his PhD in genetics and became interested in gangliosides (a group of complex lipids that are present in the gray matter of the human brain), completing a postdoctoral fellowship at Yale, under the mentorship of Dr. Robert Yu, a world leader in gangliosides, especially those related to multiple sclerosis. He received a research career development award and was appointed assistant professor of biology at Yale. He became interested in cancer and began to look at gangliosides in cancerous tumors as a side project. Lipid biochemistry became an important and eye-opening new component of his work. As a post-doc, he wanted to do some work on the ketogenic diet for epilepsy in mice but was turned down—the reviewers advised him that the ketogenic diet was "passé."

Seyfried left Yale to teach neurobiology at Boston College, even though he had never taken a class in the subject. In contrast to his relatively meager lab at Yale, his new lab at Boston college was "palatial," and he had plenty of students interested in working with him in this field. He began to pile up grants and to publish prolifically, amassing nearly two hundred published papers. His research focused mainly on epilepsy and gangliosides, and he became a leader in the field.

One day a student named Marianna Todorova approached him about attending a meeting sponsored by The Charlie Foundation on the ketogenic diet for epilepsy. He repeated to her what his Yale reviewers had said, that the ketogenic diet was passé, but he approved her participation anyway. He was so impressed with the information she brought back that they studied the ketogenic diet in mice with epilepsy and found that it worked. He and Marianna attended a "think tank" group event on the ketogenic diet for epilepsy with about twenty participants, including Dr. John Freeman and Dr. Jong Rho, leaders in the field. They also published a paper showing that the ketogenic diet lowers glucose and that this could be the mechanism for reducing seizures (Greene, 2001). Dr. Seyfried makes the point that the ketogenic diet may not stop seizures unless the blood sugar is also low.

Seyfried's interest in using caloric restriction with the ketogenic diet for cancer came in a very unexpected way. He and his lab associates met Frances Platt, PhD, who worked on lysosomal storage diseases and had found a drug that inhibits ganglioside synthesis. They were given some of the drug to study and found that it appeared to substantially shrink tumors in mice with brain cancer. The drug company gave them a sizable grant to study this further, and they looked at the drug's effect on two brain cancers: glioblastoma and ependymoblastoma. From their research, they found that the drug did not make it to the brain at all, but worked by blocking digestion of food in the stomach and, in fact, worked by restricting the amount of calories taken in by the mice. This unexpected finding set Seyfried off on a new pathway, studying caloric restriction for cancer and epilepsy. He and his key associate, Dr. Purna Mukherjee (who still works with him), studied many different diets and came to realize that caloric restriction and ketogenic diet work well together by getting ketone levels very high (he recommends aiming for 4 to 6 mmol/L) and by reducing blood glucose levels (ideally under 60 mg/dL) and this strategy is effective in treating both cancer and epilepsy (Meidenbauer, 2015). Their studies to date show that the ketogenic diet and caloric restriction target multiple pathways affecting inflammation and angiogenesis (growth of new blood vessels)—no drug can do this.

Early on, as Dr. Seyfried recognized the shifts that occur in ketones and glucose levels with these diets, he contacted some of the experts in the world of ketones, Richard Veech and George Cahill Jr. Eventually Cahill became a mentor for him of this concept. Seyfried also wondered how this nutritional approach was killing brain cancer cells and came upon a paper written by Linda Nebeling while she was working on her PhD in nursing. She published case reports of two children who had pediatric brain cancer and were very damaged by chemotherapy and radiation. Dr. Nebeling had the idea that the ketogenic diet might target the fermentation metabolism needed to drive cancer cells. In the 1930s, Otto Warburg had found that fermentation could compensate for defective mitochondrial respiration in cancer cells but was largely ignored at that time. Nebeling was given permission to treat children, who had undergone standard of care treatments but were now end-stage, with the ketogenic diet and found that they had regression of their tumors and were behaviorally improved (Nebeling, 1995). Prior to reading this paper, as a geneticist himself, Seyfried had not challenged the gene theory of cancer, but he decided to look closer at this idea. He read everything Warburg had written and soon realized that the effects they were seeing on cancer cells with the diet were operating through Warburg's theory. Seyfried also read the criticisms of

Warburg's theory and why other researchers thought he was wrong, but as he analyzed the critics' reports, he noticed that some of their work actually supported what Warburg had said—the authors hadn't analyzed their own data closely enough to see this for themselves (Otto, 2016).

Seyfried is a geneticist, and geneticists generally believed that cancer is a genetic disease, but he began to think that this idea did not make sense. He explains that most cancer cells are dependent on glucose, and Warburg had found that mitochondria are defective in cancer, and that glucose is fermented instead of going through the process of oxidative phosphorylation. He notes, though, that Warburg never mentioned the idea of using the ketogenic diet or caloric restriction for cancer. Seyfried and his associates studied the entire genome of mouse mitochondrial DNA in cancer cells, and they did not find a single mutation that was responsible for the cancer. They found that cancer occurs only if a genetic mutation disrupts the process of oxidative phosphorylation in the mitochondria. They have also found that ketogenic diet and caloric restriction will kill many different kinds of cancer cells, which puts the entire genetic mutation theory of cancer into question. For decades now, cancer research has been on the wrong track.

Somewhere along the way, one of Seyfried's students suggested that they check lipid levels, and they were shocked by the results. They found all kinds of abnormalities in lipids that were related to defects in oxidative phosphorylation in the mitochondria in tumors, specifically in cardiolipin, the signature lipid of mitochondrial that controls respiration. They started looking closely at the structure and function of mitochondria in cancer cells and confirmed that they were using glucose through a fermentation process. He firmly believes that the genetic mutations in cancer are not the cause of the cancer but rather a downstream effect of the production of reactive oxygen species (ROS) in mitochondria.

One if his own papers that caught attention reports the case of a sixty-five-year-old woman with a large glioblastoma tumor in her brain. She had undergone surgery to remove as much as possible of the tumor, but that did not eradicate the growth, and scans showed considerable edema (swelling) around the remaining areas of cancer. Shortly after the surgery, the woman started a water fast and then adhered to a strict 4:1 ketogenic diet (four grams of fat for every one gram of protein and glucose combined) with caloric restriction at 600 calories per day, while receiving standard of care treatment with chemotherapy and radiation. Two months later, the tumor and the edema associated with the cancer were undetectable by both MRI and PET scanning (Zuccoli, 2010). Unfortunately, she eventually resumed her typical diet, the tumor re-appeared ten weeks later, and she lost her life to the cancer.

As Seyfried came to understand that cancer is a metabolic not a genetic disease and began publishing his results, he realized that he was going down a dark pathway that could jeopardize his career. Because he was challenging the prevailing belief that cancer is a genetic disease, he was taking on not only the leaders in the cancer field but also the entire cancer industry—an industry that is based on treatment with lucrative drugs and radiation. After all, the cost of ketogenic diet and caloric restriction pales by comparison to the cost of the standard of care treatments for cancer; how could the cancer industry profit from that? At this point, he was a tenured professor at Boston College and was starting to lose his NIH grants. He had also found other independent studies supporting Warburg's theory that confirmed his own findings. He decided to write and publish his landmark book *Cancer as a Metabolic Disease: On the Origin, Management, and Prevention of Cancer* (2012, John Wiley and Sons, Inc., Hoboken, NY).

Seyfried gets very upset and animated when he talks about the multi-million dollar cancer industry that is based on treatment of genetic mutations and the toll this idea has taken on so many lives. He points out that every cell in a cancerous tumor has a different gene mutation and that the death rates from cancer have not gone down; to the contrary, cancer rates are increasing every year, now at more than 1,600 deaths per day in the United States and 9,000 deaths per day in China. Many physicians now agree that Dr. Seyfried is right, but they are locked into the standard of care treatments and are worried about liability should they deviate from the accepted norms.

By now, many people with all kinds of cancers have reported anecdotally that they are doing well and feel better in general using this nutritional approach, some with and some without standard of care treatments. As of early 2018, several formal clinical trials of the ketogenic caloric restricted diet as an adjunct to the standard of care are in progress or will begin soon in the United States.

Dr. Seyfried has reached outside of his own lab to collaborate with others, including Dr. Dominic D'Agostino and Dr. Angela Poff at University of South Florida, who are looking at various combinations of diet with exogenous ketones and hyperbaric oxygen, and Dr. Adrienne Scheck, who has studied the use of this nutritional approach to treating cancers in lab animals as an adjunct to standard of care treatments, such as radiation (Lussier, 2016). Seyfried and some of his collaborators have outlined and published a "press-pulse" strategy that will use the ketogenic/caloric restriction approach as a foundation while pulsing in the standard of care treatments. They hope that this will spur on clinical studies looking at this idea (Seyfried, 2017).

Seyfried's work has caught the attention of researchers in other parts of the world as well. A group of physicians in Hungary were some of the first to study his work and are getting "significant results" with a Paleo-Keto diet for cancer. Researchers in Germany now call this approach ketogenic metabolic "therapy" instead of a "diet," and they have found that it can be used to treat many different types of diseases, not just cancer and epilepsy. The ketogenic diet works wherever there is a disturbance of energy homeostasis and fasting as well as ketogenic diet can bring us back to a state of normal energy homeostasis. In China they are combining this approach with traditional Chinese medicine, and Shanghai-born Dr. George Yu, whose practice is located in Maryland, is a prime example of a physician who is embracing these concepts to treat his cancer patients with considerable success. (See Dr. Yu's story later in this chapter.)

Another point Seyfried likes to make is that Alzheimer's and cancer are opposites and yet both could respond to the ketogenic diet. Sugar feeds cancer cells, but most cancer cells cannot use ketones as fuel, so the ketogenic diet reduces blood sugar, depriving the cancer cell of fuel, while providing fuel to normal cells that can use ketones. In Alzheimer's there is the opposite problem of getting glucose as a fuel into brain cells and ketones can provide alternative fuel for the brain, effectively bypassing the problem of glucose uptake.

When asked how Boston College has reacted to him taking on and turning the cancer industry upside down, he laughs and says that they have no medical school there with physicians to challenge him on this and seem oblivious to what he is doing. He is a passionate messenger for cancer as a metabolic disease and how the ketogenic diet and caloric restriction could potentially benefit many millions of people suffering from all types of cancers. He no longer worries about the potential consequences to himself in taking punches at the hard wall that is the cancer industry. Dr. Thomas Seyfried is a survivor and his life has taken him on an incredible and important journey from fighting a war in the jungles of Vietnam to battling the war on cancer and the academic and pharmaceutical industries that profit from this disease (Seyfried, 2018).

ANGELA POFF, PHD: RISING STAR OF KETONE RESEARCH FOR CANCER

Angela Poff, born in 1988, grew up in Greenwood, Arkansas. She loved science at an early age and never really considered anything else for a career. She always wanted to do research and hoped she would discover something new. She completed her undergraduate degree in biochemistry and molecular biology at Hendrix College in Conway, Arkansas, a small liberal arts college that focuses on experiential learning. Her program included three years of research under

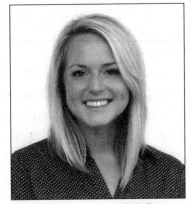

Photo 5.11. Angela Poff, PhD.

Rick Murray in developmental neuroscience, studying gene expression in dorsal root ganglia in mice. Poff was accepted to the PhD program at University of South Florida in Tampa. This is where her earlier life experience shaped what happened next. Long before she was born, her father, at only eight years of age, was diagnosed with brain tumors which were treated with radiation. The tumors returned when he was in his early thirties just a year before Angela was born and he was successfully treated again. The treatments saved his life however her father suffered a constant, progressive cognitive and physical decline from that point on. Her first step was to find a research lab to work in. She listened to presentations by various potential mentors, and the one given by Dr. Dominic D'Agostino struck a chord. He talked about the work he was doing on seizures and neuroscience, and he mentioned an idea for a side project: studying ketogenic diet and hyperbaric oxygen therapy for cancer, focusing specifically on brain cancer. Poff was intrigued by this idea, especially given her father's history.

There was no cancer research in progress at Dr. D'Agostino's lab when Angela joined, so she was involved in setting up the lab for this type of research. She worked with collaborators like Thomas Seyfried, using a metastatic model of glioblastoma in mice. Many cancers, including this particularly aggressive brain cancer, thrive on sugar, but seem to be less capable of utilizing ketones for fuel, and some tumors may even be directly damaged by ketones. They explored various ideas, such as using diabetes drugs to lower blood sugar levels, but honed in on the ketogenic diet, exogenous ketone supplements, such as butanediol and a ketone ester, specifically acetoacetate diester, and hyperbaric oxygen, alone and in various combinations. The results have been striking. They learned that exogenous ketone supplements and ketogenic diet are equally effective in shrinking and slowing tumor growth in this animal model. They also learned that there is synergy between hyperbaric oxygen and elevated ketone levels, meaning that the two strategies together are better than simply adding the effects of each strategy together. In other words, when there is synergy, one plus one is greater than two (Poff, 2014; Poff, 2016).

Poff received her PhD in 2014, completed her postdoctoral work, and continues to work alongside Dr. D'Agostino and others as a senior research associate in this very busy research lab, where numerous projects are underway to study the effects of ketogenic therapies on many different conditions. One major project is studying the idea of using "press-pulse therapy" for cancer, for example providing ketogenic diet continuously and then pulsing in treatments with hyperbaric oxygen, exogenous ketone supplements, chemotherapy and other treatments, to learn if this approach might be more effective (Seyfried, 2017). A colleague, Andrew Koutnik, is studying whether acetoacetate diester can reverse cachexia, a condition in people with cancer that involves rapid weight and muscle loss. Acetoacetate can stimulate production of muscle through a signaling mechanism of ketones and might even help people with cancer not only preserve muscle but also build new muscle. They also hope to do a clinical trial of ketogenic diet for people with low-grade glioma.

Angela Poff's father passed away after suffering a massive stroke in 2012, when she was just twenty-four and in the midst of her PhD program.

She hopes what she learns in the lab will help others so that they do not have to go through what her father and family endured.

Poff often receives communications from people seeking help with the ketogenic strategies for cancer. As a PhD and not an MD, she cannot give medical advice. She emphasizes that people should work with their personal physicians if they wish to try this type of approach and consider participating in clinical trials of ketogenic diet in conjunction with the standard treatments, which are popping up at various locations. She says it is also important to work with a nutritionist or dietitian who is trained to counsel on the ketogenic diet. By the time this book is published, clinical trials looking at the use of exogenous ketone supplements for cancer may conceivably be underway. A complete listing of clinical trials in the United States is available at www.clinicaltrials.gov (Poff, 2018).

MIRIAM KALAMIAN, EDM, MS, CNS: TURNING PERSONAL LOSS INTO ADVOCACY FOR OTHERS

Miriam Kalamian and her husband, Peter Walsh, lost their young son to brain cancer—something no parent should ever have to go through. While her son was ill, Kalamian went beyond the advice given to her by his medical providers and found a reprieve for him through implementing the ketogenic diet. She now uses the education she received in the process to help others deal with cancer and other disorders.

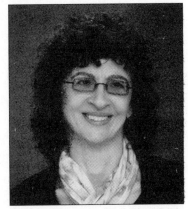

Photo 5.12. Miriam Kalamian, EdM, MS, CNS.

Miriam Kalamian was born in 1953 and grew up in an extended Armenian family in Connecticut. She excelled in science and thought she would like to be a doctor; however, like many young women of her generation, she was told by family and her school counselor that she would have to forego getting married and having children if she pursued medicine. During her sophomore year in high school, she won a science award with a prize that included a trip; however, the counselor told her she "was getting carried away with this" and took the award away, giving it to a boy in her class who also wanted to go to medical school. It was a very disappointing and unfair moment for Kalamian. Heeding the advice of her family and counselor, she took an alternative path, pursuing a master's degree in education and child studies from Smith College, where she taught for four years. After a change in administration at Smith, she returned in the mid 1980s to the family business of selling rugs and carpeting. She and her husband moved to beautiful Montana to enjoy the great outdoors in the mid-1990s and opened a similar business there.

The couple adopted their son, Raffi, from Armenia when he was two years old. He had rickets and other signs of malnutrition and a birth defect called Poland Syndrome, caused by restricted circulation through the large subclavian artery that feeds the arm; in Raffi's case, this resulted in smaller than normal right arm, hand and digits, as well as syndactyly (fusion of digits). When he was four years old, Raffi failed a vision screening, but an eye doctor falsely reassured the family that Raffi's vision was normal. The problem persisted, and eight months passed before an ophthalmologist found optic pallor (paleness of the optic nerve), which he attributed to Raffi's early poor nutrition. When the child experienced severe headaches for three days in a row, his pediatrician recommended an MRI, reassuring them that he thought a tumor was "highly unlikely." The next day the pediatrician gave Kalamian and Walsh the tragic news that Raffi did, in fact, have a brain tumor and they needed to get him to the hospital right away. The local airport was socked in due to bad weather, so they drove more than 800 miles through a blizzard to Denver Children's Hospital. At the tender age of four, Raffi was diagnosed with a juvenile pilocytic astrocytoma that was the size of an orange. The tumor had already infiltrated the surrounding tissue so extensively that it could not be removed surgically, which was devastating news to his parents. He received weekly chemotherapy treatments but developed a sensitivity to one of the drugs; before each infusion, he required administration of the very potent steroid dexamethasone, which raised his blood sugar. To make matters worse, the tumor destroyed his hypothalamus, which affected many hormones, including those related to appetite and to controlling deposition of fat. The boy gained an excessive amount of weight in a short period of time.

About two and one-half years after Raffi's diagnosis, Kalamian came across information about the ketogenic diet for cancer. She learned that most cancers thrive on sugar but cannot use ketones for fuel, and she started Raffi on the classic ketogenic diet after learning that it had been used for nearly a century for childhood epilepsy. She received support from The Charlie Foundation (see Resources), especially from other mothers and from nutritionist Beth Zupec-Kania, who has worked assiduously to establish centers for the ketogenic diet throughout the world. Zupec-Kania suggested that Kalamian give Raffi four tablespoons per day of MCT oil to help keep him in ketosis, which he tolerated very well. The couple baked keto treats with coconut oil, which is rich in MCTs. In just three months of a rigorous ketogenic diet, from April to June 2007, Raffi's tumor shrunk substantially, by 10 to 15 percent in all dimensions on a series of MRIs. His oncologist believed that the ketogenic was the only explanation for this change. He lived for six more years with the ketogenic diet as his only treatment that entire time.

After witnessing the impact of the ketogenic diet on her son's tumor, Kalamian enrolled in a master's program in nutrition at Eastern Michigan University. While taking classes, she put a "ketogenic spin" on everything she studied. She met with some resistance from professors early on but found more support from senior professors during her final year in the program. She presented a poster at the Obesity Society annual meeting in 2009, where some top-notch doctors were interested in her experience with her son. She graduated with a 4.0 GPA in 2010, completed an internship with a family health non-profit center, and passed the exam to become a certified nutrition specialist (CNS) through the Board for Certification of Nutrition Specialists, after which she started her own business.

As a certified nutrition specialist, Miriam Kalamian provides one-on-one support to people with cancer and other conditions, using mainly the classic ketogenic diet. She believes that people with Parkinson's and Alzheimer's may find more success with a less-restrictive low-carb diet that involves less calculation, weighing, and measuring. Also, some people with cancer who experience weight loss do not digest or absorb nutrients well. She may recommend, instead of the classic ketogenic diet, that they eliminate grains and added sugar, and that they practice intermittent fasting of fourteen to sixteen hours. She may also suggest that they fast before and during chemotherapy to lower blood sugar and raise ketones, potentially maximizing the effects of the treatment. Many people report that this type of fast reduces the side effects of the chemotherapy.

Kalamian's son, Raffi, lived well beyond the predictions but eventually succumbed to the tumor at age thirteen in 2013. Not long after his death, she wrote an e-book, which was published on her website in December 2013. Her practice took off after she made a presentation at the First Metabolic Therapeutics Nutritional Ketosis Conference at University of South Florida in 2016. Her updated and very comprehensive book, *Keto for Cancer,* was published in 2017 and weaves Raffi's story with information about the ketogenic diet for cancer as well as the practical nuts and bolts of adopting the ketogenic diet. She recognizes that it is hard to prove the effect of the diet on the cancer when people are also using standard treatments, however, she believes the diet often extends life. Miriam Kalamian's loss of Raffi to cancer has taken her on a path of advocacy for others. See Resources for information about her website and social media (Kalamian, 2017).

GEORGE YU, MD: WALKING THE WALK TO HELP PATIENTS

George Yu was born in Shanghai, China, in 1947. His parents, who were capitalists involved in several industries, moved out of revolutionary China, and the family lived all over the world while establishing international bases for their various businesses in South East Asia, Europe, and Latin America. George believes this mixed cultural background made him more receptive to new concepts and creative methods and more able to accept diverse ways of achieving goals.

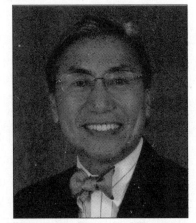

Photo 5.13. George Yu, MD.

Yu went to medical school at Tufts University in Boston, Massachusetts, and then completed a medical internship at University of Pennsylvania Medical Center and a general surgical residency at Harvard Peter Bent

Brigham Hospital. While there, he developed an acute bleeding duodenal ulcer from the stressful and busy work and was told he must have surgery immediately. A friend from Australia advised him to try Flagyl, tetracycline and Pepto-Bismol instead, a nontraditional approach. He took the uncharted therapy and was cured without surgery; his personal experience made him suspect that not all accepted therapy was correct.

His mentor at Harvard was chief of surgery Dr. Francis Daniels Moore, who was considered the world's expert on metabolism and hormonal changes after surgery and trauma. He was the first to perform a kidney transplant. Moore made a lasting impression on Yu's later career and influenced his focus. With Dr. Moore's blessing, Yu chose the unconventional career route of becoming a missionary surgeon in the Republic of the Cameroons, and later in Malawi, Kenya, South Africa, Mexico and Honduras. He gained valuable surgical experience at an early age under the guidance of some of the great Scottish surgeons, but even more importantly, he gained a much broader perspective of medicine and why certain people develop diseases.

Yu's training at Penn brought him into contact with Dr. Jonathan Rhodes, the father of hyperalimentation, who kept a dog alive for a year without using gastrointestinal bowel function. This inspired Yu to take a deeper look at providing nutrition using both gastrostomy (PEG today) and intravenous approaches, learning the pitfalls of each and the need for the proper selection of nutrition to achieve success. At Johns Hopkins, he witnessed how some symptoms of hormonal changes, such as fatigue, muscle wasting, and "hot flashes" that followed castration (as part of a treatment for metastatic prostate cancer) were similar to those experienced by menopausal women. Such changes were often associated with insulin resistance at six months post-operation, and with clinical diabetes at the one-year mark. He realized that a metabolic defect was at play. From animal research, it was discovered that, without testosterone, intracellular mitochondria become dysfunctional and swell up with vacuoles and this defect reverts to normal when you replace the testosterone hormone again.

While doing a urological reconstruction residency at Johns Hopkins, Yu met Dr. John Freeman, who was well known for his use of the ketogenic diet for drug-resistant epilepsy in children. Yu learned much more about the use of therapeutic fats from another teacher, Dr. Mary Enig, a lipid biochemist at University of Maryland, who sounded the alert that trans fats are harmful and that saturated fats, like those found in coconut oil, are not. She and Michael DeBakey, the father of coronary bypass surgery, both believed adamantly that cholesterol is an important molecule for whole-body function, especially the brain, and is not the cause of coronary vessel heart disease.

In the 1990s, Yu was assigned by George Washington University medical faculty and the National Cancer Institute to audit the Kushi Institute of Macrobiotic Diet. The macrobiotic diet was introduced to the United States in the 1950s by Michio Kushi, an immigrant from Japan. Yu reviewed about three hundred charts and noticed that on a calorie-restricted nutritional Japanese diet, when a patient's weight dropped by 10 percent, the cancer, by radiological examination, shrank at three to six months on the diet. He also noticed that the blood sugar dropped, fatty acids and betahydroxy-butyrate increased, and that there was "Visceral Defatting" (a decrease in fat around the internal organs). After seeing dramatic results of terminal cancer tumor shrinkage, he began in the early 2000s to apply intermittent calorie-restriction as a strategy in his own practice. Other mentors from his previous training at Johns Hopkins Medical Institute were Drs. Pete Pederson and Albert Lehninger, experts in biochemistry. Pederson noticed that, as a normal cell changes to a cancer cell, the metabolic functions of mitochondria deteriorate. Combining what he learned from the Kushi Institute audit with the science of cancer mitochondrial dysfunction, Yu gained even more appreciation for the importance of nutrition in clinical medicine.

For thirty-five years Yu performed pelvic and urologic reconstructive cancer surgeries, often removing part of the colon, uterus, bladder, and prostate and then reconstructing the area. He also performed adrenal, kidney, bladder and ureter surgeries. He developed a strong interest in the role of metabolism and sex hormones in disease, incorporating these concepts into his practice, and he considers himself to be a surgeon with a special focus on metabolic and endocrine factors in cancer development and treatments.

Yu has moved away from surgical treatments and now focuses his time on cancer management, including metabolic and sex hormone interventions. He takes a multi-pronged approach to tackling diseases and fine-tunes that approach to the individual. He says, "You have to use more than one tool to make a chair. A uniform theory rarely works as a solution to a clinical problem." His protocol for cancer combines modern-day medical and surgical standard of care treatments with balancing sex hormones and changing the patient's nutritional metabolism from carbohydrate to ketone metabolism, providing dense nutrition with the least calories. He uses intermittent caloric restriction with ketogenic additions, since long-term caloric restriction will affect thyroid hormones and result in sex hormone dysfunctions; testosterone levels decline, and women will lack proper sex hormone functions with arrest of menstruation depending on individual makeup. He has learned that a 10 percent weight loss is not alarming for someone with cancer. Short-term caloric-restriction, intermittent fasting, and even overnight fasting have very beneficial effects. Stephen Spindler reported on 2005 that short-term caloric-restriction can mimic the beneficial effects of long-term caloric-restriction even when used for periods as short as two weeks (Spindler, 2005). Yu also incorporates exogenous ketone supplements into the plan for certain people. He, Pedersen and Dr. Young Ko all believe that, as a cancer matures and grows, it can develop the ability to use other energy sources for further growth and metastasis besides sugar and glutamine, including other amino acids and ketones. So, a calorie-restricted ketogenic diet may not be the answer in some of these cases, as we understand more about cancer biology.

For some people, getting adequate nutrition is a serious problem, and Yu will often place a PEG (percutaneous endoscopic gastrostomy) flexible feeding tube into the stomach through the abdominal wall. This device allows people to receive nutrition using a pump that feeds ketogenic, blended foods and unpalatable supplements such as ketone esters, through a tube into the stomach.

Dr. Yu's experienced opinion is that chemotherapy, radiation, and surgery are important therapeutic tools in the treatment, but we must address the metabolic features of cancer as an adjunctive treatment. Cancer requires a cocktail—a multi-pronged approach—and the metabolic components of this protocol need to be introduced as soon as possible after the cancer is diagnosed. Dr. Yu receives emails with questions about his protocols for treating cancer from all over the world.

In November 2017, the Yu Foundation (at YuFoundation.org) organized the Tripping over the Truth Conference (TOTT), which took place in Baltimore, Maryland. The goal of the conference was to bring together leaders from the arenas of basic science and clinical science to share their work and ideas to arrive at integrated solutions to treat cancer and other medical problems. Along with forty professional researchers in basic science, cancer, and Alzheimer's disease, four famous chefs, as well as nutritionists, were brought into the conference to teach people ways to make ketogenic and calorie-restricted diets more enjoyable. More than one hundred hours of filming will be available from this conference to distribute worldwide to increase awareness of these ideas.

Dr. George Yu believes in the ancient Chinese saying that "disease starts from the mouth down." He also believes that as, a physician, you need to "walk the walk" and adopt a healthy diet and lifestyle, not only for one's own personal well-being but also to provide a good example for patients. Too many researchers don't practice what they preach, which Yu believes "totally dilutes the effectiveness of their work" (Yu, 2018).

JACOB WILSON, PHD, AND RYAN LOWERY, PHD: PERFORMANCE AND KETOSIS

Jacob Wilson, PhD and Ryan Lowery, PhD work together as a consummate team at the Applied Science and Performance Institute (ASPI), the company they cofounded in Tampa, Florida. When it comes to the world of ketones, it is hard to talk about one without talking about the other.

Jacob Wilson was born in 1983 and grew up in California. He says his family "didn't have much," but his father encouraged him to excel in school. Wilson, who had a lab coat at age five, knew that he wanted to be a

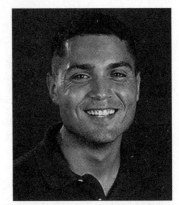

Photo 5.14. Jacob Wilson, PhD.

scientist. He and his father often performed movement experiments to see if they could improve physical performance. The younger Wilson was also into sports, including boxing, kickboxing and hockey, and was interested in improving his own cognitive and physical performance. He realized his dream to play semi-professional hockey in Canada.

Jacob Wilson's choice of majors was shaped by his desire to help his parents live "forever." He majored in nutrition as an undergraduate at California State University East Bay and then completed double master's degrees in sports psychology and exercise physiology, focusing on the skeleton and muscle. He completed his PhD at Florida State University; his dissertation was entitled, "The Effects of betahydroxybutyrate on the Cellular and Molecular Components of Muscle Across the Lifespan."

Ryan Lowery, born in 1992, grew up playing baseball, basketball, and football in New Jersey. He attended University of Tampa and played on the baseball team; they won the national championship during his junior year. His very first class was in nutrition with teacher Jacob Wilson, and they soon learned that they had a mutual interest in baseball performance research. Wilson asked Lowery to participate in a baseball velocity study and then suggested that Lowery change his major to human performance and exercise physiology. They soon became best friends and colleagues in research.

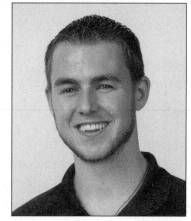

Photo 5.15. Ryan Lowery, PhD.

Together they designed a new master's program at University of Tampa in exercise and nutrition science, and Lowery was the first person ever to receive the degree.

Wilson's interest in ketones began around 2008, while he was working on his doctoral studies. While attending an Experimental Biology conference, he met Dominic D'Agostino, who had just arrived at nearby University of South Florida. They had a conversation about the ketogenic diet. Wilson had discovered through his own research that betahydroxybutyrate (HMB) prevents muscle loss inrats but learned from D'Agostino that HMB is converted to the ketone betahydroxybutyrate.

Wilson and Lowery were both aware of the use of the ketogenic diet in the world of bodybuilding, and its potential to change body composition. They attended a conference where Jeff Volek, PhD and Stephen Phinney, MD, PhD, who have published more than two hundred studies of many different aspects of low-carb high-fat diets, gave presentations on ketogenic diet and its effects on performance and strength. Volek and Phinney had not yet completed studies of ketogenic diet and resistance training, so, in 2012, Wilson and Lowery set out on their own research to learn whether a person can effectively adapt to the ketogenic diet, compared to a higher carb diet, while maintaining strength, muscle mass, and anaerobic function. They learned that the answer is "Yes" and also learned that the ketogenic diet can have favorable effects on fat mass as well. They found that people can adapt more quickly to the diet if they maintain consistent resistance training. At the molecular level, resistance training can stimulate protein synthesis to make new muscle, so that a person does not need to eat carbohydrates to make glucose in order to store glycogen in the muscles. They have also learned that keeping ketone levels elevated spares muscle when a person is losing weight.

In 2014, they were introduced by their friend Dr. Angela Poff to Brian Underwood who was putting together a company, now called Pruvit Ventures, to market ketone salts that were being developed and tested in D'Agostino's lab. Brian asked Wilson and Lowery to lead the educational piece. Not long after, they left University of Tampa to launch the Applied Science and Performance Institute (ASPI) in a beautiful location overlooking Tampa Bay.

The ASPI studies the impact of the ketogenic diet and exogenous ketones on health and performance (Wilson, 2017) and helps develop various formulations of ketone salts. They have learned that rats live longer either feeding on the ketogenic diet or taking these exogenous ketone supplements as opposed to eating a high-carbohydrate diet. They have also learned that increasing ketosis improves markers of inflammation (Kephart, 2017).

The ASPI was founded with the purpose of conducting research that would have an immediate impact on people's lives. The ASPI's facilities maintain a broad inventory of equipment designed to study many different aspects of human physical and cognitive performance as well as body composition. Every aspect of hitting a golf ball or baseball can be recorded digitally and analyzed in rooms equipped with virtual screens. An avatar of a client can be created to evaluate movement. The neurophysiology room has numerous pieces of aerobic equipment, including the mother of all treadmills, which can visually and digitally record every aspect of a person's gait. They can study and document effects of injury and recovery from injury. Staff includes experts in molecular biology, neurophysiology, sports physiology, biomechanics, food science, statistical analyses, and nutritional and supplemental therapeutics.

Institute clients range from everyday athletes trying to maximize their efforts to elite professional athletes, including thirty Major League Baseball players and forty top football players, pro hockey players and other athletes, many of them dealing with injuries. Many of these athletes try ketone salts to help with the healing process, especially when inflammation is involved. The ASPI also helps people with medical conditions such as Crohn's disease, Parkinson's, ALS, and traumatic brain injury. Concussions are a big focus for the research done here, since many athletes who have suffered concussions develop dementia while they are still in their forties. Many of them already have signs of Alzheimer's and Parkinson's disease, and they want their lives back.

Doctors Wilson and Lowery have found that the best strategy to bring about improvement for whatever the client is seeking is to combine the ketogenic diet with exogenous ketone supplements. Through the institute, Wilson and Lowery have many younger athletes working with them to improve their body composition, and the research and practice have shown that using this combined approach, athletes can gain muscle mass and lose body fat without starving. The institute's team looks forward to the day that, whenever a child or adult is involved in a sport where they could sustain a head injury, exogenous ketone supplements are available on the sidelines. They believe that everyone over thirty should take a ketone supplement to slow down the aging process.

Wilson and Lowery co-authored *The Ketogenic Bible: The Authoritative Guide to Ketosis* (2017) and set up a website, Ketogenic.com (https://ketogenic.com), which includes a plethora of creative recipes. They want to help change the reputation of the ketogenic diet as "unpalatable."

Lowery has realized his childhood dream to help his mother with her Crohn's disease—she has experienced a complete transformation while eating a lower-carb diet and taking ketone salts. His father, who dedicated his life first to the military and then to police work, has also changed to a low-carb diet and increased his exercise. Lowery says it seems as if his parents are in their thirties again. Wilson's parents, and even the family dog, are enjoying the benefits of the ketogenic diet.

(From interview with Drs. Jacob Wilson and Ryan Lowery on Dec 13, 2017.)

CHAPTER 6

THE FULL SPECTRUM OF KETOGENIC DIETS

"Humans live on one-quarter of what they eat; on
the other three-quarters lives their doctors."
—Translation of inscription on Egyptian
pyramid from around 3800 B.C.

A ketogenic diet could be defined as any diet that increases ketone levels, a state called "ketosis." It is a common misconception that a ketogenic diet mainly means eating a low-carbohydrate diet; another crucial component is eating more fat. It is possible to get into ketosis and lose weight, for example, without increasing dietary fat by eating low-carb and adequate amounts of protein while reducing calories, but without enough fat in the diet, the body will have a much greater tendency to burn muscle to provide basic energy needs, and this can result in losing critical muscle mass.

Beginning in middle age, we tend to lose a little muscle each year, and we don't want to speed that up, since muscle mass has everything to do with strength and our ability to carry out everyday functions. Also, the less muscle mass you have, the fewer calories you burn in a day. So, if you lose weight and muscle along with it, you will need to eat less to keep from regaining the weight. This probably explains the yo-yo effect that many of us experience—we lose weight and then regain the weight and end up at a higher weight than where we started out. For many people this happens over and over, and they end up bigger and bigger. The problem is that individuals are used to eating a certain number of calories, but they need fewer calories because they have less muscle—as a natural result of aging, as a result of dieting patterns that cause muscle loss, or both—making it very difficult to maintain the weight loss. Healthy dietary fats can be our friend on a low-carb ketogenic diet by increasing our body's tendency to use fat for fuel rather than muscle.

Another crucial factor is that, when you are using diet alone (i.e., with no ketone supplements) to get into and stay in ketosis, you will be most successful if you maintain a ketogenic ratio of fat to protein plus carbs for *each* meal and snack. This is probably the hardest part of the ketogenic diet for most people. If you decide to have some of your daily allotment of carbs as a snack, like an apple, without eating fat at the same time, it could reduce your level of ketosis or even knock you completely out of ketosis.

To recap, at least three important factors will determine whether your diet results in ketosis:

- the combined number of grams of carbs and protein you eat per day.
- how much fat you eat (and what type of fat).
- the combination of fat and protein plus carbs you eat at each meal and snack.

THE SPECTRUM OF KETOSIS

There is a wide spectrum of ketosis, from mild to moderate to "deep" ketosis, depending on the level of ketones in the bloodstream (Figure 6.1). Someone in deep ketosis could have blood levels ten times higher than someone in mild ketosis. Where you choose to fall in that spectrum will depend on what your goals are as well as your age and health status. For example, a middle-aged person who wants to prevent later memory impairment, or an elderly person who already has memory impairment, might aim for mild ketosis with levels of 0.5 to 1 mmol/L through eating a low-carb diet, supported with coconut oil and/or MCT oil at each meal. A young, healthy adult looking for more energy, better sleep, improved mental focus, and perhaps some fat loss might aim for ketone levels in the 1 to 3 mmol/l range. A person with a serious medical condition, such as epilepsy or cancer might want to reach levels of 4 to 6 mmol/l. An elite athlete might wish to achieve ketone levels in the "optimal" range as a baseline and use an exogenous ketone supplement before a workout or competitive event to push ketone levels higher for an extra burst of energy.

Two people can eat the same combinations and amounts of foods and yet have different responses in their ketone levels, so it is often a matter of experimentation to find out what works best for you. In this chapter, we will begin with a review of the four standard ketogenic diets that have been used to treat people with epilepsy for many years but now are proving to be useful for people with other conditions as well. For example, the classic ketogenic diet is now used by many as an adjunct to standard treatments or when standard treatments are no longer work-

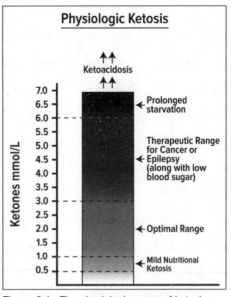

Figure 6.1. The physiologic range of ketosis begins at about 0.5 mmol/L. Above 7 mmol/L ketoacidosis requiring medical intervention could occur. [Graphic design by Joanna Newport.]

ing for people with cancer. The low glycemic index diet and the modified Atkins diet could be very helpful to people with diabetes to control their blood sugar and reduce or even wean off some of their medications. The MCT oil diet could be beneficial to someone with a progressive neurologic condition, such as Alzheimer's or Parkinson's disease, multiple sclerosis, or amyotrophic lateral sclerosis (ALS or Lou Gehrig's disease). It is very important to consult with your physician before embarking on a radical new diet, such as a ketogenic diet.

FOUR STANDARD KETOGENIC DIETS FOR EPILEPSY

There are four standard ketogenic diets used currently for patients with epilepsy that result in ketone levels in the moderate to high range. The Charlie Foundation has a very helpful diagram on their website (https://charliefoundation.org/) showing the relative percentages of fat, carbohydrates and protein in each of the four standard diets (see Figure 6.2).

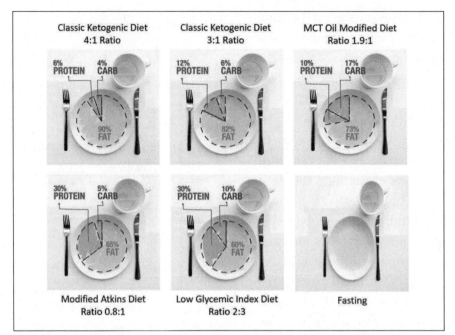

Figure 6.2. Comparison of ratios of the macronutrients fat, protein, and carbohydrates for the classic ketogenic diet, the modified ketogenic diet, the MCT ketogenic diet, the modified Atkins diet, and the low glycemic index diet, as well as intermittent fasting. * 50 percent MCT / 21 percent LCT; MCT stands for medium-chain triglycerides, LCT stands for long chain triglycerides. With permission from The Charlie Foundation: https://charliefoundation.org/diet-plans.

The Classic Ketogenic Diet

For decades, the classic ketogenic diet was used mainly in the treatment of epilepsy, but more recently it has been adopted for use by people with cancer, children with autism (especially when seizures are involved), and people with rare enzyme defects that affect their ability to use glucose as a fuel, such as GLUT 1 deficiency syndrome, which affects the ability of glucose to enter the brain. It is extremely important to work with a nutritionist who is educated and experienced in the use of the classic ketogenic diet due to the complex nature of the calculations involved for an individual to get each meal and snack right and avoid the potential immediate and long-term problems that can occur with the diet.

In the classic ketogenic diet, 80 to 90 percent of calories come from fat, and the other 10 to 20 percent come from protein and carbohydrate combined. Protein is limited because it can be converted in the liver to carbohydrate, generating about one-half gram of glucose for each gram of protein eaten when carbohydrate stores have been used up, through gluconeogenesis. At the same time, it is necessary to provide enough protein to prevent the breakdown of muscle and other tissues in the body, the so-called lean body mass. For children with seizures on a ketogenic diet, protein is strictly calculated to allow for preservation of muscle and for adequate growth.

One way of looking at the classic ketogenic diet is to consider the "macronutrient ratio." The strictest form of the diet is a 4:1 ratio of the number of grams of fat to the combination of protein and carbohydrate grams. Fat has roughly 9 calories per gram, and protein and glucose each contain about 4 calories per gram, so this works out to a diet that is about 90 percent of total calories as fat. The slightly less strict 3:1 ratio works out to 87 percent of total calories as fat and the 2:1 ratio is about 82 percent fat. It is very important to get enough protein from the diet and this does not leave much wiggle room for carbohydrates.

For most conditions treated with this diet, the goal is to push the ketone levels to at least 3 mmol/L or even higher depending on the condition and the individual's response to the diet. Dr. Thomas Seyfried, a geneticist who has studied the ketogenic diet for both epilepsy and cancer, believes that levels of 4 to 6 mmol/L are required for people with cancer and that it also is crucial for these patients to simultaneously reduce blood glucose level to about 60 mg/dL or less. The expectation is that the elevated ketone levels will provide fuel to the brain and other organs and prevent the symptoms that would often occur when the blood glucose is this low. It is very important to work with your doctor when aiming for low blood sugars in this range and for this reason. (See Dr. Thomas Seyfried's story in Chapter 5.)

For success with the classic ketogenic diet, the total number of calories needed per day must be carefully calculated to allow for adequate growth in the infant and child or maintenance of weight in an adult, and these figures can vary significantly depending on age, weight, and level of activity. The amount of protein needed is based on age and body weight and considers the need for growth in the infant and child. For example, in a young infant, 1.52 grams of protein per kilogram of body weight is needed per day; for a ten-year-old this drops to 0.95 grams per kilogram of body weight; for an adult a minimum of 0.8 grams per kilogram of body weight may be required to maintain muscle mass. The diet needs to include adequate vitamins and minerals and the amount of sugar and other nutrients in medications and supplements need to be factored in as well. On top of that, many foods contain a combination of fat, protein, and carbohydrates and this needs to be accounted for when planning every meal and snack to maintain the desired ratio. This involves carefully weighing and measuring foods. It cannot be stated often enough that this is all so complex that it is well worth undertaking this strict diet with the help of a nutritionist who is educated and experienced in using the diet.

For young infants who are not yet eating solid foods, ketogenic formulas have been developed—a godsend for families dealing with seizures. For everyone else, arriving at a basic set of recipes will make the diet easier to maintain overall, but one of the big challenges is to avoid the monotony of eating the same meals and snacks day in and day out. Fortunately, a number of companies have developed ketogenic drinks, meals, flours, and other products and recipes to go along with their products that can make life easier (See the Resources section in the back of this book). The package label usually indicates the macronutrient ratio in the product. Recipes have been developed and shared by The Charlie Foundation and Matthew's Friends, as well as by websites dedicated to the ketogenic diet, such as https://ketogenic.com, with a macronutrient breakdown for each recipe.

Another very helpful tool for planning meals, the Ketodietcalculator, was developed by Beth Zupec-Kania, a consultant for The Charlie Foundation (ketodietcalculator.org). This tool is used by thousands of people around the world with an ever-growing database. Nutritionists can use the tool to calculate the energy requirements and macronutrient ratios needed by their clients and plan meals; the nutritionist can allow the client to access the database as well to plan meals for themselves (Zupec-Kania, 2008).

For decades the classic ketogenic diet for epilepsy was started with a fast while the patient was closely monitored in the hospital. It is still initiated for some patients this way, but now, many patients work closely with a nutritionist outside of the hospital to get started. In this scenario, the diet might be started at a 1:1 ratio of grams of fat to grams of protein and carbs the first day, then move to 2:1 the second day, and eventually 3:1 or higher the third day and thereafter.

Thanks to the Internet and social media, support groups are springing up around the world for those utilizing the ketogenic diet, allowing them to connect and share. Several good books provide extensive information on the science behind the ketogenic diet and its implementation for epilepsy, and other conditions. Here are two:

- Kossoff, Eric H., MD, John M. Freeman, MD, Zahava Turner, RD, and James E. Rubenstein, MD. *Ketogenic Diets: Treatments for Epilepsy and Other Disorders.* 5th ed. New York, NY: Demos Medical Publishing, 2011.
- Masino, Susan A., PhD. *Ketogenic Diet and Metabolic Therapies.* New York, NY: Oxford University Press, 2017.

The MCT Oil Ketogenic Diet

In 1966, studies by Drs. Hashim, VanItallie, and Bergen revealed that medium-chain triglycerides (MCTs) are absorbed directly from the intestine into the portal vein leading to the liver and are then partly converted in the liver to ketones (Bergen, 1966). This occurs regardless of what type of meal a person eats. Therefore, including MCT oil in the diet at each meal and snack could help push up the blood ketone levels and sustain ketosis. Use of MCT oil in infants and children came into use not long after, when it was reported in 1971 that MCT oil was well tolerated by premature infants and that they absorbed more fat when they were given MCT (Tantibhedhyangkul, 1971). Not long after this report was published, the 60 percent MCT oil diet was introduced in 1971 by Peter R. Huttenlocher, MD. This brilliant alternative to the classic ketogenic diet serves as a way to maintain ketone levels while allowing more protein and carbohydrate into the diet. Focusing on offering more of a variety of foods, this diet showed good results in eliminating or reducing seizures. In this diet, 60 percent of the total calories come from MCT oil, which works out to about 6.6 grams of fat for each 10 grams of protein and carbohydrate combined, or a 2:3 ratio (Huttenlocher, 1971).

A big drawback to the 60 percent MCT oil diet is that some people experience bloating, diarrhea, or other intestinal symptoms when taking this much MCT oil and a modification of the diet was later developed at John Radcliffe Hospital in Oxford, United Kingdom, by Ruby Schwartz, MD and her colleagues. The modified version reduces the MCT in the diet from 60 to 30 percent of total calories in the beginning, allowing the other 30 percent of fat in the diet to come from longer-chain fats, like those in olive oil or corn oil. The MCT oil is then very slowly increased as tolerated to 45 or 50 percent of fat calories if ketone levels are not high enough and seizures are not controlled.

MCT oil and coconut oil, which contains MCTs, are often used now in meal planning for the classic ketogenic diet as well as other modifications of the diet to help sustain a baseline of ketosis. Sometimes MCT oil and/or coconut oil are simply added to the existing diet to introduce mild ketosis.

The Low Glycemic Index Diet (LGIT)

The low glycemic index diet was developed by David J. A. Jenkins, DM, in 1981. It was originally used in working with diabetics, was found to work for other conditions, and even became a fad diet at the time (Jenkins, 1981). It came into use for treatment of drug-resistant epilepsy in children, called the low glycemic index treatment or LGIT, in 2002 as an alternative to the classic ketogenic diet. The LGIT allows 40 to 60 grams per day of carbohydrates, with emphasis on portion control, as well as eating carbohydrates together with fat and protein to lower the glycemic impact (Pfeifer, 2005). (See side box for explanation of glycemic index and glycemic load. Also see Table 6.1. Glycemic Index and Glycemic Load Chart for Common Foods.)

Since it is well known that rising glucose levels and falling ketone levels can rapidly provoke a seizure in someone who is on the ketogenic diet for epilepsy, the concept of the LGIT is to prevent dramatic fluctuations in blood glucose levels that can occur after a meal. Fat represents about 60 percent of the calories in this diet as opposed to 80 or 90 percent fat in the classic ketogenic diet, and protein is about 30 percent of total calories with 10 percent as carbohydrates. Another advantage is that the diet can be initiated outside of the hospital and does not usually begin with a fast. (For more information see: https://www. epilepsy.com/learn/treating-seizures-and-epilepsy/dietary-therapies /low-glycemic-index-treatment.)

Table 6.1. Table of common foods showing the glycemic index, typical serving size, number of carbohydrates, and glycemic load for each serving.

Food	Glycemic Index high > 70 med: 56–70 low < 56	Serving Size	Carbs Per Serving (grams)	Glycemic Load Per Serving high > 20 med: 11–20 low < 11
All-Bran™ cereal	38	1 cup	23	9
Apple juice	40	1 cup	30	12
Apples	38	1 medium (138g)	16	6
Asparagus	8	6 spears	4	1
Baked Potato	85	1 medium (173g)	33	28
Banana	51	1 medium	26	14
Banana	52	1 large (136g)	27	14
Bean sprouts	25	1 cup (104g)	4	1
Broccoli; steamed	6	1 cup	4	2
Brown rice	55	1 cup (195g)	42	23
Brown rice (boiled)	55	1 cup	33	18
Cabbage; raw	6	1 cup	7	1
Carrots; raw	47	1 large (72g)	5	2
Cashew nuts	22	1 oz	9	2
Corn on the cob	53	1 ear	29	15
Cornflakes	81	1 cup	26	21
Dates, dried	103	2 oz	40	42
Doughnut	76	1 medium	23	17
French Fries	75	½ cup	29	22
Glucose	100	50 g	50	50
Grapefruit	25	½ large (166g)	11	3
Green beans; boiled	28	½ cup	5	1

Food	Glycemic Index high > 70 med: 56–70 low < 56	Serving Size	Carbs Per Serving (grams)	Glycemic Load Per Serving high > 20 med: 11–20 low < 11
Green peas; boiled	48	¼ cup	6	3
Honey	55	1 tbsp (21g)	17	9
Ice cream	61	1 cup (72g)	16	10
Jelly beans	78	1 oz	28	22
Kidney beans; boiled	28	1 cup	25	7
Lentils, dried; boiled	29	1 cup	18	5
Lowfat yogurt	33	1 cup (245g)	47	16
Macaroni and cheese	64	1 serving/ cup (166g)	47	30
Oates, dried	103	2 oz	40	42
Oatmeal	58	1 cup (234g)	21	12
Oranges; raw	48	1 medium (131g)	12	6
Pancake	67	6" diameter	58	39
Peanuts	14	4 oz (113g)	15	2
Pearled barley; boiled	25	1 cup	42	11
Pears, raw	38	1 medium	11	4
Pizza	30	2 slices (260g)	42	13
Popcorn	72	2 cups (16g)	10	7
Potato chips	54	4 oz (114g)	55	30
Puffed rice cakes	78	3 cakes	21	17
Raisins	64	1 small box (43g)	32	20
Russet potato (baked)	76	1 medium	30	23
Rye, pumpernickel	41	1 slice	12	5
Skim milk	31	8 fl oz	13	4

Food	Glycemic Index high > 70 med: 56–70 low < 56	Serving Size	Carbs Per Serving (grams)	Glycemic Load Per Serving high > 20 med: 11–20 low < 11
Snickers bar	55	1 bar (113g)	64	35
Soda crackers	74	Qty: 4	17	12
Spaghetti	42	1 cup (140g)	38	16
Spaghetti, white; boiled 15 min	44	1 cup	40	18
Spaghetti, whole wheat; boiled	37	1 cup	37	14
Spinach; steamed	6	1 cup	7	2
Sugar (sucrose)	68	1 tbsp (12g)	12	8
Tomatoes; raw	6	1 cup	5	1
Watermelon	72	1 cup (154g)	11	8
White bread	70	1 slice (30g)	14	10
White rice	64	1 cup (186g)	52	33
White rice (boiled)	64	1 cup	36	23

Glycemic Index and Glycemic Load

The *glycemic index* was developed by David J. A. Jenkins, DM and associates in 1981 (Jenkins, 1981). Its original intent was to help diabetic patients make healthier food choices and so avoid the marked increases in blood sugar levels that occur after eating certain types of carbohydrates (See Figure 6.5). Working with five to ten healthy test subjects, researchers tested subjects' blood sugar levels before and at frequent intervals for two hours after eating glucose (the glucose tolerance test). For comparison, they also tested subjects' blood sugar levels before and after eating an equivalent amount of various other carbohydrate foods, including other sugars like sucrose, fructose and maltose, many different types of vegetables, breads, rice, pastries, pasta, cereals, beans, fruits and fruit juices, dairy products. They calculated the average area under the curve for glucose and for each of the other foods. Using glucose as the comparison point, they assigned a value of 100 to the average response to glucose and calculated the average responses to other foods as a comparison. They named the value glycemic index (GI). Basically, the higher the GI for a given food, the faster and higher the blood sugar rises after consuming it. A food is considered to have a high GI at 70 or above, a medium GI at 56 to 69 and a low GI at 55 or below. Generally speaking, whole grain flours and rice tend to have a lower GI than refined versions, whole fruits have a lower GI than fruit juices, and lentils are quite low in the GI ranks.

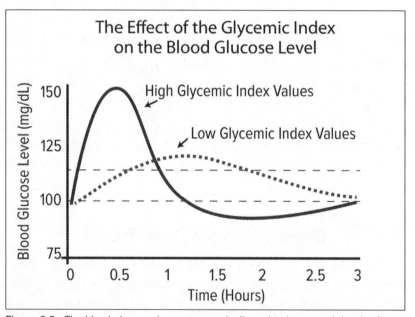

Figure 6.5: The blood glucose rises more gradually and to lower peak levels after eating a low-glycemic-index food compared to a high-glycemic-index food.

Several problems arise with this idea: A given individual might respond differently to a particular food than the people in the study; the actual portions eaten may be considerably larger or smaller than the amounts used to calculate the GI; the GI does not taken into consideration the impact of other foods eaten at the same time that could affect the increase in blood sugar levels after the meal. A food could have a low GI, but, if a large portion is eaten, the impact on the blood sugar could be greater than the GI would predict. Also, if a piece of white bread is smothered with butter, the blood sugar response could be blunted compared to just eating the bread. Also, the impact on insulin levels is not considered in the GI calculation.

The concept of the *glycemic load* (GL) was developed to correct for differences in portion sizes and is calculated by multiplying the number of grams of carbohydrate in the portion of the food eaten times the food's GI and then dividing by 100. This compares the effect on blood sugar of 1 gram of the food compared to 1 gram of glucose. An extensive listing showing the GI, average portion sizes, and GL for hundreds of international foods can be found at ajcn.nutrition. org/content/76/1/5.full.pdf. (Also see Table 6.1. Glycemic Index and Glycemic Load Chart for Common Foods.)

The Modified Atkins Diet (MAD)

The modified Atkins diet (MAD) was developed as an alternative to the classic ketogenic diet in the early 2000s at Johns Hopkins by pediatric neurologist Erik Kossoff, MD, who reported in 2003 that ketones levels remain high and many children with epilepsy respond well to this diet (Kossoff, 2006). The modified Atkins diet does not limit protein, though people who use this diet tend to average about ½ gram per pound of body weight, and the diet also encourages liberal fat intake. Foods do not need to be weighed and measured, with the exception that carbohydrates are monitored closely and are restricted for the first month to 10 grams per day and then gradually increased to between 15 and 20 grams per day. MAD averages out to about 65 percent of total calories as fat, 30 percent as protein, and 5 percent as carbohydrates for most people on this diet. This diet can also be started outside of the hospital and without a fast. (https://www.epilepsy.com/learn/treating-seizures-and-epilepsy/dietary -therapies/modified-atkins-diet.)

BEYOND THE CLASSIC KETOGENIC DIET

For those of us who do not have serious medical conditions, we can choose from a full spectrum of ketogenic dieting, depending on what our goals are. For anyone who is very young or old, for anyone pregnant or breast-feeding, or for anyone who has a medical condition, I strongly advise that you read Chapter 6 and consult with your health-care provider before taking steps toward adopting a serious ketogenic diet.

Most people who want to go keto should probably aim for the mild to optimal range of nutritional ketosis, somewhere between 0.5 and 3 mmol/L levels of ketones (see Chapter 9 on Monitoring for Healthy and Not-So-Healthy People for ways to measure your ketone levels to tell if you are in ketosis). Ketogenic diet expert Beth Zupec-Kania of The Charlie Foundation says that people who are willing to "clean up their diet" are more likely to be successful with maintaining a ketogenic diet, so that is a good place to start. For her this means moving to a whole food diet or ancestral-type with healthy fats at each meal and free of added sugar, sugary drinks and foods. I can't agree more. She finds that many people feel better just with these changes. You'll find more detail about how to get started with this in Chapter 2.

A QUICK LOOK AT U.S. GOVERNMENT RECOMMENDATIONS

In my research for this book, I reviewed many different sources of information to understand where the current guidelines for eating come from and how the so-called experts arrived at their calculations. Since so many people are diabetic or pre-diabetic (three-quarters of adults by age seventy-five in the United States) and/or overweight and likely insulin-resistant to some degree, I find it helpful to think in terms of diabetes and what impact sugar has on us. I found a huge discrepancy between the widely held beliefs—what we have been told to eat by groups like the American Heart Association and even the American Diabetes Association—and what the Institute of Medicine has put forth as the recommendations for dietary intakes.

For decades, high-profile groups have promoted a very-low-fat diet that is quite high in carbohydrates. When searching the Internet for recommendations for how much fat to eat, a common answer that comes up is 20 to 35 percent, and that figure reportedly comes from the National Institutes of Health. For people who have diabetes, the idea that that they should eat only 20 to 35 percent of their calories as fat and 45 to 65 percent of their calories as carbohydrates, as recommended by some high-profile groups, means more insulin and/or oral medications to control blood sugar and more damage to tissues from excessive sugar intake. For a typical person who eats about 2,400 calories per day, 45 percent of total calories comes to 1,080 calories or 270 grams of carbohydrates. At 65 percent of calories as carbohydrates this equates to a whopping 1,560 calories or 390 grams of carbs per day or the amount of sugar in ten 12-ounce cans of Coca-Cola.

For the past few years, I have made home visits to take care of many elderly people and even middle-aged people who live with a variety of chronic health conditions. Some take fifteen to twenty different medications every day, often including insulin and one to three oral diabetic medications. The damage to their bodies from diabetes, from so much sugar and so much medication, is eye-opening and I cringe when I see what many of them are eating. While some have just given up and eat whatever they want, many others believe they are following what they have been instructed to do—eat a high-carb, low-fat diet!

Through the National Institutes of Health Office of Dietary Supplements, the National Food and Nutrition Board of the Institute of Medicine has put forth an extensive series of recommendations for dietary intake, including one for energy and macronutrient intakes. All of these reference books can be downloaded in PDF form for free at https://ods.od.nih.gov/Health_Information/Dietary_Reference_Intakes.aspx. As I read through sections of the massive 1,332-page *Dietary Reference Intakes for Energy, Carbohydrate, Fiber, Fat, Fatty Acids, Cholesterol, Protein, and Amino Acids* (National Academies Press, 2005), I was greatly impressed with the comprehensive evidence-based approach taken to arrive at each of their recommendations for every age group, as well as for pregnant and breastfeeding women. It was quite clear that the groups making these recommendations were well aware of glucose and ketones as fuel for the brain and other organs, and the authors have cited research by many of the ketone experts mentioned in this book. They looked closely at the energy requirements of the brain and the body as a whole, taking into consideration the contributions of both glucose and ketones and alternative pathways to make glucose. They discuss studies step-by-step to provide justification for their calculations.

For both men and women of all ages, on page 290 of their book, the Institute of Medicine states that their Recommended Daily Allowance of carbohydrate is 130 grams. Yet, the guideline put out by the American Diabetes Association for diabetics allows for two to three times this much carbohydrate, for example, if someone eats a typical 2,400 calorie diet. The Institute of Medicine recommends 0.8 grams of protein per kilogram of body weight per day for both men and women, equal to what is used for adults in the classic ketogenic diet but somewhat less than what some keto experts recommend (1.1 gm/kg/day). What stood out to me, though they have very specific recommendations for intakes of specific types of fats, on page 481 they state, "A Tolerable Upper Intake Limit (UL) was not set for total fat because of the lack of a defined level at which an adverse effect, such as obesity, can occur." I have to admit that I was a bit shocked when I read that statement, as it was unexpected. Furthermore, on page 295, they state, "Sugars such as sucrose (e.g., white sugar), fructose (e.g., high-fructose corn syrup), and dextrose that are present in food have been associated with various adverse effects. These sugars may be either naturally occurring or added to foods." This statement was not at all surprising to me.

Using the Institute of Medicine formula for calculating energy requirements, or how many total calories a person should consume in a day, an average-size active young adult could easily arrive at 2,400 calories. So, I decided to calculate how much fat would be in a 2,400-calorie diet for a person who weighs 150 pounds (68 kilograms), using their recommended daily allowances for protein and carbohydrate. At 0.8 grams of protein per kilogram per day (54 grams) and 130 grams of carbohydrate per day, the combination of protein and carbohydrate equals about 736 calories (proteins and carbohydrates are each about 4 calories per gram). Subtracting 736 calories from 2,400 calories, that leaves 1,664 calories for fat. At 9 calories per gram of fat, that amounts to 185 grams of fat which would be equivalent to 13 tablespoons of oil or about 63 percent of total calories as fat! This is a far cry from the low-fat diet that has been drilled into us for so many years. The point here is that the numbers put forth by the most researched authority just don't add up to a "low-fat diet."

On the other hand, something I am quite mystified about is the complete lack of any mention of medium-chain triglycerides in the *Dietary Reference Intakes,* even though they have been used in infant formulas for many years. This book was written in 2005 and with increasing use of coconut oil and MCT oil in the United States, I hope that will change soon.

MOVING TOWARD A HIGHER-FAT, LOWER-CARB DIET

Many people are going the keto route for better health and not necessarily to lose weight. But if you have ever been on a diet to lose weight you are probably familiar with counting calories and keeping track of grams of carbohydrate, fat and protein.

To get into ketosis purely from diet (without supplementing with medium-chain triglycerides) requires consistently eating fewer carbs, less than 60 grams per day for most people, and possibly fewer than 20 or 25 grams per day for someone with type 2 diabetes. People who are able to manage this can expect to be rewarded with lower blood glucose and insulin levels and all of the beneficial effects of simply eating less sugar. To compensate for eating fewer carbs and, therefore, fewer calories and, to avoid burning important muscle, eating adequate protein and healthy fat is also very important. Protein requirements are easy to calculate, are based on your weight and will stay the same for you regardless of how much carb and fat you decide to eat. Calculating how much carbohydrate and fat to eat is quite a bit more complicated. A physically active person who engages in bodybuilding or frequent vigorous exercise could probably double the amount of protein eaten without an issue.

If you have been mainly focused on eating low-carb up until now and think you have been on a ketogenic diet, the discussion that follows might surprise you.

CALORIES VERSUS GRAMS

There are two ways to consider how much fat versus how much carbohydrate you're consuming. One is to look at the relative percentages of calories from fat, protein, and carb compared to total calories. To help visualize this, Figure 6.3 illustrates what happens to the number of calories as fat and the number of calories as carbs when the percent of fat in the diet is increased, while keeping protein at the same level. In this example, a 150-pound (68 kilogram) adult is eating 2,400 calories per day, which could be a typical amount for a healthy, young, active adult who is not trying to lose weight. At 0.5 grams of protein per pound of body weight per day, protein remains the same at 75 grams, which equals about 300 calories. On a very-low-fat diet (20 percent of calories from fat), the number of calories from fat would be 480, and for carbohydrate 1,620 calories. On a very-high-fat diet (80 percent of calories from fat), the number of calories from fat would be 1,920 and from carbohydrate 180 calories.

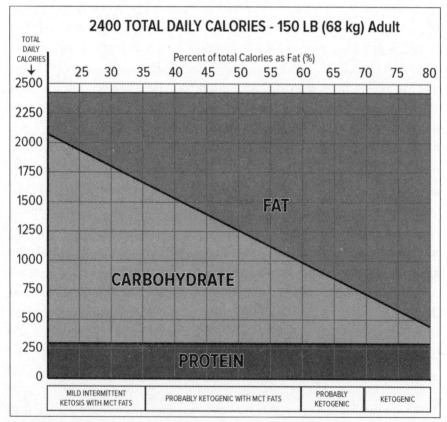

Figure 6.3. Example of the changes that occur in the relative number of calories from fat, carbohydrate, and protein when the percent of total calories as fat increases from 20 to 80 percent at 2,400 calories per day in a 150-pound person.

Another way to look at fat versus carbs as the percentage of fat increases is to look at the number of grams of each macronutrient you're consuming. Figure 6.4 illustrates this point, again using a 2,400-calorie diet for a 150-pound (68-kilogram) person and providing 75 grams of protein per day. Since fat is so much denser in calories than carbohydrate and protein, there are overall fewer total grams of food in the diet and the top line trends down as the percent of total calories as fat increases. In this example, eating 20 percent of calories as fat, a person would eat 53 grams of fat and 405 grams of carbohydrates, quite substantial. At 50 percent fat, this would amount to 133 grams of fat and 225 grams of carbs. At 80 percent fat, 213 grams of fat and 45 grams of carbs. If you convert 213 grams to how much fat you would eat in a day, this is equivalent to 15 tablespoons of oil!

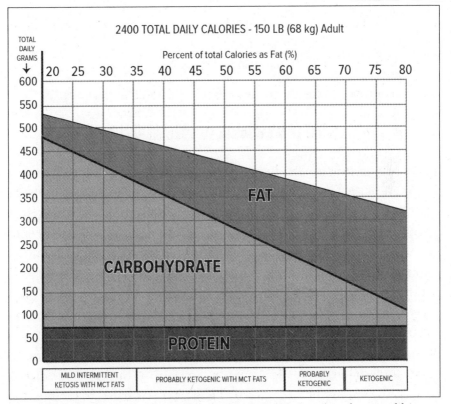

Figure 6.4. Example of the changes that occur in the relative number of grams of fat, carbohydrate and protein when the percent of total calories as fat increases from 20 to 80 percent at 2400 calories per day for a 150-pound person.

In other words, to get and stay in ketosis using diet alone, an average-size healthy young active adult eating an average amount of calories to maintain weight would need to consistently eat about 75 grams of protein, at least 210 grams of fat and 45 to 50 grams of carbs.

If the amount of dietary fat needed to get into ketosis is unthinkable to you, then you might consider trying some other strategies to increase ketone levels, such as

- adding medium-chain triglycerides to the diet, which could allow for sustained mild to moderate ketosis while eating a more moderate amount of fat and more carbs
- fasting overnight to start the day in ketosis, followed by a ketogenic meal
- exercising vigorously
- taking exogenous ketone supplements to provide temporary ketosis or boost your level of ketosis
- adding branched chain amino acids and/or caffeine.

Each of these strategies is covered in more detail in Chapter 7.

WHAT IF MY GOAL IS TO LOSE WEIGHT?

Many people look to the low-carb ketogenic diet for weight loss, so 2,400 calories per day is well above the range they are looking for. On the other hand, if you weigh around 250 or 300 pounds, you could lose weight at 2,400 calories, so this may be a good place to start. As you lose weight, you will need to reduce your total calorie intake by a couple hundred calories per day periodically to keep the weight loss going, since it will require fewer calories per day to keep your body running at your lower weight. If you weigh around 200 pounds, you might find good results at 1,800 calories per day and then bump down to 1,600 calories if you reach a plateau. Remember that it is very important to consult with your physician before undertaking a drastic change in diet, such as the ketogenic diet. It is especially important for both type 1 and type 2 diabetics to monitor the blood sugar closely and work with their physician, since the blood sugar will likely drop and insulin or other medications may need to be adjusted accordingly.

To make it easy to plan your diet, Table 6.2 provides a chart showing how many grams of fat and the combined number of grams of protein and carbs you would eat for diets of 1,600, 1,800, 2,000, 2,400 and 2,800 calories per day. This chart will work, no matter how much you weigh. To use the Quick Reference Table for Macronutrients for Moderate to High-Fat Diets, proceed as follows:

1. Multiply how many pounds you weigh by 0.5 = number of protein grams to eat daily; OR Multiply how many kilograms you weigh by 1.1 = number of protein grams to eat daily.

   (Example: Someone who weighs 200 pounds [91 kilograms] would eat 100 grams of protein per day.)

2. Select the desired number of total calories per day at the top of the chart.

   (Example: 1,800 calories/day)

3. Under the total number of calories/day you have selected, choose the percentage of fat you are considering on the left side of the chart.

   (Example: 65 percent fat at 1,800 calories per day)

4. Find the number of grams of fat and the combined grams of protein and carbs.

   (Example: At 65 percent fat and 1,800 calories per day, this would be 130 grams of fat and 157 combined grams of protein and carbs.)

	QUICK REFERENCE CHART FOR MACRONUTRIENTS FOR MODERATE TO HIGH FAT DIETS									
	1600 CALORIES/DAY		1800 CALORIES/DAY		2000 CALORIES/DAY		2400 CALORIES/DAY		2800 CALORIES/DAY	
	FAT (grams)	PROTEIN & CARBS (grams)	FAT (grams)	PROTEIN & CARBS (grams)	FAT (grams)	PROTEIN & CARBS (grams)	FAT (grams)	PROTEIN & CARBS (grams)	FAT (grams)	PROTEIN & CARBS (grams)
40% FAT	71	240	80	270	89	300	107	360	124	420
45% FAT	80	220	90	247	100	275	120	330	140	385
50% FAT	89	200	100	225	111	250	133	300	156	350
55% FAT	98	180	110	203	122	225	147	270	171	315
60% FAT	106	160	120	180	133	200	160	240	187	280
65% FAT	115	140	130	257	144	175	173	210	202	245
70% FAT	124	120	140	135	155	150	187	180	218	210
75% FAT	133	100	150	113	166	125	200	150	233	175
80% FAT	142	80	160	90	177	100	213	120	249	140
85% FAT	151	60	170	68	189	75	227	90	264	105

Table 6.2.

5. To figure out the total number of carbs to eat per day, subtract the number of protein grams you arrived at in Step 1 from the total combined grams of protein and carbs.

(Example: At 65 percent fat and 1,800 calories per day, you would subtract your protein of 100 grams from the 157 combined grams of protein and carbs and you would arrive at 57 grams of carbs.)

6. So, in this example, a person who weighs 200 pounds eating an 1,800-calorie diet with 65 percent fat would eat daily:
   - protein 100 grams
   - carbohydrate 57 grams
   - fat 130 grams

These levels of fat, protein, and carbohydrates could support ketosis, even more so if you are eating fewer calories than you burn—meaning it could get you on your way to weight loss. If you are not in ketosis after four or five days, you could try increasing your fat to 70 percent, which would bring your carbohydrate intake down to 35 grams per day. As an alternative you could try 1,600 instead of 1,800 calories per day.

For someone who is diabetic and weighs 200 pounds, with your doctor's help and close monitoring, you could aim for about 72.5 percent fat. You would average the fat grams for 70 percent and 75 percent, which would be 145 grams fat, and average the "protein and carbs" grams, which would be 124; subtract 100 grams of protein, leaving you with 24 grams carbs.

PLANNING AND PREPARING MEALS AND SNACKS

After you have decided how many calories you would like to eat per day and what percentage of those calories you would like to eat as fat, you can begin to build meals. Table 6.3 Quick Reference Table for Macronutrients for Meal Planning provides a look at the macronutrient composition of meals containing various percentages of fat; the breakdown of grams of fat and combined grams of protein and carbs are shown for meals that are approximately 400-, 500-, 600-, 700- and 800-calorie meals. If you wish to eat a 200-calorie snack, you can simply divide the grams of fat and combined grams of protein and carbs by a factor of 2. If you want a

450-calorie meal, you could aim for midway between the gram figures for 400 and 500 calories in the table.

QUICK REFERENCE CHART FOR MACRONUTRIENTS FOR MEAL PLANNING									
	400 CALORIE MEAL		500 CALORIE MEAL		600 CALORIE MEAL		700 CALORIE MEAL		800 CALORIE MEAL	
PERCENT CALORIES AS FAT	FAT (grams)	PROTEIN & CARBS (grams)	FAT (grams)	PROTEIN & CARBS (grams)	FAT (grams)	PROTEIN & CARBS (grams)	FAT (grams)	PROTEIN & CARBS (grams)	FAT (grams)	PROTEIN & CARBS (grams)
50% FAT	22	50	28	63	33	74	39	87	44	100
60% FAT	27	39	33	50	40	60	47	70	53	80
70% FAT	31	30	39	37	47	44	54	53	62	60
80% FAT	35	21	44	26	53	30	62	35	71	40
90% FAT	40	10	50	13	60	15	70	18	80	20

Table 6.3.

Once you have figured out how many grams per day of fat, protein, and carbohydrate you are going to eat, the next step is to figure out how to turn them into ketogenic meals. There are relatively few foods that are just fat, just carbs, or just protein, so this part of planning your diet becomes more complicated. If you need help with this, and especially if you have a medical condition, such as epilepsy or cancer, a nutritionist who is educated and experienced in the ketogenic diet could help you work out the very strict ratios of fat, protein, and carbs needed for success.

Several excellent books contain recipes that spell out the macronutrient grams and calories per serving, which could make your planning much easier. My mouth waters when I look at the beautiful photos accompanying the recipes in *The Ketogenic Bible: The Authoritative Guide to Ketosis* by Drs. Jacob Wilson and Ryan Lowery, who are featured in Chapter 5. This book has invaluable information and advice on every aspect of ketosis written by keto experts who have worked closely with professional athletes and many others at the Applied Science and Performance Institute in Tampa, Florida. You'll also find numerous excellent recipes at Ketogenic.com.

Another book I recommend is *Keto for Cancer* by keto nutritionist Miriam Kalamian, whose story is featured in Chapter 5. Even though the book is geared toward people dealing with cancer, the innumerable tips it contains will help anyone who wishes to go on a ketogenic or low-carb diet.

When you begin to plan your own meals and snacks, one item you will need to get started is a good online reference, such as the USDA Food Composition Database at https://ndb.nal.usda.gov/ndb/ or a book showing the gram counts of fat, carbohydrates, and protein for a variety of foods. My favorite is *The Nutribase Complete Book of Food Counts* by Corrine T. Netzer (2017, 9th edition, Dell), but you'll find many more to choose from. You can find nutrient information for many foods by doing a search for the food, followed by the words "nutrition facts," for example, "cashews nutrition facts."

Some other items you will need are a good kitchen scale that accurately measures down to a small number of grams; measuring cups, including a small 1- or 2-ounce cup; and measuring spoons.

MAKE A LIST AND SAVE YOUR PLANS

It is helpful to start by making a list of the foods you normally like to eat for snacks and at mealtime. You can figure out the number of fat, protein, and carb grams per serving of each of these foods from the references you have chosen and from package labels and begin to build a foundation for meal planning. Most people eat a relatively limited number of different meals and snacks, so it will not take too long to arrive at a basic group of meals that you can rely on and not have to calculate over and over. Write each food and meal down to make your life easier. After a while some of these will become second nature and, if not, you will have your notes to look back at.

BUILDING A DAY OF MEALS

The easiest way to plan a day's worth of meals, is to begin by figuring out how much and what types of proteins you want to eat. You will start by calculating how much total protein you want to eat per day.

Multiply your weight in pounds by 0.5 grams per pound (or your weight in kilograms by 1.1 grams per kilogram) = grams of protein per day. For example: A person who weighs 160 pounds (or 74.5 kilograms) would plan for 80 grams of protein per day.

Now you can go to your own reference or look at Table 6.4 below to find a list of proteins and approximately how many grams of protein are in each serving. For example, if you weigh 160 pounds and want to eat 80 grams of protein per day, your protein choices over the course of the day could be:

- three eggs and 1 ounce of grated cheese with breakfast
- 3 ounces of turkey for lunch
- 3 ounces of chicken for dinner
- 1 ounce of nuts and 1 ounce of cheese for snacks

If you are a very active muscular 160-pound person, you could consume more protein and perhaps even double the portion sizes of each of these protein food items.

Many of the foods on the list in Table 6.4 include carbohydrates and fats as well, which are not noted, and this, of course, makes your planning more complicated. This is where journaling will help you accumulate an easy reference for yourself.

Once you figure out how many grams of protein you are going to eat and note how many grams of fat and carbs are in each of these foods, you can continue to build a plan for each meal by adding other foods.

The next step is to figure out how many grams of carbs you want to eat. So you can now go to Table 6.2 and use this table, as described in more detail under "What if My Goal Is to Lose Weight?" Decide how many calories you want to eat per day and what percent fat you want to eat and find the total grams of protein and carbs to eat per day. Subtract your grams of protein from the total, and you will have the number of grams as carbs to eat per day. You can then use this number to build the meals and snacks you wish to eat.

Table 6.4 contains a list of net grams of carbohydrates per typical serving of common foods. Net grams of carbohydrates are the total carbohydrates minus the grams of fiber and grams of sugar alcohols, neither of which impact the blood sugar or insulin levels. You will quickly see that one serving of some of these foods will use up your entire allotment of carbs for the day. Table 6.5 contains a list of serving sizes that you can use to add foods with carbs that you enjoy but in more reasonable amounts that will help you stay in keto territory. You can use this list to decide what carbs you might like to eat, but don't forget to also look up how many grams of fat and protein are in each of these foods and factor these into your totals.

The next step is to figure out how much fat to add to your day's worth of meals. Look again at Table 6.2 in the column for how many total calories you plan to eat and the percent of total calories as fat and find the total number of grams of fat to eat for the day. If any of the foods you selected when deciding on your proteins or carbs contain any fat, then you can subtract these grams of fat from your total. Once you have arrived at how many grams of fat you will eat for the day, you will then need to figure out how many grams of fat to eat at each meal to keep that meal ketogenic. The ratio of fat to carbs and protein combined needs to be at a ketogenic level for each meal and snack to stay in ketosis if you are doing this with food alone and without the help of adding medium-chain triglycerides to the diet and/or using exogenous ketone supplements.

If all of this sounds complicated, you are right! A true ketogenic diet is far from easy to calculate and maintain long term, but it is possible with determination and good math skills or the help of a knowledgeable nutritionist.

Adding medium-chain triglyceride oil or coconut oil to your diet could allow you to use a lower percent of fat in your diet overall to get into and stay in ketosis. These oils could help you sustain a level of nutritional ketosis if they are consumed as part of at least two or three meals per day. You may need to experiment to find out what works for you.

If you are getting discouraged while reading this, a couple of ideas appear at the end of this chapter that may make planning a little easier. In addition, the next chapter offers more strategies for "going keto."

Table 6.4: PROTEIN CONTENT OF COMMON FOODS

# GRAMS PROTEIN PER SERVING (+/– 1 GRAM)	PROTEINS FOOD AND SERVING SIZE
25	3 ounces of cooked beef, pork, poultry, lamb, or tuna 1 cup cottage cheese or ricotta cheese
21	3 ounces of most fish (except tuna and cod) or lobster 1 cup boiled green soybeans
15	3 ounces cod, crab, or shrimp 1 cup plain Greek yogurt
8	2 tablespoons peanut or almond butter
7	1 ounce hard cheese
6	1 egg 8 ounces of milk 1 ounce soft cheese, such as brie or blue cheese 1 to 1½ ounces nuts ½ cup most beans
2 or less	½ cup most cooked vegetables or 1 cup leafy green vegetables ⅓ cup undiluted coconut milk or 1 ounce grated coconut
0–1	Nearly all fruits, 1 medium or typical serving

Table 6.5: CARBOHYDRATE CONTENT OF COMMON FOODS

# NET GRAMS CARBOHYDRATE PER SERVING (+/– 1 GRAM)	CARBOHYDRATES (SUGARS AND STARCHES) FOOD AND SERVING SIZE
51	1 medium white potato (flesh and skin)
42	½ cup white flour
41	1 cup long grain brown or white rice, cooked
40	½ cup whole wheat flour 1 cup cooked white or whole wheat egg noodles or pasta 8 ounces "fruit on bottom" yogurt
38	Three 4-inch pancakes
36	1 cup most beans (except green string beans)

# NET GRAMS CARBOHYDRATE PER SERVING (+/– 1 GRAM)	CARBOHYDRATES (SUGARS AND STARCHES) FOOD AND SERVING SIZE
32	1 cup cooked corn
30	1 large (6½" diameter) whole wheat pita
28	½ cup granola 1 medium sweet potato ¼ cup raisins
26	1 medium banana 1 cup cooked oatmeal, cream of rice, or cream of wheat
25	8 ounces orange juice 1 cup of many cold cereals 1 cup "old fashioned" oatmeal, prepared
22	2 slices most white or whole wheat bread 1 medium pear 1 cup boiled peas 1 cup acorn squash, baked
17	1 medium apple 1 cup regular plain yogurt
15	1 tablespoon agave, corn syrup or honey
14	8 ounces Gatorade sports drink ½ cup grapes
13	1 medium nectarine
12	1 tablespoon table sugar 1 cup full-fat cow or goat milk 1 medium orange 1 cup full fat Greek yogurt ½ cup blueberries
10	8 ounces tomato juice or V-8 vegetable juice
7–9	1 medium peach, fig ½ medium grapefruit 1 cup halved strawberries 1 ounce cashews

# NET GRAMS CARBOHYDRATE PER SERVING (+/– 1 GRAM)	CARBOHYDRATES (SUGARS AND STARCHES) FOOD AND SERVING SIZE
5–6	1 cup cottage cheese or ricotta cheese ½ cup blackberries ½ cup sliced beets ½ cup boiled onions 1 cup cherry tomatoes or 1 medium tomato 1 whole lime or lemon
2–4	1 medium apricot ½ cup raspberries 1 medium avocado 4 asparagus spears 1 ounce almonds, peanuts, Brazil nuts, walnuts, or macadamias ½ cup cooked broccoli or cauliflower ½ cup green or string beans, or turnips ½ cup chopped bell or sweet peppers 1 cup boiled, chopped kale or other "greens" 1 cup chopped cucumber or celery 3 ounces lobster 1 tablespoon catsup or sweet relish
0–1	1 whole egg 1 ounce hard or semi-soft cheese 3 ounces shrimp or crab 1 tablespoon butter, cream, half-and-half, or sour cream 1 cup most lettuces, spinach, other leafy greens and cabbages 1 medium carrot or radish 1 cup cooked yellow or zucchini squash 1 ounce olives 1 ounce pecans or pistachios 1 tablespoon mayonnaise, mustard, dill relish, or vinegar
0	Fish, beef, pork, poultry, or lamb Coconut oil, MCT oil, all other oils, butter and lard

Table 6.6: REDUCED SERVING SIZES OF SOME HIGH-CARB FOODS

# NET GRAMS CARBOHYDRATE PER SERVING (+/- 1 GRAM)	SOME HIGH-CARBOYDRATE FOODS REDUCED TO SMALLER PORTIONS FOOD AND SERVING SIZE
30	1 whole grain medium bagel (3-inch diameter)
25	½ medium white potato (flesh and skin) 1 glazed doughnut (only if you must!)
20	½ cup cooked whole wheat egg noodles or pasta ½ cup most beans (except green string beans) ½ cup long grain brown or white rice, cooked
15	½ large (6½-inch diameter) whole wheat pita ½ medium whole grain bagel (3-inch diameter for whole bagel)
14	3 cups microwave popcorn ¼ cup granola ½ medium sweet potato
13	½ medium banana 4 ounces orange juice ½ cup regular cream of wheat, prepared
12	1 medium orange ½ cup baked potato, flesh only One 4-inch pancake
11	1 slice whole wheat bread (1 ounce)
10	¼ cup long grain brown rice, cooked ½ medium pear
9	¼ cup cooked corn 1 medium peach ½ medium apple ½ cup regular plain yogurt
7	½ cup boiled peas
6	½ cup plain Greek yogurt
4	½ cup halved strawberries
3	½ cup raspberries ½ cup ricotta cheese or cottage cheese

NATURALLY KETOGENIC FOODS

As you are building your list, it is helpful to know that some foods are naturally ketogenic by virtue of the ratios of fat, protein, and carbohydrate found
in them. Some of these foods would be great to use as ketogenic snacks. If
the food is packaged, be sure to double-check the nutrition label to make
sure the manufacturer hasn't added some surprise ingredients, such as sugar
(and most ingredients ending in *-ose*). If the fat content of a food is higher
than what you are aiming for, no worries; it will be more ketogenic, not
less. For example, a fresh 7-ounce avocado has 29 grams of fat (29 x 9 = 261
calories), 17 grams of carbs, and 4 grams of protein (21 x 4 = 84 calories). If
you divide 261 calories as fat by 345 calories for the whole avocado, there is
75 percent fat, making it naturally ketogenic if you eat it by itself. If you put
some mayonnaise on it, the percent of fat content will be even higher. So, a
whole avocado could be a great snack or a side dish in one of your meals.

Here are some naturally ketogenic foods by virtue of their high fat
content:

- any pure natural oil, MCT oil, butter, cream, ghee, lard, mayonnaise,
  many salad dressings (100 percent or nearly 100 percent fat).
- coconut milk, undiluted (88 percent fat - do not use "lite" versions;
  see recipe to dilute)
- nuts (Macadamias 89 percent, pecans 86 percent, walnuts 83 percent,
  almonds 76 percent, cashews 66 percent fat)
- olives (85 to 91 percent fat).
- full-fat sour cream (85 percent fat)
- cream cheese (80 percent fat)
- avocado (75 percent fat)
- sunflower seeds (74 percent fat)
- full fat string cheese (69 percent fat)
- eggs (64 percent)

MAKE IT KETO

Many foods easily can be made "keto" by simply adding ½ to 1 tablespoon (7 to 14 grams) of oil, butter, cream, mayonnaise or a high fat

salad dressing. Foods that come to mind are yogurt, ricotta cheese, cottage cheese, milk, salads, any vegetable side dish, soup, chili, rice ,and hot cereals.

For example, I like Greek yogurt a lot and often eat it for breakfast or a snack. The brand I use, per ½ cup serving, has 11 grams of fat (99 calories as fat), 6 grams of carbs (24 calories as carbs), and 8 grams of protein (32 calories as protein). The total calorie count for this snack is 155. If we divide 99 calories of fat by 155 total calories x 100, this works out to 64 percent of calories as fat. If we stir in just one more tablespoon (14 grams) of MCT or olive oil to the yogurt, adding 126 more calories as fat, we divide the new total of 225 calories as fat by 281 total calories and now have a snack that is 80 percent of total calories as fat, now within the ketogenic range. If you add some macadamia nuts or pecans or even a few berries you will still be in ketogenic territory.

Let's use a higher-carb example. Maybe you like oatmeal and don't really want to give it up. If you make plain whole grain oatmeal with water, a half-cup serving of oatmeal would have only 2.3 grams fat (about 21 calories) with 16 grams of carbs and 4 grams of protein (64 calories of carbs and protein. If you divide 21 calories by the total calorie count of 85, this comes to just under 25 percent fat. However, if you eat the oatmeal with 4 teaspoons of butter, coconut, MCT or other oil mixed in, or one-quarter cup of cream (20 grams of fat), you would add 180 more calories as fat, bringing the total calories to 245. When you divide the new total of 201 calories as fat by 245 total calories x 100 you arrive at 76 percent fat, which is much closer to ketogenic territory. If you would rather not add the fat to your oatmeal, you could add it to your coffee or tea instead, as long as you drink it at the same time as the meal is eaten. If you eat this with a couple of eggs cooked with coconut oil or butter, you have a great keto breakfast.

WRITE IT ALL DOWN

Ultimately, the time and effort you spend up front planning meals and snacks and then making notes will save you time later. You can also make life easier by finding recipes on the many good keto websites out there, like Ketogenic.com.

CHAPTER 7

OTHER STRATEGIES TO HELP YOU GO KETO

"You have to use more than one tool to
make a chair. A uniform theory rarely works
as a solution to a clinical problem."
George Yu, in 2018

Besides manipulating the ratios of fat, carbohydrate, and protein in your diet to increase your ketone levels, other strategies exist that can propel you into ketosis and support and enhance your efforts to stay there. If you adopt several of these strategies on a consistent basis, they could begin to add up to higher average level of ketones. How high that average is will vary from person to person and will depend on your age, personal metabolism, health status, the diet you choose, and consistency in staying on that diet. You can expect to see fluctuations in ketone levels throughout the day following meals, changes in level of activity, exercise, caffeine use, use of medium-chain triglycerides and/or coconut oil, and use of exogenous ketone supplements. (See Figure 7.1.) (Figure 7.1 also shows the typical ketone level that occurs in diabetic ketoacidosis, a worry that some people, including physicians, may have if they are unfamiliar with the many benefits of normal "physiologic" ketosis.)

Some of these strategies can be used independent of diet to produce mild to moderate or intermittent temporary ketosis but could also be used in conjunction with the diet to further enhance ketosis for those wanting higher ketone levels.

KETOGENIC STRATEGY :	KETONE LEVELS mmol/L:
Caffeine →	0.2 to 0.3
Coconut Oil →	0.3 to 0.5
Vigorous Exercise →	0.3 to 0.5
Overnight Fast →	0.3 to 0.5
MCT Oil →	0.3 to 1.0
Branched Chain Amino Acids →	0.3 to 1.0
Ketone Mineral Salts →	0.5 to 1.0
Classic Ketogenic Diet →	2 to 6
Starvation →	2 to 7
Ketone Esters (Oral or IV) →	2 to 7 or higher
Diabetic Ketoacidosis →	10 to 25

Figure 7.1. Strategies to increase ketone levels. The value for the ketone level is for each strategy alone. Combining strategies could boost ketone levels higher. Ketoacidosis levels are considerably higher than what occur using these strategies or combinations of these strategies.

Pseudoketosis—A Confusing Concept

There is a confusing term called *pseudoketosis* that some have misconstrued to mean ketosis that comes from taking a supplement and not from a ketogenic diet. The word *pseudoketosis* would be equivalent to "false ketosis." I found just one citation on PubMed.gov and, in this case, the term *pseudoketosis* was used to indicate a false positive test result in which an elevation of paraldehyde, which is not a ketone, caused a lab test to register as elevated ketones. Another definition of *pseudoketosis* referred to a urine test showing presence of "large" ketones when the blood pH and glucose levels were normal. This would more properly be called pseudoketoacidosis. When a person takes an exogenous ketone supplement, like ketone salts or ketone esters or 1,3-butanediol, the betahydroxybutyrate is the very same naturally occurring molecule that occurs when the liver converts fatty acids to ketones. There is nothing false about the resulting ketosis that occurs. The current formulations of exogenous ketones provide temporary, but not false, ketosis.

You will find many good reasons to consider overnight and short intermittent fasting as well as increasing the frequency, duration, or intensity of your exercise. More work needs to be done to confirm whether the same metabolic changes that occur with the ketogenic diet also occur with other short-term strategies, such as use of caffeine, coconut oil, MCT oil, and exogenous ketone supplements, but there is some lab-animal research, case reports, and small human clinical trials suggesting that they might. There are also studies that show the benefit of an intervention without directly connecting the results to an increase in ketone levels. For example, at least one study has shown that forced bicycling using a specialized bicycle that can be set to a specific speed to force the person to exercise decreases or temporarily eliminates tremors in Parkinson's disease, but ketone levels were not monitored, and we can only surmise that ketones might play a role in this phenomenon (Shah, 2016). An interesting video and story on this can be viewed at http://www.theracycle.com/articles/parkinsons-bike-study.aspx. Studies of ketogenic health interventions often hone in on one particular benefit, or set of benefits, such as improvements in memory and cognition, or in physical performance, but may not look at markers of inflammation, for example. Also, many studies look at the short-term effects of an intervention, such as a single dose or use of the intervention for several weeks, rather than at long-term benefits of periodically repeating these strategies.

Having said all of that, here are some of the many good reasons to use one or more strategies to increase ketone levels. Ketosis can potentially

- provide ketones as alternative fuel for the brain and other organs (except the liver)
- increase your energy level
- improve your behavior, sleep, and mood (e.g., reduce anxiety and depression)
- slow down brain aging and atrophy by increasing formation of new brain cells and the connections between brain cells
- enhance your cognitive performance—mental focus, concentration, ability to carry out daily activities, learning, and memory

- enhance your physical performance by preserving muscle and improving strength and coordination
- promote anti-aging by removing damaged cells, promoting growth of new cells, and repairing DNA.
- protect your brain and other cells from damage by free radicals/ reactive oxygen species
- reduce inflammation and its effects on the brain and other tissues, such as walls of arteries and joints
- reduce your aches and pain
- lower your resting heart rate and blood pressure
- help you lose fat by decreasing appetite and increasing use of fat as fuel
- help you overcome insulin resistance and reverse type 2 diabetes and pre-diabetes
- help you avoid or reverse metabolic syndrome and avoid the long-term complications of these conditions
- possibly prevent or slow down or even reverse the progress of cancer, Alzheimer's, Parkinson's, autism, and other neurodegenerative diseases.

In the rest of the chapter, we will go into more detail about the strategies listed in Figure 7.1 with the exception of starvation and the classic ketogenic diet which were discussed previously in the book in Chapters 4, 5 and 6.

FASTING

Intermittent fasting, sometimes for days or even a week or longer, was a way of life for our hunter-gatherer ancestors and still is for many people living in our world today due to lack of available food or intentionally, as a religious practice or for perceived health benefits. The process of evolution allowed for human survival as a species through metabolic adaptations to these periods of feast and famine. Specifically, the ability for the brain and other vital organs to easily switch from using glucose to ketones for fuel makes survival possible in the face of starvation, as long as the body has fat to burn. Fasting to stop seizures was documented thousands of years before the modern day classic ketogenic diet and has also been used since ancient times deliberately for religious reasons and in some populations for the recognized benefits to cognition and physical health (See Figure 7.2).

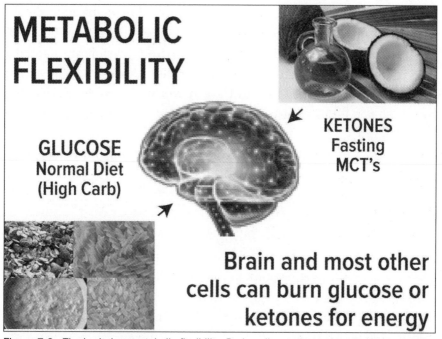

Figure 7.2. The brain has metabolic flexibility. Brain cells can instantly switch from using glucose to ketones for fuel.

There are numerous ways to approach fasting to stimulate an increase in ketone levels, and the results will depend on which approach or combination of approaches you choose. During any fast, it is important to drink plenty of water and other sugar-free, calorie-free fluids to prevent dehydration. Use of fluids with caffeine is controversial and is an individual decision, but consideration should be given to the slight bump in ketone levels that occurs after taking caffeine. (See Caffeine)

It is also possible to lose important electrolytes, including sodium, potassium, chloride, calcium, and magnesium from your body during a fast of twenty-four hours or longer. These can be partly replenished by consuming liquids such as broth or bottled water that contains electrolytes and vitamins; adding sea salt or Himalayan pink sea salt to water; or using an electrolyte supplement. If you are not a big fan of plain water, adding a small amount (1 to 3 teaspoons) of lemon or lime to the water or using sparkling water can help.

Also, people who are diabetic or pre-diabetic, taking insulin or any other diabetes medication, or otherwise prone to hypoglycemia should exercise caution when undertaking any type of fast. It is quite likely that your blood sugar and insulin levels will drop, possibly substantially during a fast and close monitoring of your blood sugar and adjustment of your medications may be necessary. If you are at risk for developing hypoglycemia for any reason, please work with your doctor should you decide to fast.

Let's take a look at the various types of fasts that could be beneficial in maintaining a state of ketosis.

Water Fast

Water fasting (consuming only water or calorie-free and caffeine-free liquids) is the quickest way to get into ketosis and for nearly one hundred years has been the starting point for the classic ketogenic diet for children with drug-resistant epilepsy. The Johns Hopkins Hospital's longtime protocol for the classic ketogenic diet begins with a thirty-six-hour fast, during which time some children stop having seizures, apparently due to the metabolic changes that occur from increasing ketones and/or reducing blood glucose levels. Other protocols have emerged and fasting may or may not be used to initiate the classic ketogenic diet these days.

It is possible to continue a water fast for many days as long as there is adequate hydration and replacement of minerals and vitamins; the downside, however, is that you will likely lose muscle mass with a prolonged fast, which is not in your long-term interest.

Overnight Fast

In building your foundation for ketosis you could start with an overnight fast by not eating food (fasting) for ten to fourteen hours or more overnight. That is how long it takes the average person who is resting to use up the glycogen stored in the liver and start breaking down fat as fuel, which will be partly converted to ketones. If you exercise during that time, you will use up glycogen stores sooner and head into ketosis more quickly. Generally, the longer you fast, the higher you can expect your ketone level to be. If you are not in ketosis at the start of your fast, by ten hours or so of overnight fasting, the betahydroxybutyrate level could be at 0.3 mmol/L or a little higher, providing a starting place to build on the rest of the day.

Extended Overnight Fast

This would involve fasting for eighteen or more hours a day and eating any solid foods or liquids that contain calories, like smoothies, within a window of time of six hours or less, perhaps reducing to two meals per day. This would likely increase ketones at least temporarily and decrease the total quantity of food you eat. The ketone levels could be sustained if ketogenic meals and snacks are chosen. Be sure to factor enough protein into the meals; a protein infused carb-free water could help.

Fat Fast

You could break the overnight fast with a fat fast, eating only fat for your first meal and possibly your second. Some ways to do this would be to drink coffee or tea with liquid or powdered MCT oil, coconut oil powder, coconut milk diluted with water, butter and/or cream, or by eating a ketogenic "fat bomb" (Several fat bomb cookbooks are available and the Recipe section of this book has a few ideas too). A ketogenic fat bomb is a very high-fat, very-low-carb snack or treat formed into the shape of a ball, small muffin, or popsicle. The fat bomb can be savory or sweetened with stevia, erythritol, or another artificial sweetener. One of my favorites is a combination of half coconut oil and half unsweetened baker's dark chocolate melted and blended together with a small amount of honey and stevia plus erythritol to taste. The mixture is poured into the wells of an ice cube tray and placed in the refrigerator to harden. Peanut butter, unsweetened grated coconut, or nuts could be added for variety. (See "Coconut Fudge" in the Recipe section.)

Intermittent Fast

An intermittent fast is one in which you interrupt your usual eating pattern by greatly reducing your intake for one or more days on a regular basis. You can accomplish this in any number of different ways; here are just a few ideas:

- Try a water fast for twenty-four to forty-eight hours once a week or once a month.
- Intermittent caloric restriction: Decrease your total daily calorie intake to 500 or 1,000 calories once or twice a week, every other day, or two days on/five days off. You could take this all as one meal or divide it up throughout the day. You will achieve higher ketone levels if your 500 to 1,000 calories are calculated carefully to be ketogenic. In this case, the grams of fat would need to be at least double the combination of grams from carbs and protein, so getting enough protein on an alternate day fast would be difficult if you are closer to the 500-calories-per-day range. Cutting out carbs completely would be the easiest way to get more protein.
- Ketone salt fast: In early 2018, Pruvit Ventures introduced an idea they call the 60-Hour Keto Reboot, a once-a-month liquid fast. This fast lasts sixty hours, during which servings of betahydroxybutyrate ketone salts, and broth and teas containing betahydroxybutyrate are interspersed throughout the day, as well as a supplement to promote DNA repair.

Cyclic Ketogenic Diet

This type of diet consists of eating a ketogenic diet for five or six days per week and then taking a break while eating a higher carb diet for two days. The problem with this type of diet is that it can take several days to get back into the nutritional ketosis range of 0.5 mmol/L or higher, so you would not be in ketosis most of the time. On the other hand, if you are creative, you could try to combine this with an extended overnight fast on the nights between the higher-carb day or days and/or take MCT oil or ketone salts on the higher-carb days to see if you are able to sustain or quickly get back into ketosis. I am not aware of any studies of this and you could find out if this works for you by monitoring your ketone levels closely. (See Chapter 9.)

My Personal Experience with Fasting

For most of my life, I have had a fear that if I didn't have a snack shortly before bedtime I would wake up hungry during the night and not be able to get back to sleep. For several decades, my evening snack was a high-fiber cereal with skim milk, but I sometimes did wake up hungry in the middle of the night and was not able to get back to sleep. When I transitioned to a low-carb diet, I found that I did not wake up hungry if my snack consisted of an ounce or two of full-fat cheese or some plain full-fat Greek yogurt (or ricotta cheese) with grated coconut and a few nuts. I began to eat the low-carb, high-fat snack earlier in the evening to allow for a twelve hour or longer overnight fast, broken in the morning with a fat-only drink (coffee plus coconut and MCT oils or powder, sweetened with stevia), and discovered that I was able to go several more hours without wanting to eat something solid.

In early 2018, I was inspired by others who were fasting regularly to try it for myself and decided to try Pruvit Ventures 60-Hour Keto Reboot, a liquid fast, drinking only water with lemon or sea salt, broth, tea and two servings per day of ketone salts containing sodium, potassium, calcium, and magnesium. I expected to be ravenous at some point, but much to my surprise, I experienced only a few twinges of hunger that were quenched with another round of broth, lemon water, or ketone salts. I was especially worried that I would have trouble sleeping but slept like a log. I was a bit light-headed during the last couple of hours of the forty-eight hour fast in spite of drinking plenty of fluids, but this sensation went away shortly after breaking the fast with cheese and some coconut and MCT oil.

EXERCISE

Most of us have heard in the news that staying physically active with regular exercise can reduce the risk of developing dementia. How does this work? Ketosis could provide the answer. We talked about exercise earlier in the book in the historical context of research on post-exercise ketosis at the beginning of Chapter 5 and from the 2018 review article by Mark Mattson and others in Chapter 3, where there was discussion of the many signaling pathways affected by metabolic switching from glucose to ketones as primary fuel during intermittent fasting and exercise.

Another important study to discuss here was conducted at Sherbrooke University in Canada. Dr. Cunnane and his associates studied ten people (four men and six women) with mild Alzheimer's who participated in a twelve-week aerobic program and had lab studies as well as ketone and glucose uptake PET scans at the beginning and end of the study. The program consisted of walking at a moderate pace of about 2.5 (0.4 km) per hour on a treadmill, gradually working up to forty minutes three days per week during the first six weeks. Testing revealed that this moderate exercise tripled blood ketone levels to an average of 0.6 mmol/L and at the same time nearly *tripled ketone uptake in the brain*. Glucose uptake in the brain did not change (Castellano, 2017).

More intense and/or prolonged exercise could potentially increase ketone levels even more and sustain them longer. Eating a ketogenic meal, perhaps containing coconut and/or MCT oils prior to the exercise could potentially result in even higher levels of ketosis (needs to be studied to confirm). The combination of an overnight fast and exercise in the morning prior to eating could further increase ketone levels as well.

CAFFEINE

It is already well known that caffeine increases the basal metabolic rate and stimulates energy use. Dr. Stephen Cunnane and his associates have now learned that caffeine is a ketogenic agent in humans. They studied two men and eight women with an average age of thirty-three and gave them caffeine, dosed at either 2.5 mg/kg or 5 mg/kg of body weight (about 150 or 300 milligrams for the average participant). The study found that, between two and four hours after the caffeine dose, there was an increase of the ketone betahydroxybutyrate by 88 percent for the lower caffeine dose and by 116 percent for the higher caffeine dose. The increase in ketone levels of around 0.2 to 0.3 mmol/L is equivalent to what is seen after an overnight fast (Vandenberghe, 2017).

COCONUT OIL, PALM KERNEL OIL, AND MCT OIL

If you are otherwise eating a standard higher carbohydrate diet, incorporating oils with medium-chain triglycerides into your diet could help get you into mild ketosis and sustain it if you take the oils several times per day. It is a great strategy to provide a baseline for your other efforts. In modifications of the classic ketogenic diet for treating epilepsy, larger amounts of MCT oil are used (ranging from 30 to 60 percent of total calories) to enhance and support ketosis—potentially allowing for more protein and carbohydrate in the diet.

The most widely available natural oil that contains medium-chain triglycerides (MCTs) is coconut oil, which is the richest natural source at nearly 60 percent. Palm kernel oil (not red palm oil) is a close second at about 54 percent. Supplemental MCT oil is a clear, colorless, and odorless oil, extracted either from the coconut meat or from the center of the palm kernel and refined to remove the heavier longer-chain triglycerides. It comes in liquid and powder forms. The outside orange pulp of the palm tree fruit is used as a source of red palm oil, which contains many other beneficial nutrients but only a miniscule amount of MCTs. A few other natural oils such as babassu oil (55 percent MCTs) and ucuhuba butter (13 percent MCTs) contain relatively high quantities of MCTs but are not widely available in the United States. Also, human milk and the full-fat milk of other mammals, such as goats, cows, and sheep, contain MCTs, as well as the butters and creams and full-fat yogurts, kefirs, and cheeses made from them.

Most commercial infant formulas around the world contain coconut oil or palm kernel oil along with other oils such as soybean to try to mimic the fats in human breast milk. Many formulas also contain MCTs, particularly those made for premature newborns and children and adults who have problems with malabsorption from the bowel. For example, some commercial food replacement shakes marketed to the undernourished, to the elderly, and to bodybuilders contain MCTs. Some medications and vitamin products contain MCT oil to improve absorption. Please see Table 7.1 for a list of some of the many foods containing MCTs. Some of these foods also contain tiny amounts of short-chain fats, which are fatty acids with less than six carbons in the chain and are ketogenic as well.

If you have not used MCT oil, coconut oil, or palm kernel oil before, and especially if you have been eating a low-fat diet or no longer have a gallbladder, it is important to know that trying to incorporate oils too quickly in the diet can have intestinal consequences, such as diarrhea (sometimes explosive), gassiness, bloating, and possibly even nausea and vomiting. Begin slowly, as outlined in the Quick Start guidelines in Chapter 2, and increase the oils in your diet as tolerated, adding some to each meal and snack, ½ to 1 teaspoon (2.5 to 5 grams) at a time, or even less if you find you are overly sensitive. If this amount is tolerated without a problem, then increase your dosage by this same amount every two to three days as tolerated. If there is some diarrhea, back off to the previous level, wait for several days, and then increase even more gradually.

The remainder of this section goes into more detail about specific oils, some of the beneficial substances they contain, strategies for incorporating them into your diet, and other topics.

Coconut Oil and the Special Properties of Lauric Acid

Coconut oil is quite different from the usual oils in the typical Western diet, such as soy, corn, olive, peanut and canola oils, which contain no MCTs. Nearly 60 percent of the fats in coconut oil are the MCTs C6, C8, C10, and C12. (C6, C8, etc., is shorthand for how many carbon atoms the fat molecule contains.) Recall that MCTs are partly converted to ketones in the liver, and the rest are used immediately as fuel rather than being stored as fat. Most of the MCT (and about half of the total fat) in coconut oil is lauric acid (C12). Lauric acid has some properties of MCTs and some properties of long-chain triglycerides (LCTs); for example, some of it is not taken up directly by way of the portal vein to the liver like C8 and C10, but rather is packaged into fat globules for digestion like LCTs. How much is taken to the liver may depend on what else it is eaten with. Also, lauric acid is not nearly as ketogenic in the liver as C8 (tricaprylic acid).

Table 7.1: FOODS WITH SHORT- AND MEDIUM-CHAIN FATTY ACIDS

Fats and Oils	Grams per 0.5 fluid ounce (approximately 3 tsp or 15 ml)
Coconut oil	8.3
Babassu oil	7.7
Palm kernel oil	7.5
Goat butter	2.4
Ucuhuba butter	1.8
Cow butter	1.6
Nutmeg butter	0.4
Shea nut butter	0.24
Lard	0.04

Creams and Cheeses	Grams per 1 fluid ounce (approximately 6 tsp or 30 ml)
Goat cheese	2.0
Feta cheese	1.4
Cow cream (heavy)	1.3
Cream cheese	1.0
American cheese	0.85
Mozzarella	0.78

Milks and Cottage Cheese	Grams per 8 fluid ounces (approximately 1 cup or 240 ml)
Goat milk	1.7
Infant formula	1.0
Cow milk (full-fat)	0.9
Human breast milk	0.78
Cottage cheese (full-fat)	0.78

Note: The following commonly eaten fats and oils contain no short- or medium-chain fatty acids: canola, cod liver, corn, fish, flaxseed, olive, peanut, safflower, soybean, and sunflower oils, as well as margarine.

Source: U.S. Department of Agriculture National Nutrient Database for Standard Reference, Release 23. Agricultural Research Service (www.ars.usda.gov/nutrientdata), 2010.

However, evidence suggests that lauric acid may be ketogenic directly in the brain.

The Nisshin OilliO Company Group, LTD, based in Tokyo, Japan, has produced MCT oil for about forty years, originally as a by-product of separating oils for other purposes. The company's research revealed the thermogenic properties of MCTs. For many years, they have marketed an oil in the United States, called Healthy Resetta Oil, that combines medium- and long-chain fats on the same triglyceride molecule. This oil has the health seal of approval from the government since it is not stored as fat and can, therefore, prevent accumulation of fat when substituted for other oils. Researchers at the Nisshin OilliO Group wanted to understand how coconut oil could bring about improvement in my husband, Steve, and others, even though blood levels of ketones are not very high after consuming it compared to pure, supplemental MCT oil. They conducted a two-part experiment to try to find out, with interesting results (Nonaka, 2016).

For Experiment 1 they fed seven-week old Sprague-Dawley rats one of the following three oils by placing it through a tube into the animal's stomach:

- coconut oil, which was about 46.7 percent lauric acid (C12), 8.3 percent C8, and 6.4 percent C10
- high-oleic sunflower oil, which contained no MCTs
- pure MCT oil, which was about 73.9 percent C8, 35.8 percent C10, and just 0.3 percent C12 (lauric acid).

They took blood samples to measure total ketone bodies, total triglycerides, and total free fatty acids before the oil was given and again at two and four hours after. They found that MCT oil substantially and significantly increased total ketone body levels as well as the area under the curve (which gives a good idea of how much total ketone was produced), whereas there was not much difference in these measurements between coconut and sunflower oil. The total plasma triglycerides and total free fatty acid levels and areas under the curve were increased at two and four hours for sunflower oil more than for coconut oil, but lower for MCT oil.

When they looked at the individual fatty acids, C8 and C10 levels were slightly but significantly higher at two and four hours for MCT oil compared to coconut and sunflower oil. Something that stood out was that levels of C12 (lauric acid) from coconut oil were substantially higher with almost no change at two and four hours (14.7 ± 3.0 grams per 100 grams versus 14.8 ± 3 grams per hundred grams), suggesting that lauric acid levels are sustained at high levels in the blood for a number of hours after consuming coconut oil.

In Experiment 2, cultures of KT-5 mouse astrocytes (brain cells that nourish nearby neurons as one of their functions) were used and one of the following was added to each set of cultures:

- vehicle (non-ketogenic substance to serve as control) alone
- vehicle plus oleic acid (C18:1) at 50 μL or 100 μL
- vehicle plus caprylic acid (C8) at 50 μL or 100 μL
- vehicle plus lauric acid (C12) at 50 μL or 100 μL

Total ketone bodies in the individual cultures were measured after four hours. The difference in total ketone body levels between vehicle and oleic acid (C18:1) was significant at 100 but not at 50 μL, but for both lauric acid (C12) and for caprylic acid (C8), the total ketone bodies were significantly higher both at 100 μL and at 50 μL. A notable finding here is that all three of these fatty acids, C8, C12, and C18:1 (the predominant fat in olive oil), were oxidized to produce ketones in astrocytes but required a larger amount for C18:1 to do so.

Considering the information from these two experiments together, the researchers made the following points:

- Most of C8 and C10 is absorbed via the portal vein to the liver and oxidized in the liver without entering the bloodstream outside of the liver. So it is unlikely that C8 and C10 would be present in the bloodstream long enough to cross the blood-brain barrier and stimulate significant ketone production directly in astrocytes in the brain.
- C18:1 enters the peripheral circulation when it is consumed; however, it does not cross the blood-brain barrier well and would not have much opportunity to reach astrocytes in the brain directly as C18:1.

- Lauric acid (C12) is partially absorbed by the portal vein, but most enters peripheral circulation and stays elevated much longer than C8 or C10 in the blood. It is therefore more likely that lauric acid would produce ketogenesis directly in astrocytes in the brain than C8 or C10, assuming it does cross the blood-brain barrier.

The researchers point out that their findings need to be confirmed in human astrocyte cultures, since the study was conducted in mouse astrocytes. Likewise, a study needs to be conducted to confirm whether or not lauric acid (C12) crosses the blood-brain barrier and, therefore, is able to reach astrocytes in the brain. They concluded from this study that lauric acid (C12) "directly and potently" stimulates ketone production *in vitro* (in the lab), but the same effect needs to be confirmed *in vivo* (in the living organism). Since one important function of astrocytes is to supply nearby neurons with fuel, it is conceivable that astrocytes supply neurons with ketones produced within the astrocyte itself. If this hypothesis holds up *in vivo*, it could at least partly explain how coconut oil appears to bring about improvement in people with Alzheimer's or Parkinson's disease.

Lauric acid appears to have cancer killing properties as well. Dr. Rosamaria Lappano and her associates published a report in 2017 of their experiments showing that lauric acid caused the death (called apoptosis) of breast and endometrial cell cancers, and they found several metabolic and gene expression changes occurring in the cells that could explain this phenomenon. They also mention a study showing similar results for colon cancer and another in which women with breast cancer who ate coconut oil during chemotherapy experienced improved "global quality of life" (Lappano, 2017; Fauser, 2013; Law, 2014).

Fabian Dayrit is a biochemist in the Philippines who has studied and written about coconut oil extensively. He published a review paper in 2015 that provides exquisite detail of the biochemistry of the fats in coconut oil, with special attention to lauric acid, which is about half the fat in coconut oil. For those who want an intense understanding of this complex subject, I recommend reading the entire article (Dayrit, 2015), which includes complete references.

In addition to the unique properties bestowed by its medium-chain triglycerides, which are discussed in more depth below, here are a few other important properties of the fats in coconut oil.

- About 4 to 6 percent of the fat in human breast milk is lauric acid. Lauric acid is also about 50 percent of the fat in coconut oil.
- Coconut oil is more water soluble and is absorbed more quickly from the bowel than long-chain fat oils due to the positioning of lauric acid within the triglyceride molecules of coconut oil: 54 percent is in the *sn*-2 (middle) position, and 46 percent is on the *sn*-1 or *sn*-3 (outside) positions.
- A study of C10 through C18 fatty acids showed that lauric acid is the most rapidly absorbed of these fats into the dermis (the thick layer of tissue in the skin that contains blood vessels, nerve ending, oil glands and hair follicles), which may explain why coconut oil is rapidly absorbed on the skin as well, making it a great non-greasy moisturizer and medium for massage and essential oils (Kezutyte, 2013). Lauric acid and coconut oil are widely used in skin products.
- In addition to containing the fatty acids categorized as triglycerides, coconut oil contains diglycerides and monoglycerides, including the very antimicrobial monolaurin. Both lauric acid and monolaurin have been shown to kill microbes that cause disease through several different mechanisms, including numerous bacteria, viruses, fungi (such as candida), and protozoa. Just a few of the bacteria that are vulnerable to lauric acid are those that cause acne, dental cavities, and stomach ulcers. Furthermore, as lauric acid is digested, relatively large amounts of monolaurin are released. The monoglyceride C10, which is also found in coconut oil, is antimicrobial but not quite as active as C12. Lauric acid blocks toxins released by certain bacteria. Amazingly, at the same time, the fats in coconut oil support the growth of normal gut bacteria.
- Lauric acid easily crosses through the mitochondrial membrane and does not require carnitine to accomplish this as the LCTs do. In the liver, much of the lauric acid is beta-oxidized to
  - produce citric acid to enter the energy-generating TCA cycle and make ATP there.

- produce ketones, which can be used directly by mitochondria in cells outside of the liver to produce ATP.
- A meta-analysis of sixty controlled clinical trials showed that lauric acid increases both total cholesterol and HDL (so called "good") cholesterol in such a way that it results in a more favorable total cholesterol to HDL ratio (Mensink, 2003). Populations who have coconut oil as a staple in their diet do not have high rates of heart disease, and evidence suggests that it may be beneficial against atherosclerosis.
- Lauric acid and the other MCTs may help maintain the homeostasis (normal functioning) in cell membranes through effects on peroxisome proliferator-activated receptors (PPAR), which regulate cell development and metabolism.
- Lauric acid and the other MCTs are "potent activators" of a compound called thermogenin (UCP1) that increases thermogenesis (body heat production) through brown fat.
- Among the dietary fatty acids with twelve or more carbons in the chain (C12 and above), lauric acid contributes the least to accumulation of bodily fat.

COCONUT OIL, CHOLESTEROL, AND THE LIVER—SOME NEW INFORMATION

In May 2018, researchers Chaturthi Senanayake and Nimanthi Jayathilaka at University of Kelaniya in Sri Lanka reported very interesting findings relevant to this discussion to the American Oil Chemists Society 2018 conference (Jayathilaka, 2018; Senanayake, 2018). They studied the effects of four different diets on Wistar rats, each of which contained one of the following fats: soybean oil, coconut oil, butter, and margarine. The researchers reported that coconut oil resulted in the least amount of fat accumulation in the rat livers and the highest anti-oxidant activity. Coconut oil also resulted in, far and away, the highest HDL and the lowest LDL cholesterol levels and the lowest triglyceride levels, and it tied with soybean oil for the lowest total cholesterol level. The presenters attributed these findings to the predominance of medium-chain fatty acids in coconut oil compared to the other fats.

The Unique Properties of Medium-Chain Triglycerides

There is a common misconception, perpetuated mainly by the American Heart Association, that all saturated fats are bad and should be avoided. Medium-chain fatty acids are saturated fats but are metabolized differently in the body than longer-chain saturated fats. They have special properties that may result in significant health benefits.

Medium-chain triglycerides (MCTs) are molecules that consist of three (tri-) of the same medium-chain fatty acid molecule linked together by a glycerol molecule. The medium-chain fatty acid molecules consist of chains of six (C6) to twelve (C12) carbon atoms. The length of the carbon chain affects the various properties of each fatty acid. All of the medium-chain fatty acids are fully saturated fats, meaning that all available docking sites are occupied by hydrogen atoms, but they behave very differently than the longer-chain saturated fatty acids (see Figure 7.3).

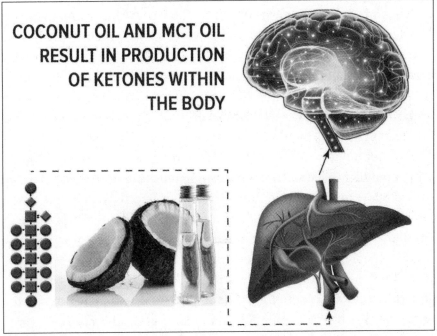

COCONUT OIL AND MCT OIL RESULT IN PRODUCTION OF KETONES WITHIN THE BODY

Figure 7.3. The medium-chain fatty acid caproic acid (C6). All medium-chain fatty acids are fully saturated, meaning that all docking sites that can be occupied by hydrogen atoms are occupied.

Table 7.1: **NOMENCLATURE AND MOLECULAR STRUCTURE OF THE MEDIUM-CHAIN FATTY ACIDS.**

Abbreviation based on # carbon atoms in chain	Chemical Structure	Common Names
C6	$CH_3(CH_2)_4COOH$	caproic acid hexanoic acid
C8	$CH_3(CH_2)_6COOH$	caprylic acid octanoic acid
C10	$CH_3(CH_2)_8COOH$	capric acid decanoic acid
C12	$CH_3(CH_2)_{10}COOH$	lauric acid dodecanoic acid

MCTs are produced in the human in the mammary glands of lactating women, making up 10 to 17 percent of the lipids in breast milk. After weaning, a baby's MCTs must come from food, so for the infant, to mimic breast milk, MCTs are added to nearly every infant formula in the United States as coconut oil and/or palm kernel oil and as MCT oil in formulas made for premature newborns and for infants and children with malabsorption issues. MCT oil is a human-made product usually extracted from coconut or palm kernel oil. Most over-the-counter brands contain a formulation that is primarily C8 and C10 with minimal amounts of C6 and C12. Newer liquid coconut cooking oils contain larger amounts of lauric acid. A product called Carrington Farms liquid coconut cooking oil in the United States and Laurin in other areas is produced by Chemrez in the Philippines and contains 31 to 36 percent lauric acid. It is also possible to buy almost pure C8 over the counter but is more likely to cause diarrhea in some people (www.parrilloperformance.com).

A number of differences between MCTs and the longer-chain triglycerides (LCTs) account for MCTs' efficiency in conversion to fuel for immediate use by brain, muscles, and other organs and, as a result, provide significant health advantages. Unlike the LCTs, MCTs do not require digestive enzymes (lipases and bile salts) to break them apart, or packaging into chylomicrons to be transported, and they are easily absorbed directly from the intestine and taken by way of the portal system to the liver, rather than into the lymphatic system. Along with this easy absorption, MCTs appear to enhance absorption of other substances such as calcium, magnesium, and amino acids, potentially providing a nutritional advantage for those who have an immature bowel, such as premature newborns, as well as people with impaired fat metabolism and malabsorption syndromes, such as biliary cirrhosis, Crohn's disease, regional enteritis, celiac disease, or pancreatitis. (See Figure 7.4.)

Unlike LCTs, MCTs do not require carnitine for oxidation, and they easily pass through the mitochondrial membrane without enzymes or a shuttle system. Once in the mitochondria, they enter metabolic pathways to produce acetyl-CoA, which is either oxidized by way of the tricarboxylic acid cycle or further converted to ketones. Alternatively, acetyl CoA can be transported into the cytoplasm of the hepatic cell and used for new synthesis of long-chain fatty acids.

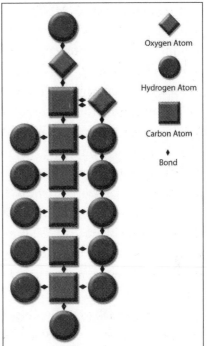

Figure 7.4. Medium-chain triglycerides are taken from the gut by way of the portal vein to the liver where they are partly converted to ketones, which can be used by the brain and most other organs (except the liver where they are made) as fuel.

MCTs provide about 8.3 kilocalories per gram compared with 9.0 kilocalories for LCTs and, since they are converted directly to fuel for immediate use, are not stored as fat. For this reason, MCTs are useful for people who have increased energy needs, such as those recovering from surgery, severe injuries or burns, or dealing with cancer. They are also used in people who have difficulty absorbing other fats from the bowel (malabsorption syndromes). MCTs also have been shown to increase physical endurance, and, coupled with the increased immediate energy availability, would be useful to those who desire to enhance their athletic performance, as well as the elderly or frail who, very literally, wish to have more energy.

Compared to LCTs, MCTs are relatively thermogenic, meaning that they increase the metabolic rate and therefore burn more calories. A number of studies in animals and people have shown that, when equivalent amounts of either MCTs or LCTs are added to the diet, or when a high-fat diet rich in MCTs is eaten compared to a low-fat diet, much less fat is deposited by those consuming the diet high in MCT oil (Papamandjaris, 1998). Also, MCTs appear to suppress appetite, resulting in fewer calories consumed. The net result is that a diet rich in MCTs could be useful as a weight loss or weight maintenance strategy—*so long as they are substituted for other fats and/or carbohydrate in the diet and not simply added to the existing diet.*

Another unique property of MCTs is that they significantly increase the utilization of glucose that is mediated by insulin, both in diabetics and non-diabetics, thereby potentially providing improved glucose control in the diabetic person and in people with other conditions that are complicated by insulin resistance.

This leads back to further discussion of the use of MCTs, and the resultant ketones from their metabolism, as alternative fuel for the brain, skeletal and cardiac muscle, and other organs. Recall from Chapter 3 that ketones can readily be used as an alternative fuel, bypassing the early steps required for glucose metabolism and entering the energy-generating tricarboxylic acid cycle (aka Krebs cycle) to produce acetyl-CoA and ultimately ATP. When glucose is not readily available to burn as fuel, or when stores have been used up, such as during prolonged fasting or while running a marathon, ketones can provide alternative fuel. They can also serve this function when glucose is ineffectively transported across the cell membrane, as in cells that are insulin resistant, since insulin is required for glucose to enter cells. For the diabetic, this could provide some protection from the eventual organ deterioration that often occurs, affecting the eyes, kidneys, skin and other organs.

In recent years, MCT oil and coconut oil become standard fats for use in the ketogenic diet for epilepsy and have come into popular use for people with Alzheimer's disease, other dementias, Parkinson's disease, ALS, and other neurodegenerative diseases that are characterized by decreased glucose metabolism in the affected areas of the brain and/or peripheral nervous system. The idea here is that dietary ketosis through consumption of MCTs may effectively bypass the problem of insulin resistance and result in improved function and survival of the affected cells. Relatively small studies of MCT oil in Alzheimer's disease and mild cognitive impairment have shown improved memory and cognitive performance in nearly half of people who are given MCT oil, and several larger studies of MCT oil are in progress. In addition, MCT oil has been shown to protect cognition in brittle type 1 insulin-dependent diabetics during severe hypoglycemic episodes (Page, 2009).

The many unique properties of MCTs make a strong case for incorporating coconut oil, MCT oil, and other sources of MCTs in the diet on a daily basis. These substances can provide a baseline level of ketosis if taken consistently several times per day—potentially a very good strategy to support your ketogenic diet. More information is coming out about the individual MCTs. For example, C6 is even more ketogenic than C8; C10 has direct and indirect anti-seizure effects and increases the number of mitochondria (energy producing organelles) in cells (Augustin, 2018).

See a complete set of references for this section under "Chapter 7: Special References for MCT Oil."

Mixing Coconut and MCT Oils

About two months after starting Steve on coconut oil, once we received the results of his ketone levels, we began experimenting with mixing MCT oil and coconut oil. When Steve took just coconut oil in the morning, his ketone levels peaked at about three hours but had returned to nearly normal after eight to nine hours, just before dinner time. With just MCT oil, Steve's ketone levels went higher, peaked at about ninety minutes, but were gone within three hours. I reasoned that a mixture of MCT and coconut oil should result in steadier, higher ketone levels overall that lasted longer. If he took this mixture three to four times a day, some ketones should always be circulating and available to his brain.

You may wonder, why not just use MCT oil? If you use just MCT oil without coconut oil several times a day, the ketone levels may fluctuate up and down more than they would with coconut oil alone or with a mixture of coconut and MCT oils. Also, some fatty acids that are contained in whole coconut oil are not found in MCT oil, and I believe they might have contributed to the improvements in Steve and others. For example, the lauric acid in coconut oil kills certain types of viruses, such as those that cause fever blisters. Several groups of researchers have found evidence of the herpes simplex virus type 1 that causes fever blisters in the beta-amyloid plaques in the brains of people with Alzheimer's, especially those with the ApoE4 gene like my husband (Wozniak, 2010; Itzhaki, 2016). Before Steve started taking coconut oil, he was regularly fighting fever blisters, sometimes for several weeks at a time; once he was on daily coconut oil, these episodes were much less severe and less frequent, with just four episodes over six years. The fever blister outbreaks coincided with other infections and setbacks, adding more weight to the idea that this virus may have contributed to Alzheimer's disease progression, at least for Steve.

Well then, why not just use coconut oil? Many people have reported to me that they have seen improvements in their loved ones with Alzheimer's once they started using coconut oil by itself. Steve had a dramatic improvement using just coconut oil for the first two months. I don't know for certain if there is any additional benefit to adding the MCT oil, so I see no problem with using just coconut oil for this dietary intervention. One of the reasons to consider adding MCT oil would be to achieve higher levels of ketones. In the Axona (MCT oil) studies, people with higher ketone levels tended to have more improvement in cognitive function (Reger, 2004; Constantini, 2007 and 2008). Only a portion of MCT oil is converted to ketones, so the remaining medium-chain fatty acids could potentially be used by neurons as an alternative fuel. Bottom line: the more MCT oil one can tolerate, the more ketones and MCTs will be available to the brain. Much more needs to be learned about exactly what medium-chain fatty acids do.

Another point to consider is that by mixing MCT and coconut oil in a 4:3 ratio, the long-chain saturated fatty acids are reduced to about 10 percent of the total fat. Recent studies are finding less and less evidence that saturated fat and high LDL or total cholesterol levels are the culprits in heart disease. But for those who are still worried about possible health issues related to saturated fats, this mixture of MCT and coconut oil offers an alternative to using an equivalent amount of just coconut oil.

MCT and coconut oil, when mixed together, stay liquid at room temperature and can safely be stored at room temperature. Both MCT and coconut oil have a shelf life of at least two years. The 4:3 (MCT to coconut) combination is a light, creamy, tasteless and nearly odorless oil that works well when added to many different foods—hot, warm or cold—unlike coconut oil alone, which hardens when it comes into contact with cold food. The blend can be used to cook on the stove at low heat (less than medium) and in the oven when mixed into foods at up to 350°F. You can also add the mixture to coffee or tea, milk, smoothies, soup, cottage cheese or ricotta cheese, vegetables, or salads.

As is the case with either coconut oil or MCT oil by itself, when too much of the blended oils is taken too soon, there may be a laxative effect (or worse!), so it is a good idea to start with a small amount, such as ½ to 1 level teaspoon once or twice a day. Increase every two or three days as tolerated and take with other foods to lessen the chances of intestinal distress. If a problem occurs, cut back to the previous level for one or two weeks before trying to increase again.

In 2017 the Pruvit company approached me about producing a specialized blend of MCT and coconut oils that would be available commercially. While experimenting to find the right combination to help Steve, I had settled on the 4:3 ratio of MCT to coconut. I also added soy lecithin to the mixture in an attempt to provide Steve with important brain phospholipids, specifically phosphatidylcholine. For the commercial product, I found a source of pure, concentrated phosphatidylcholine extracted from lecithin. Pruvit formulated the combination, which was released on the market in late 2017 under the name MCT//143. It is a proprietary blend of organic virgin coconut oil, medium-chain triglycerides (MCTs) from coconut oil, and phosphatidylcholine. It contains more than 85 percent medium-chain triglycerides (C6 through C12) and less than 10 percent long-chain saturated fats.

Phosphatidylcholine (PC) is a phospholipid that is a major component (more than 50 percent) of cell membranes and is particularly abundant in the brain. PC is involved in whole-body energy regulation. The choline component of PC is essential for normal function of all cells and assures the structural integrity and signaling functions of cell membranes. PC is further metabolized to the major neurotransmitter acetylcholine, which is involved in memory and other important brain functions. PC is involved in the formation of sphingomyelin, important to myelin formation. Higher PC levels are associated with higher HDL and lower LDL cholesterol levels, and lower homocysteine levels (high homocysteine levels are associated with heart disease and strokes). Human milk is rich in choline, which is critical to normal fetal brain development. PC is reduced in the brains of people with Alzheimer's and some other types of memory impairment. PC transports essential omega-3 fatty acids such as DHA and EPA into the brain. PC is also important in heart, liver, lung, and muscle health.

More information about coconut oil and MCT oil, including questions and answers, can be found in the Addenda.

BRANCHED-CHAIN AMINO ACIDS

Amino acids, the building blocks of protein, are partly converted either to glucose or to ketones when they are metabolized. Three branched-chain amino acids—leucine, isoleucine, and valine—are ketogenic and have been used as supplements by bodybuilders for many years to help build and maintain lean body mass.

More recently, due to their ketogenic propensity, branched-chain amino acids have been used in studies of childhood epilepsy and autism. An interesting study by Athanasios Evangeliou, a Greek pediatrician, and others added branched-chain amino acids to the ketogenic diet of seventeen children with seizures. This additive proved helpful to the children, whose conditions were not responding well to the diet alone, and resulted in three of the children becoming seizure free and five more experiencing a reduction in the number of seizures by a factor of 50 to 90 percent. In addition, the extra protein from the amino acids meant they could reduce the ratio in their diets of grams of fat to combined grams of protein and carbohydrate (from 4:1 to 2.5:1) without lowering the ketone levels, allowing the children to have a more versatile, satisfying diet (Evangeliou, 2009).

Another laboratory study showed that, like lauric acid, leucine rapidly stimulates production of ketones in astrocyte (specialized brain cell) cultures, even when glucose is present in adequate amounts to provide fuel for the astrocytes. Researchers found increased levels of the ketone bodies betahydroxybutyrate and acetoacetate in these astrocyte cultures containing leucine as well as alpha-ketoisocaproate. Alpha-ketoisocaproate is in a pathway of metabolism that leads to production of hydroxymethylbutyrate, some of which will go on to form more betahydroxybutyrate, cholesterol, and other substances (Bixel, 1995).

Based on this evidence, supplementing with the branched-chain amino acids leucine, isoleucine, and valine as one of your strategies could help increase ketone levels not only in the plasma but also—potentially—in the brain astrocytes as well.

Branched-chain amino acids are widely available in health food stores and on Internet sites. Websites for bodybuilders suggest doses of 5 to 15 grams per day for someone who is 150 pounds. One caution is that high levels of branched-chain amino acids in the blood may interfere with tryptophan getting into the brain. Tryptophan is a precursor for serotonin, which regulates mood and sleep, so taking too much branch-chained amino acid could possibly have a negative impact on mood and sleep. This speaks to how complex metabolism is, particularly in the brain, and how upsetting the balance by taking too much of a good thing could have negative consequences. If you decide to try this as an additive, my advice is to start with a small amount, such as 2 to 5 grams and increase as tolerated if you wish.

EXOGENOUS KETONE SUPPLEMENTS

As explained early in the book, endogenous ketones are those that are made inside the body, and exogenous ketones are those that originate outside the body. When you fast, exercise, eat a low-carbohydrate diet, or consume coconut or MCT oil, your body produces endogenous ketones. Current formulations of exogenous ketone supplements, by comparison, contain one of the identical ketones made and used by the body either: betahydroxybutyrate or acetoacetate; perhaps future exogenous ketone supplements will contain a combination of these two ketones. There are many other ketones in nature that do not have effects on our metabolism akin to betahydroxybutyrate and acetoacetate. For example, a supplement called raspberry ketones was popular several years ago and was promoted to help lose weight; that particular ketone is found in the raspberry—as well as some other berries—and is a component of their fragrances but has nothing to do with the ketones involved in making ATP and affecting other signaling pathways in our metabolism.

As of early 2018, true exogenous ketone supplements for humans include ketone salts and ketone esters. Conceivably, other types and combinations could be developed in the future. These supplements provide a rapid increase in ketone levels, sometimes referred to as "instant ketosis," that is not sustained for very long. The levels peak somewhere between thirty and sixty minutes after the supplement is consumed, drop significantly an hour later, and are back to normal after several more hours. A question that comes up is whether sustained-release forms of these supplements might be more (or less) beneficial. The answer is not known at present.

My Personal Experience with Exogenous Ketone Supplements

I have considerable personal experience with both ketone salts (for myself) and with the betahydroxybutyrate/butanediol ketone ester (for my husband, Steve; I also tried several doses myself). The ketone ester had profound effects for Steve, reversing certain Alzheimer's symptoms during the first hours, days, and weeks of taking it and sustaining his improvements for about twenty more months before he experienced serious setbacks again. For me, taking ketone salts every day combined with a high-fat, low-carb diet in mid-2016 helped me lose more than 30 pounds of fat over about four months. I travel extensively and like to try new foods wherever I go, which could easily put the fat back on my body. Using the ketone salts daily has curbed my appetite and made it much easier to maintain the weight loss. I must say that I sleep very well, never feel as if I need a nap in the middle of the afternoon, have no aches or pains, and just feel good at age sixty-six. My blood pressure is low at about 105/65, and my fasting blood sugar and insulin levels are in the normal range. One serving (one packet—about 19 grams) of KetoOS/Max increases my betahydroxybutyrate level by 1 mmol/L from the baseline level.

Ketone Salts

Ketone salts are nutritional supplements that as of early 2018 have not been evaluated or approved by the FDA to treat any medical condition. That said, there is plenty of scientific evidence that raising levels of ketones in the body can provide alternative fuel to the brain, reduce inflammation, and burn fat. Countless people taking ketone salts have reported increased energy, endurance, focus, mental clarity, improved mood and sleep, fewer aches and pains, and fat loss.

Betahydroxybutyrate ketone salts were developed and tested at the University of South Florida in the labs of Dominic D'Agostino and burst onto the scene in January 2016. They were first sold to the public by Pruvit Ventures, a U.S. company using a multi-level marketing model, which has been the leader in increasing awareness and education on the subject of ketones and the use of ketone salts. In their Keto OS/Max products, 90 percent of the betahydroxybutyrate is the D- form, which is believed to be more bioactive than the L- form and appears to raise ketone levels more (see Chapter 3 for more information). A number of other companies are currently marketing the 50/50 mixture, which is less expensive to make, and most of these contain the ketone salts mainly as sodium and potassium. This is worth investigating directly with the company before choosing a product.

A big concern that many people have about taking the ketone salts is the high sodium content. Pruvit has reduced the sodium and potassium content of some of their products substantially by adding magnesium and calcium forms of the ketone salts and carefully testing and adjusting the ratios of these to help replace the loss of these minerals that naturally occurs in the process of keto-adaptation (see Chapter 10). They also add other interesting high-quality substances to their products to further promote and support the effects of ketosis, such as MCT oil, fermented branched-chain amino acids, and a compound called AC-11 that appears to promote DNA repair. The ketone salts are "salty" as might be expected and somewhat bitter, but careful attention to flavoring makes the salts very drinkable. There are even flavored broths and teas containing the ketone salts. Also, the salts come with and without caffeine. Caffeine alone can give a slight boost to the ketone level. (See the section on caffeine earlier in this chapter.)

Taking 8 to 10 grams of betahydroxybutyrate as non-racemic ketone salts can quickly, but temporarily, increase ketone levels from the baseline by about 0.5 to 1 mmol/L or more, depending on the individual. Betahydroxybutyrate blood ketone testing strips measure only the D- form of betahydroxybutyrate at present, so they might underestimate the total betahydroxybutyrate present in the blood as both the D- and L- forms. (See Chapter 9 for more about monitoring ketosis.)

The big limitation to how much ketone salts can be taken in a day are the salts themselves, and they may not be safe for everyone. A full serving of ketone salts, as recommended by the sellers, can contain between 925 and 1,600 milligrams of sodium and up to 500 milligrams of potassium. The daily value of sodium recommended by the FDA is 2,300 milligrams (about 1 teaspoon of table salt), so taking just one serving of ketone salts would not leave much room for either salt in other foods eaten the rest of the day nor the sodium that often turns up in medications that most people, including doctors, may not think to include in calculating their salt intake. It is possible to work with a knowledgeable dietician or nutritionist to factor the amounts of sodium, potassium, calcium, and magnesium into the diet, and this is especially important if you have a medical condition.

Some people are very sensitive to sodium and may already have high blood pressure related to their sodium intake. Taking the salts in this case could significantly increase blood pressure. Some people report water retention with puffy feet and hands when using the salts. People who take diuretics (water pills) and/or potassium supplements already have difficulty maintaining a normal balance of their electrolytes and mineral levels and the balance could be upset if taking ketone salts.

Also, the blood sugar and insulin levels drop when ketone levels go up and this holds true when taking ketone salts. The change in blood sugar level can occur rapidly, over an hour or less, so people who have high blood sugar or episodes of low blood sugar, such as with pre-diabetics, diabetics, and especially people who take insulin and/or oral diabetic medications, need to be aware that changes in blood sugar can occur when taking the salts and can result in potentially serious symptoms.

The large amounts of salts could be a big problem for pregnant women who already have a natural expansion in their plasma volume of 50 percent and have a tendency to go into ketosis more easily than non-pregnant women, and for the elderly who have a lower daily requirement for salt, and for infants and children who generally need less sodium, potassium and other minerals than adults (their needs are based on how much they weigh). Ketone salts have not been studied in pregnant women, in the elderly, or in young healthy infants and children. Please see Chapter 8 for more information on ketogenic diets and supplements in these special groups of people.

The point here is that anyone who has a medical condition or is very young or elderly should use ketone salts with caution, beginning with small amounts such as a teaspoon or two, and, in my opinion, *only with support and monitoring by their personal physician*. If you fall into one of these categories, you and your doctor must weigh the risks and benefits. For an adult with Alzheimer's or Parkinson's, or a child with epilepsy or autism, the benefits could greatly outweigh the risk, so use of the ketone salts should not necessarily be ruled out.

I do not at present recommend using the ketone salts in pregnant women since the effect of acutely raising ketone levels on the developing fetus is not known and in the two studies that exist, just one case report on two people and the other in mice, suggest that there could be a problem (see Chapter 8).

As of early 2018, just a few studies of the use of ketone salts in people (two of which are discussed later in this chapter) have been published; however, other studies are in progress, and numerous reports will have been released by the time this book is published.

Ketone salts are not new and have been used in the past in research, although mainly outside of the United States. I found an article on PubMed. gov from 1961 that was published in Russian on the synthesis of the sodium salt of betahydroxybutyrate from acetoacetate ester, which indicates that a ketone ester was already available at that time (Kondrashova, 1961).

I became quite excited when Richard Veech sent me a very encouraging report on the use of betahydroxybutyrate ketone salts. The study was performed by Johan Van Hove, MD, PhD, and his associates and was published in April 2003 in the *Lancet* entitled "D, L-3-Hydroxybutyrate Treatment of Multiple Acyl-Coa Dehydrogenase Deficiency." They reported successful treatment of three young children with the sodium salt of betahydroxybutyrate. The three children each had a very rare enzyme defect called multiple acyl-CoA dehydrogenase deficiency (MADD). People with this defect are unable to use fat to produce energy once they have used up their stores of glucose. One of the three was paralyzed and near death at two years of age and had a nearly complete reversal to walking and talking nineteen months after beginning treatment with ketones. Similar improvements occurred in the other two children who were treated with the ketone compound.

The Van Hove study provides important evidence that ketones and ketone salts could be used to treat a life-threatening disease and even reverse the effects of a disease without serious side effects. It is important to note that while some improvements occurred during the first days, other improvements occurred over many months. Another exciting point is that the levels of ketones reached in this study were relatively low—0.3 mmol/L—similar to the levels we measured in Steve after consuming coconut oil (Van Hove, 2003). These results suggested that the comparable, relatively low level of ketosis achieved using MCT oil and coconut for my husband, Steve, might lead to ongoing improvement in his Alzheimer's symptoms as this level of ketones did in the children with the enzyme defect over a period of many months.

While it is tempting to start with a whole serving of ketone salts in hopes of seeing maximum benefits right away, I suggest for elderly people, children, and those with medical conditions—who all need approval of and to be closely monitored by their physician—to start with 1 or 2 level teaspoons per day, which would be equal to about 1/8 to 1/4 of a serving. Then, if no issues arise (e.g., intestinal distress), you could increase by the same amount every few days until arriving at ½ to 1 full serving per day. The total amount could be divided into smaller portions throughout the day.

It is very important that the person taking ketone salts drink plenty of water and other clear liquids. Ketone salts can have a dehydrating effect in some people, especially in the beginning. Also, ketones can suppress appetite, which is great if you need to lose weight. If you are very thin, however, you might consider adding more calories to your diet with calorie-dense naturally ketogenic foods such as coconut oil, coconut milk, olive oil, butter, cheese, cream cheese, cream, avocado, and nuts.

Ketone Esters Versus Ketone Salts

An ester is a molecule made by combining an acid with an alcohol. The ketones betahydroxybutyrate and acetoacetate are acids, which means that taken alone they would be harmful to the stomach and esophagus; therefore they are not good candidates to use as supplements to increase ketone levels. However, combining one or both of them with an alcohol to make a ketone ester would essentially neutralize the harmful acid, creating an exogenous ketone supplement that could be well tolerated.

Biochemically speaking, the peak levels of ketones that can be achieved with ketone salts are dampened due to rate-limiting factors in the chemical pathways that affect how quickly they can be metabolized. By contrast, the sky is the limit with ketone esters, which are metabolized rapidly. A 2017 study by Brianna Stubbs, PhD, and others reported that, when equal amounts of betahydroxybutyrate were consumed in salt versus ester (as BHB/BD ester) forms, the peak ketone level was higher with the ketone ester than with the ketone salt—2.8 versus 1 mmol/L on average. The doses of the ketone ester and ketone salts used in the study were based on the weight of the individual participant (3.2 mmol.kg^{-1}) and would equal a dose of about 20 grams of BHB for a person who weighs 154 pounds (70 kg). The ketone salt product used in the study was a 50/50 mixture of D- and L- betahydroxybutyrate. Since then, at least one company (Pruvit Ventures) has begun to produce a $\geq$90 percent mixture of D- to L- beta-hydroxybutyrate salts, which would likely result in a higher peak level. Also, it is noteworthy that in the Stubbs study, this dose of BHB/BD ester resulted in an average drop in blood pH from 7.41 to 7.31 and in bicarbonate level from 23.6 to 17.0, reaching the lowest levels at about one hour after taking the drink and still had not returned to baseline an hour after that (two hours after taking the dose); these changes could be metabolically significant and indicate that the acid load from the ester is not immediately compensated for by the body's ability to buffer it for a period of time possibly lasting two or more hours. This drop in pH did not occur with an equal amount of betahydroxybutyrate as ketone salts, remaining around 7.4, with bicarbonate no lower than 20 at any time in the study (according to Figure 3 of the report, but exact data was not provided in the paper). Surprisingly, the glucose level dropped about equally for both the ketone ester and the ketone salts: from 5.7 mmol/L (102.6 mg/dL) to 4.8 mmol/L (86.4 mg/dL) one hour after the dose. Also unexpected in my view, the sodium and chloride levels increased more with the BHB-BD ester than with the ketone salts and the potassium level dropped about equally (Stubbs, 2017). My own results measuring BHB levels after taking ketone ester versus non-racemic ketone salts yields similar results. Following 8 grams of the BHB/BD ester my BHB level increased by 1.3 mM/L as opposed to an increase of 1 mM/L after taking an equal amount of BHB as the non-racemic ketone salts.

Athletic performance studies with the BHB/BD ester have yielded some intriguing results. A set of five studies of thirty-nine elite athletes were conducted under the direction of Dr. Kieran Clarke of Oxford University (Cox, 2016):

- Experiment 1. Exercise intensity altered the metabolism of nutritional ketosis. The athletes each took the same amount of BHB-BD ester based on their weight (equivalent to about 40 grams for a 154-pound/70 kilogram person) on two different occasions at two different levels of exercise intensity (randomized), 40 percent of W_{max} and 75 percent of W_{max}. At complete rest, the betahydroxybutyrate (BHB) levels increased to > 5 mmol/L, whereas during the exercise experiments, the BHB level increased to about 3 mmol/L just before the experiment began and dropped during the experiments by 1 mmol/L more for the high-intensity exercise than for the low-intensity exercise. They calculated that BHB was oxidized more rapidly with higher intensity exercise (75 percent of W_{max}) compared to lower intensity (40 percent of W_{max}).

- Experiment 2. Ten athletes were each tested on three different randomized occasions, once receiving the BHB-BD ester, another time a carbohydrate drink, and a third time a high fat drink. The BHB-BD was given ten minutes before the start of the exercise, and a smaller dose was taken forty-five minutes into the exercise. The amounts of BHB-BD ester given were based on weight and would be equivalent to 40 grams for a 154-pound (70-kilogram) person before onset of exercise and about 13 grams at forty-five minutes into the exercise. The carbohydrate and fat drinks were equal in calories to the BHB-BD drink. The exercise consisted of one hour of constant load cycling at 75 percent of W_{max}. They found that blood lactate levels were significantly lower at thirty and forty-five minutes with the BHB-BD drink compared to the other two drinks. They also found that ketosis resulted in lower glucose levels and suppressed the rise in free fatty acids compared to the other two drinks. BHB and other metabolites were measured in skeletal muscle taken by biopsies before and after one hour of bicycle ergometer exercise after receiving the BHB-BD, the carbohydrate, or the high fat drinks. BHB levels in the muscle were three-fold higher after the BHB-BD drink just before the exercise and two-fold higher after one hour of exercise compared to the other two drinks. Even though muscle glucose was higher initially with the carbohydrate drink, the glucose level was significantly higher at the end of exercise with the BHB-BD drink. Several glycolytic intermediates were lower pre-exercise with the BHB-BD drink, and all of the intermediates measured were lower after one hour of exercise and this was in proportion to the skeletal muscle concentration of BHB. Researchers concluded that these findings suggest that ketosis suppresses skeletal muscle glycolysis and that this would explain the lower lactate levels as well reported in Experiment 2. Also, branched-chain amino acids increased during exercise for all drinks, however, leucine and isoleucine were 50 percent lower for the BHB-BD drink than for the other two drinks.

- Researchers also performed several experiments in which BHB-BD ester was given along with carbohydrates, compared to a drink with carbohydrates alone or a drink with nicotinic acid. They found that there appeared to be synergy when the carbohydrate and BHB-BD were combined, with higher intramuscular BHB and hexose levels, compared to carbohydrate alone.

- In another experiment seven athletes exercised for two hours at 70 percent of W_{max} after receiving the BHB-BD ester with carbohydrate compared to carbohydrate alone. Testing suggests greater lipid oxidation with a drop in intramuscular lipids by 24 percent with the BHB-BD plus carbohydrate drink compared to just a 1 percent drop with the carbohydrate only drink.

- Eight athletes each performed two blinded bicycle exercise trials with either BHB-BD with carbohydrate or carbohydrate alone. Each workout consisted of an hour-long ride at a steady state workload at 75 percent of W_{max} immediately followed by a 30 minute time trial for maximum distance. The athletes had an average performance improvement of 2 percent in distance covered while taking the BHB-BD plus carbohydrate drink versus the carbohydrate alone.

After completing all five experiments, the researchers concluded that "ketosis may alter substrate competition for respiration, while improving oxidative energy transduction under certain conditions, such as endurance exercise. Consequently, nutritional ketosis may help unlock greater human metabolic potential."

Status of Commercially Available Ketone Ester Products

The BHB/BD ketone ester[2] was created by Richard Veech and tested in elite athletes by Kieran Clarke. It is currently recognized by the FDA as safe in healthy individuals for athletic performance. Toxicity testing in healthy people to obtain what is known as "generally recognized as safe" certification, or GRAS certification, and studies of its use in Alzheimer's and other neurologic conditions could be in progress soon.

A dose of 25 to 35 grams of the BHB/BD ester can raise ketone levels to the 5 to 7 mmol/L range (or higher) within thirty to sixty minutes, comparable to those that occur during starvation. We found that my husband's levels easily reached these levels at these doses (see Figure 7.5.)

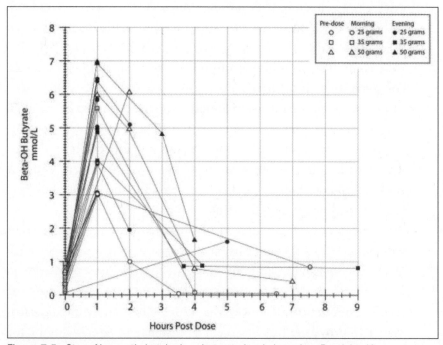

Figure 7.5. Steve Newport's betahydroxybutyrate levels based on Precision Xtra meter readings at various dose of ketone ester.

2　Technically, (R)-3-hydroxybutyl (R)-3-hydroxybutyrate, which is a combination of non-racemic betahydroxybutyrate and 1,3-butanediol.

In early 2018, two companies HVMN (pronounced "human") at https://hvmn.com/ and Ketoneaid at http://ketoneaid.com are launching commercially available versions of this ester, both marketed to athletes for performance enhancement, with a 25-gram serving size. On the HVMN website, the company reports studies showing that when its ketone ester is taken before exercise, there is a decrease in the breakdown of intramuscular glycogen and protein compared to taking carbohydrates alone; during a workout, the D-betahydroxybutyrate is anti-inflammatory and reduces exercise-induced oxidative stress that can damage cells; and post-workout, taking the ketone ester could expedite the re-synthesis of glycogen by 60 percent and protein by double, allowing faster recovery (Cox, 2016; Holdsworth, 2017; Vandoorne, 2017; Stubbs, 2017; Clarke 2012). The Ketoneaid company has recently improved the taste of their product by adjusting the pH and adding a subtle flavor and recommend diluting it by at least double with water. They have found that chasing it with sparkling water reduces the after-taste. They are also developing a new energy drink, tentatively called Ketone Water (ketonewater.com, available in 2019) that contains a unique molecular combination of betahydroxybutyrate, butanediol, and mineral salts that greatly reduces the bitter taste.

Possible Issues with Supplemental Ketone Esters

With higher ketone levels come potentially bigger problems related to some of the side effects of ketones, notably a rapid drop in both blood sugar and insulin levels that could be quite detrimental to someone who is diabetic and is taking insulin or oral medication to lower blood sugar. In theory, the high ketone level should protect the brain and prevent a seizure and other symptoms from happening if the blood sugar drops too low, however, that may not be the case. My husband, Steve, had already been taking the ketone ester for about three years but had his first seizure about one hour after taking the ketone ester, around the time the ketone levels should have been peaking. The severe seizure, which involved his whole body and interfered with his breathing, lasted for about twenty minutes and was followed by another. Thanks to emergency services arriving quickly, he survived but was never the same after that. I strongly believe that the Alzheimer's or Lewy body brain pathology caused the seizure and not the ketone ester, but it did not prevent it in his case.

My gut feeling (based on personal experience) about the ketone ester is that it needs to be made in a sustained release form to keep BHB and glucose levels more stable. It may be unnecessary to reach ketone levels of 4 or 5 mmol/L to bring about improvement in someone with Alzheimer's or Parkinson's. After a couple of years of Steve's taking the ketone ester, we noticed that his level of awareness would sometimes fluctuate between doses. He was taking 25 grams three times a day. When the dose was wearing off, he would "disappear" into another world but would literally sigh and reappear within 15 or 20 minutes of taking the next dose of the ester. If the goal is to match the 150 grams of ketones per day that are produced during starvation, it should be considered that ketones are being produced continuously in that situation, and dividing 150 grams of supplemental ketone ester into multiple doses per day might not produce the same results. Using a sustained release formulation could provide a steady, more consistent elevation of ketone levels, meaning that less—possibly considerably less—might be required to fill the gap in the energy supplied to the brain that occurs in people with mild cognitive impairment, Alzheimer's disease, and Parkinson's disease.

Another major drawback to the BHB/BD ketone ester is its overwhelming "jet fuel" taste. Food scientists need to tackle this problem before the ester is used in clinical trials to avoid high levels of dropout rates.

For an excellent review of everything you ever wanted to know about therapeutic uses of ketones and the ketone esters, I suggest you read an article by Sami Hashim and Theodore VanItallie in the *Journal of Lipid Research* titled "Ketone Body Therapy: From the Ketogenic Diet to the Oral Administration of Ketone Ester" (Hashim, 2014).

1,3-BUTANEDIOL

A ketogenic substance called 1,3-butanediol is an alcohol that has mainly been used as a solvent for food flavoring and as a humectant (drying agent) in pet food, tobacco, and cosmetics. It is partly converted to betahydroxybutyrate after consumption. It is one of the substances used to make the BHB/BD ester and has been subjected to research studies in past decades. While it is possible to increase ketone levels significantly and could be used as an exogenous ketone supplement, its established use is in much smaller amounts for the purposes mentioned above. Clinical studies using larger doses of 1,3-butanediol in humans should be performed to assure that it is safe at these amounts before it comes into widespread use.

I encourage you to get creative in combining strategies to achieve and maintain a deeper state of ketosis. You could start by fasting for ten to fourteen hours (or more) overnight. When you do eat, add coconut oil, MCT oil, or a product like Pruvit KetoKreme or MCT//143 to your fully caffeinated coffee. Later, prepare a vegetable, egg and cheese omelet cooked in coconut oil. Fry up some bacon to go with it—who doesn't like bacon! Eat low-carb for the rest of the day, making sure to include healthy fats as a very important part of this strategy (see Chapters 2 and 6).

Engage in vigorous exercise to sustain increased ketone levels for up to eight or nine hours. Ketone uptake nearly triples in the brain following just thirty minutes of brisk exercise, such as walking on a treadmill. But be aware that if you eat a high-carb meal before the exercise, ketone levels might not increase at all.

Taking an exogenous ketone supplement alone while eating a high-carb diet could be counter-productive to achieve the health benefits you desire. Instead, consider building a strong foundation for ketosis by transitioning to a high-fat, low-carbohydrate diet adding MCT and/or coconut oil to help sustain ketone levels. Then build on this foundation by adding an exogenous ketone supplement, which will provide "instant ketosis" and boost your ketone levels further. For me, one serving of KetoOS/Max, which is 90 percent D-betahydroxybutyrate, increases my betahydroxybutyrate level by 1 mmol/L within one hour. Ketones are known to suppress appetite, and many people who take ketone salts confirm this—a great advantage if you are trying to lose or keep off fat.

What I hope you've gained from this chapter is the knowledge that you can pick and choose the ketone-raising strategies that will fit into your lifestyle and will help you reach your goals.

CHAPTER 8

CONSIDERATIONS FOR SPECIAL POPULATIONS
Moms, Children, Seniors, People with Cancer or Other Medical Conditions, and Pets

Before getting into the details about ketosis for special groups, I want to make it clear that these suggestions are my opinion based on what I have learned. They should not be taken as medical advice. You must consult with your personal health-care provider or your pet's veterinarian (especially if the pet has a medical condition such as diabetes or cancer) before making a major transition in diet. Feel free to take information about my suggestions to the health-care provider for discussion.

PREGNANT AND BREASTFEEDING WOMEN

I do not recommend that pregnant women use ketone salts or ketone esters since the effect of acutely raising ketone levels on the developing fetus is not known. Studies of the use of ketone salts or esters in pregnant or lactating women do not currently exist, and there likely never will be any prospective studies due to the risks involved. (A prospective study is one in which the participants take the supplement, for example, versus a placebo, and are followed over time to look for effects.) As an example of why there is concern, when ketone esters are consumed in healthy adults at a dose of 20 grams, acute temporary acidosis lasting at least two hours can develop and this would likely result in temporary acidosis for the fetus as well as in the pregnant woman (Stubbs, 2017).

Many metabolic changes occur during pregnancy and the pregnant woman has a natural tendency to develop ketosis more quickly than a non-pregnant woman when fasting (Rudolf, 1983). The expectant mother needs more calories to support her own metabolism as well as that of the rapidly growing fetus. While many women fear gaining too much weight during the pregnancy, this is not the time to begin a moderate to strict ketogenic diet that could potentially result in weight loss, even though mostly through losing fat. An exception might be a pregnant woman with epilepsy whose is having seizures and has not previously been on a ketogenic diet as treatment; in this case, consideration should be given to try one of the modified diets, such as the low glycemic index diet (LGIT) and moving to the classic ketogenic diet only if the modified ketogenic diet is not successful in reducing the seizures.

Another consideration to starting a ketogenic diet during pregnancy is that fat tends to store toxins that people have been exposed to for many years, such as medications, pesticides and airborne chemicals, and burning off fat that results in weight loss could release some of those toxins and potentially affect the fetus. This can occur during breastfeeding as well.

Also, while on a ketogenic diet, there is a tendency to lose water that could possibly lead to dehydration and also to a loss of minerals that are vitally important, such as sodium, potassium, calcium, and magnesium; an imbalance in these minerals could affect the mother and fetus. In addition, the ketogenic diet can result in a mild chronic metabolic acidosis, which could have consequences for mother and fetus.

There are very few studies of the ketogenic diet during pregnancy to provide guidance, and the results are worrisome. Two studies performed in mice by Sussman and others and reported in 2013, looked at the strictest ketogenic diet (the human equivalent of a 4:1 diet) compared to a standard mouse diet (Sussman, 2013; Sussman 2015).

In the first study, the mice on the ketogenic diet had more trouble conceiving and had smaller litter sizes; the authors speculate that the problem could have been the high levels of ketones, however, the smaller amount of protein in the ketogenic diet could also explain this. In the second study, during lactation, some of the mouse mothers on the ketogenic diet developed ketoacidosis and died. The mammary glands of the mice on the ketogenic diet were underdeveloped and produced less milk.

The mice who were born to the mothers on the ketogenic diet and were fed milk from a mouse on the ketogenic diet compared to the standard diet did not grow as well and had a tendency toward smaller brain size overall with certain areas of the brain that were smaller (the cortex, hippocampus, corpus callosum, fimbria, and lateral ventricles) and areas that were larger (hypothalamus and medulla). Sussman discusses the point that the fetal brain can use ketones and needs ketones for normal development, however, excessive levels of ketones could have a detrimental effect, citing other studies showing that elevated ketone levels in the mouse fetus affect metabolism of amino acids and other important substances in the brain.

The authors concluded that the changes they saw in the brain could result in functional and behavioral changes that may become apparent later. They conducted a third study to look at mice as young adults whose mothers were on the ketogenic diet while the mice pups were in the womb; these mice pups were fed a standard diet after they were born. These mice showed less depression and anxiety, along with more activity, but had smaller brains with differences in specific areas of the brain compared to mice whose mothers were on a standard diet throughout pregnancy and who themselves were fed a standard diet after birth and in later life (Sussman, 2015).

In 1983, Dr. Mary Rudolf wrote an extensive review of the considerable information that was already accumulated at that time on ketosis during pregnancy and ketosis in the fetus. She notes that, in general, non-pregnant women go into ketosis during fasting earlier than men and that this is even more exaggerated in the pregnant woman. She cites studies reporting that a pregnant woman who fasts will triple her ketone levels in eighteen hours and achieve high ketone levels of 4 mmol/L or more by two and a half to three days of fasting. Ketones are easily transmitted across the placenta as is glucose. The blood sugar also drops more quickly and to lower levels than in a non-pregnant woman, which is reflected in the fetus, who will experience blood sugar levels at least 10 mg/dL lower than the mother's. While the fetus uses ketones as fuel and as building blocks for lipids in the brain, including formation of protective myelin around nerves, lung, skin, and possibly other tissues, excessive levels of ketones could potentially be harmful.

Another metabolic change that occurs during the later part of the pregnancy is the development of insulin resistance, meaning that it takes higher levels of insulin for glucose to enter cells. Some women develop gestational diabetes that usually goes away after the pregnancy, but results in high glucose and insulin levels while pregnant. When the mother's glucose level is high, the developing baby's glucose level is high as well and the baby's pancreas puts out higher levels of insulin in response. This sets up the baby for developing very low blood sugar shortly after birth since the baby's pancreas is overproducing insulin, and the pancreas can take several days or even weeks to readjust. Worries about the possibility of seizures and brain damage from low blood sugar sends many babies to the newborn ICU during the first hours of life.

In her review, Dr. Rudolf also discusses diabetic ketoacidosis in pregnancy, which carries a very high mortality for the baby and high rates of brain damage when the child survives. She mentions one study showing that, when ketones were present in the urine of non-diabetic mothers, this condition appeared to have a negative effect on the neuropsychological development of the infant. She points out that there are other metabolic derangements going on in diabetic ketoacidosis that could explain the adverse effects on the fetus, so it is not certain whether high levels of ketones alone would have adverse outcomes. Her opinion was that it is prudent to avoid ketosis during pregnancy, stating, "Regardless of whether ketones *per se* have adverse effects, they, at least, appear to be clinical markers for an unfavourable environment for the fetus" (Rudolf, 1983).

As of early 2018, very little information on the use of ketogenic diets during pregnancy in humans is available. I could find only one article from 2016 reporting outcomes of two women on a ketogenic diet for epilepsy. The first patient was twenty-seven years old and was started on the classic ketogenic diet during pregnancy due to frequent seizures. The diet included MCT oil, and carbohydrates initially were kept at 75 grams and then lowered to 47 grams per day. Her blood ketone levels ranged from 0.2 to 2.6 mmol/L and her pregnancy had a good outcome with normal growth and development of the fetus that continued through the follow-up period at one year of age. The second patient was thirty-six years old, and she was consuming a modified Atkins type ketogenic diet, with carbohydrates restricted before pregnancy to 20 grams, which was increased during pregnancy to 30 grams. She had 2 to 4+ ketones in her urine (no blood measurements were reported). She had seizures during the pregnancy and was on an anticonvulsant that was increased due to more frequent seizures. Her baby had mild deformities of both ears, but normal hearing, and normal neurologic development at eight months of age. It is uncertain what caused the ear deformities: the diet, the medication, or neither (Van der Louw, 2016).

Regarding the ketogenic diet while breastfeeding, there is just one case report in which a strict ketogenic diet seemed to be the only factor leading to ketoacidosis, and it is concerning. This case report was on a thirty-two-year-old breastfeeding mother whose baby was ten months old. The mother ended up in the emergency room with nausea, vomiting, heart palpitations, trembling, and cramps in her extremities. She had started a strict ketogenic diet to lose weight about ten days earlier, eating less than 20 grams of carbohydrate per day, and she had lost about 9 pounds. Her ketone levels were 7.0 mmol/L, her blood was acidic with a low pH of 7.20 (7.35 to 7.45 is normal), her blood sugar was low at 68 mg/dL (no other tests suggested diabetes). She recovered with treatment within several days. The authors mention other reports of breastfeeding women developing ketoacidosis related to fasting, having infections, breastfeeding twins, or after having bariatric surgery (reconstruction of the stomach and bowel to reduce the amount of food the stomach can contain; von Geijer, 2015).

Another case report from 2017 considered a twenty-seven-year-old average size (BMI 23.0) breastfeeding mother whose baby was eight weeks old. The patient said that for two years she had eaten a diet she described as "safe ketosis" with carbs at 10 percent (about 20 grams per day), protein at 20 percent, and fat at 70 percent of calories. She developed gastroenteritis (nausea and vomiting) and was unable to eat for about four days and presented to the emergency room with fever, aches, malaise, and disorientation. She had severe (life-threatening) acidosis with blood pH 7.021 and bicarbonate extremely low at 5.1 mmol/L. Her blood betahydroxybutyrate ketone level was 5.4 mmol/L, and she had "large" ketones in her urine (acetoacetate). Her blood sugar was 120 mg/dL, ruling out diabetes. She was successfully treated in the ICU and advised to eat more carbohydrate and more calories. This case illustrates that an illness could tip an otherwise healthy breastfeeding mother on a ketogenic diet into serious ketoacidosis (Sloan, 2017).

The National Academies Press published a massive 1,332-page book in 2005 under the umbrella of the National Institutes of Health Office of

Dietary Supplements through the National Food and Nutrition Board of the Institute of Medicine, called *Dietary Reference Intakes for Energy, Carbohydrate, Fiber, Fat, Fatty Acids, Cholesterol, Protein, and Amino Acids,* which provides guidelines for recommended intakes of each of these nutrients by age group, as well as in pregnancy and lactation, and provides the evidence in detail leading to each recommendation. In pregnancy and lactation, for each nutrient they consider how much is needed by the mother and by the fetus or breastfed newborn to come up with their recommendations. This is the source used for the suggested amount of carbohydrates, proteins, and fats discussed below. This very practical and informative book can be downloaded for free at https://ods.od.nih.gov /Health_Information/Dietary_Reference_Intakes.aspx.

The Institute of Medicine recommends that the estimated average requirement (EAR) for carbohydrate for a pregnant woman between the ages of fourteen and fifty years of age is 135 grams per day and the recommended daily allowance (RDA) is set at 130 percent of the EAR at 175 grams per day. The EAR is an average, but the RDA covers the needs of 97 to 98 percent of people. So, if you are a small person carrying one baby, 135 grams may be adequate, but if you are tall and are carrying twins you might want to aim for closer to 175 grams per day. For breastfeeding women, the EAR for carbohydrates starts at 160 grams, and the RDA is 210 grams per day. The discussion of how they arrived at these numbers includes an extensive analysis of scientific studies, including the published review by Mary Rudolf discussed above, and work by many others who studied the fuels used by mother and baby during pregnancy and lactation, including glucose and ketones, and how much each of these fuels contributes to the energy used by the brain and by the whole body.

Suggestions for Pregnant and Breastfeeding Women

The bottom line here is that very little information is available about the effects of a ketogenic diet, and studies on the use of ketone salts or esters during pregnancy or while breastfeeding do not exist. There are concerns with use of a strict 4:1 ketogenic equivalent (4 grams of fat for every one gram of protein and carbs combined) in pregnant and lactating mice, which can give us an idea, but not a definite answer since humans and mice are very different animals. Pregnant women are prone to developing ketosis and low blood sugar more quickly, and metabolic changes that affect the mother are often reflected in the fetus. The fetus is capable of using ketones as fuel for the brain and other organs and also uses ketones as building blocks for lipids in the brain and other tissues, so mild ketosis, which is common throughout pregnancy and while breastfeeding, is unlikely to be harmful. Women are also prone to developing insulin resistance and even gestational diabetes later in the pregnancy.

I tend to agree with Dr. Rudolph's position in her 1983 review, that prudence is warranted and deliberate fasting or other strategies to increase ketones to moderate or high levels during pregnancy and while breastfeeding should be avoided unless and until there is clear information that this practice is safe for the mother and developing fetus. It is unlikely we will get answers to these questions in the near future, but we may begin to see case reports of use of ketone salts and esters from women who decided to do this on their own. Mild to moderate intensity exercise for thirty minutes, like walking or swimming, can mildly increase ketones and may have health benefits for the pregnant mother. Coconut oil slightly increases ketone levels and has been used throughout history as a staple in the human diet in tropical parts of the world, so it is unlikely that a slight elevation of ketones from eating coconut oil would cause a problem for the mother or the fetus. Medium-chain triglycerides are present in human breast milk, and MCT oil, coconut oil, and palm kernel oil have been used directly in infant formulas for nearly forty years, so it is unlikely that consuming any of these in moderation during pregnancy or while breastfeeding would be harmful to the mother or the fetus.

I believe the best approach to eating during pregnancy is to stay away from a moderate to strict ketogenic diet (or any other weight loss diet) and instead aim for reducing excessive sugar and choosing carbs wisely. Some strategies to decrease excessive carbohydrate intake and eat healthier are outlined in Chapter 2. The pregnant woman should eat a moderate amount of carbohydrate, between 135 and 175 grams per day, depending on her size and how many babies she is carrying. From the middle third of the pregnancy onward, more calories are needed to support the growth of the fetus. While breastfeeding, the same advice applies, except now the growing baby's demand for energy will increase with age and producing breast milk requires a lot of calories. So, while breastfeeding, the carbohydrate intake should be increased, ranging from 160 to 210 grams per day, depending on how large the mother is and how many babies she is feeding.

For pregnant and breastfeeding moms, please consult your physician or a dietician to determine how many calories and other nutrients you need, since this varies quite a bit from person to person, depending on your size and your activity level.

Guidelines for Diet During Pregnancy and Breastfeeding

Carbohydrates: (Counting carbs can help prevent excessive sugar intake)

During pregnancy: Aim for 135 to 175 grams per day, depending on your size and number of babies.

During breastfeeding: Aim for 160 to 210 grams per day, depending on your size and number of babies.

Protein:

During pregnancy: At least 0.5 grams per pound you weigh per day (1.1 grams/kg/day)

During breastfeeding: At least 0.6 grams per pound you weigh per day (1.3 grams/kg/day)

Fat: The Institute of Medicine does not have specific recommendations for total fat in the diet and did not set a "tolerable upper limit" because there is a lack of evidence showing adverse effects from eating too much fat. They state that the average fat intake for women is 30 to 33 percent of calories. For example, if you eat 2,000 calories per day, this would translate and range of 600 to 660 calories, or around 70 grams of fat per day (about 5 tablespoons of oil), including the fat naturally contained in foods. There are recommendations for pregnant and breastfeeding women to get adequate DHA omega-3 fats from fish and/or supplements. There are DHA supplements from algae on the market for this purpose.

Avoid: Fruit juices, sugary soft drinks and other sugary beverages, sweets (pastries, cakes, pies, cookies, candy), added sugar (table sugar, honey, agave, syrup and high-fructose corn syrup in packaged food and drink), foods made with refined grains (white flour, white rice). Also, in pregnancy it is recommended to avoid fish that may contain mercury, as well as handling raw meat or eating raw dairy products that may carry pathogens like toxoplasmosis or listeria.

Eat in moderation:

- Dairy: one serving at meals.
- Fruit: one to three portions per day. (Consider low-sugar fruits like berries.)
- One serving per meal of whole grain bread (2 slices), whole grain rice, or whole grain cereals (½ to 1 cup) or starchy foods such as beans and potatoes. Eat along with some proteins and fats to further reduce glycemic load.

Eat: Three meals per day and two or three snacks, combining protein, carbs, and healthy fats at each meal whenever possible. For carbohydrates focus on vegetables and choose a variety of colors and types of vegetables, including leafy greens and non-leafy vegetables.

Drink: Plenty of water and other non-sugary fluids. Drink tea and coffee in moderation.

Sugar substitutes: FDA considers sugar substitutes to be safe in pregnancy in small amounts including stevia, sucralose, saccharin, aspartame, erythritol, xylitol, and others.

CHILDREN

The classic ketogenic diet has been used for nearly one hundred years to treat drug-resistant epilepsy in infants and children, with several less-strict modifications of the diet appearing within the past forty years. More recently, the diet is being used for children with a number of other conditions, such as cancer, autism, and rare enzyme deficiencies affecting utilization of glucose. While the ketogenic diet has brought about considerable improvement for numerous children with these conditions, there are sometimes adverse effects such as poor growth and poor bone mineralization, occasionally leading to fractures, kidney stones, metabolic problems, such as chronic metabolic acidosis and electrolyte or mineral imbalances. These adverse effects have occurred in some cases even with the best nutritional counseling.

There are many studies now of ketogenic diet in children with a variety of medical problems, most abundant for epilepsy, and some of these focus on the adverse effects and potential ways to treat or prevent them. Use of ketone salts and ketone esters with very close monitoring by the child's physician and nutritionist could become a tool to help maintain ketosis when used in conjunction with the ketogenic diet.

On the other hand, I have not been able to find any studies or case reports of the use of the ketogenic diet in healthy infants and children and whether the diet affects growth or results in other adverse effects. The brain in the infant is capable of using ketones for fuel. The infant also uses ketones as building blocks for proteins in the brain and other tissues. However, glucose is an important fuel for the brain, which is a very active organ requiring a large share of the calories taken in by the baby or child. In the newborn, the brain uses up to 74 percent of the energy consumed.

Considering the lack of information either way and the complications potentially affecting growth in children who are on the diet for a medical reason, I cannot recommend using a ketogenic diet that results in moderate to high levels of ketones for a healthy child. As physicians we are taught to always consider the risks and benefits of any therapy, and in the case of a healthy child, the risks of using a moderate to strict ketogenic diet probably outweigh the benefits.

Depending on what the mother eats, breast milk has about 40 to 50 percent of its calories as fats, about 40 to 50 percent as carbohydrates, and about 9 percent protein. Breast milk has about 10 to 17 percent of its fats as medium-chain triglycerides (C6 to C12), the higher percent found in the milk of a mother with a premature newborn. The newborn who is exclusively fed breast milk goes into ketosis within hours of birth, and this continues for at least a few days until the mother's milk is established.

Breast milk is a complex living tissue with thousands of substances, such as lipids packaged inside of membranes made of important brain phospholipids, antibodies, hormones, and healthy bacteria that just can't be duplicated in infant formulas. Newborn intensive care units are turning to human donor milk, and fortifiers derived directly from breast milk, that is tested for infection and pasteurized. Studies are showing significantly lower rates of some serious complications when 100 percent breast milk and breast milk-derived fortifiers are used. Discharge home happens considerably sooner on average when breast milk is used in the tiniest premature newborns instead of infant formulas, which contain about one hundred ingredients by comparison to the thousands in breast milk. For example, there are more than 160 known oligosaccharides (complex sugars) with many different functions in breast milk, but only one has been synthesized for use in some infant formulas. So, whenever possible, breast milk is the best food for the infant, ideally exclusively, for the first six months of life before solid foods are introduced.

After six months of age, introduction to a variety of tastes and textures of vegetables, will make it more likely for the child to like these foods later and be willing to try new foods. Also, persistence, trying the same food six or eight times before giving up, will result in acceptance and a more well-rounded diet. It is easier than ever to make foods for infants in the home kitchen. If you are eating healthy vegetables, you can easily puree some for the baby with a NutriBullet or other blender.

My recommendations for older infants and children are very similar to those for the pregnant or breastfeeding mothers. Instead of looking to the ketogenic diet for answers, focus on providing your child with a well-balanced, healthy diet, with a moderate amount of carbohydrates, plenty of protein to grow on, and healthy fats. Also, steering away from fruit juices and sugar-sweetened beverages, and limiting other sweets like candy, cake, and sugary cookies to very special occasions can go a long way to teaching the child good food habits that could lead to a healthier adulthood. There are many books and websites with recipes for lower-sugar foods. Many of these are geared toward the ketogenic diet, and there is every reason to include some of these foods in the child's diet even if the child is not on a ketogenic diet in general. (See Chapter 2 for ways to reduce simple sugars and added sugars in the diet.)

During a fast, ketone levels increase rapidly in a child and even more rapidly in an infant and reach high levels days sooner than in a fasting adult. (See Figure 8.1.) Young children often sleep ten or twelve hours at night without eating and are very likely in mild ketosis at least part of the time, so intermittent mild ketosis is likely not harmful and may even be beneficial. Children tend to be very active, often engaged in vigorous activity for prolonged periods, and likely are in mild ketosis when this happens. I have not been able to find any studies in children to support this, but there are a number of studies of post-exercise ketosis in adults. (See Chapter 7.)

The Institutes of Medicine *Dietary References for Intake* includes recommendations for carbohydrate intake in children of all ages based on a thorough review of the evidence accumulated and including intense study of the fuels used by the brain and body as a whole, including glucose and ketones. These recommendations could be used as a guide to help the

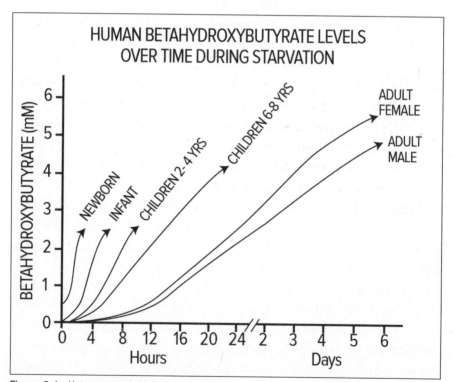

Figure 8.1. Ketones reach high levels much sooner in infants and children than in adults during starvation, and women reach higher levels faster than men. (Cahill, 2006).

parent know how much carbohydrate is needed for their child's normal growth and allow them to set a limit so that the child does not receive too much sugar. The institute states that the average intake of carbohydrates from birth to six months of age is 60 grams per day, and 95 grams per day for infants seven through twelve months. For children one through eighteen years, they state the estimated average requirement for carbohydrates is 100 grams per day, and the recommended daily allowance is 130 grams per day, which will cover the needs for 97 to 98 percent of children in this age group. Again, no upper intake is listed for fat.

The institute continues to recommend these same amounts for both men and non-pregnant and non-breastfeeding women throughout adult life. While the institute states that there are no known adverse effects of consuming large amounts of fat, they say that there *are numerous adverse effects* from consuming too much sugar and have dedicated a substantial number of pages to discussing them.

Autism

During the past three decades, the number of children diagnosed with an autism spectrum disorder (ASD) has rapidly increased. Some of the common symptoms include problems with social communication, language deficits, anxiety, and repetitive behaviors. The percent of children who are overweight or obese has been steadily rising at the same time, suggesting that there may be a connection. In one study, there were more than twice as many children with autism who were overweight or obese than in a control group (from information at autismspeaks.org and the U.S. Centers for Disease Control). In another study, absence of breastfeeding resulted in much higher odds (2.48 times higher) of a diagnosis of autism than in children who were breastfed for more than six months (Schultz, 2006).

At least one study reported improvement of symptoms in autistic children with the ketogenic diet. This study included forty-five children diagnosed by standard criteria between the ages of three and eight years old. They were divided into three groups of fifteen and received the modified Atkins diet, a gluten-free casein-free diet, or a diet labeled "well-balanced nutrition" (the control group). All patients received neurological examinations and anthropometric measurements, and were assessed with the Childhood Autism Rating Scale (CARS) and Autism Treatment Evaluation Test (ATEC) scales both before and six months after starting the diet. Both special diet groups showed significant improvement in ATEC and CARS scores in comparison to the control group. However the children on the modified Atkins diet also scored better results for cognition and sociability compared to gluten-free casein-free diet group (El-Rashidy, 2017).

In the case of children with autism, the benefits of a ketogenic diet could potentially outweigh the risks, so it is worth considering with a physician's approval and monitoring and help from a qualified nutritionist experienced in ketogenic diets.

SENIORS

A major worry among seniors as they grow older is fading memory and whether or not this will lead to dementia, such as Alzheimer's disease. Loss of muscle strength is also a big problem, since it can affect one's ability to carry out everyday functions as simple as getting up from a chair. Evidence is beginning to accumulate that at least some elderly people who do not yet have dementia can benefit from increasing their ketone levels through the ketogenic diet or by taking MCT oil; benefits may include better cognitive performance and perhaps even greater muscle strength. When my husband, Steve, improved after taking coconut oil and MCT oil, we saw not just cognitive improvements, but his tremors virtually went away. After about two months on this new diet, his slow, stiff gait returned to normal, and he was able to pick up his feet and run again.

Dr. Stephen Cunnane of Sherbrooke University in Canada has been performing glucose and ketone PET scans on healthy younger and older adults, as well as on people with mild cognitive impairment and Alzheimer's disease. He has confirmed that the areas of the brain affected by Alzheimer's show decreased glucose uptake but that these same areas take up ketones normally, a profound finding that supports the idea that ketones could provide alternative fuel to the brain. He has found that there is an energy gap in the brain in older people without dementia. This gap, which is the difference between how much energy the brain needs and how much energy the brain actually receives, is greater in people with mild cognitive impairment and even more so in people with Alzheimer's disease. (See Chapter 5 for Dr. Cunnane's story and related references.) He has found that ketones supply about 3 percent of the energy to the brain all throughout adulthood. Furthermore, while the young adult is able to meet the energy needs of the brain, there is an energy gap of about 7 percent in cognitively normal older adults, and this gap is higher when there is memory impairment. He has learned through PET scan studies that taking 30 to 45 grams per day of MCT oil could fill in the energy gap. This was reported at the Alzheimer's Association International Conference in July 2017 and will likely be published by the time this book is in print (Croteau 2018 B, in press). Dr. Cunnane and associates have also learned that walking on a treadmill for forty minutes three times a week triples ketone uptake to the brain in people with Alzheimer's, and this would very likely apply to healthy older adults as well. This is discussed in more detail under Exercise with citations in Chapter 7.

In early 2018, there are studies in progress using ketogenic substances such as MCT oil, a strict classic ketogenic diet, and the MCT oil modified ketogenic diet in people with mild cognitive impairment. While there is a good chance the classic ketogenic diet will prove to be beneficial, the main problem is that it takes a highly motivated patient as well as a highly motivated caregiver and supportive family to maintain a strict ketogenic diet for the long haul. One slip up can stop ketosis immediately, and it can take days to get back up to the desired ketone level. The MCT oil diet still requires considerable motivation but allows more carbohydrate and can help maintain at least a baseline of ketosis even if a meal with too many carbs creeps in here and there. Coconut oil can be part of this diet and would confer the benefits of lauric acid not found in MCT oil (see Chapter 7). One problem with the MCT oil diet is that many people, as many as 20 to 25 percent of patients, experience diarrhea or other intestinal discomfort even with amounts of MCT as small as 5 or 10 grams (1 or 2 teaspoons). It is possible to overcome this by starting with a very small amount, such as 2 grams two or three times a day with food and increasing very slowly. In most cases, there is no rush, so gradually adding MCT oil to the diet could ultimately provide good results. Most people (but not all) tolerate coconut oil more easily than MCT oil; mixing MCT and coconut oil could work well for many people. (See Chapter 7.)

If the ketogenic diet isn't practical for your family, adding coconut oil and/or MCT to the usual diet could be helpful for some people by mildly increasing ketone levels. MCT oil (C8 or a combination of C8 and C10 are widely available) is extracted from coconut oil or palm kernel oil. MCT oil is more ketogenic. However, lauric acid (C12), which constitutes about half the fats in coconut oil, appears to stimulate ketone production in the brain cells called astrocytes, is anti-microbial, and has anti-cancer properties. (See Chapter 7.) My belief and personal practice is that both coconut and MCT oil are each probably beneficial for different reasons for prevention and improvement for age-related memory problems and even for mild, cognitive impairment and Alzheimer's disease in some people. Why some people respond, and others do not, is a mystery at present.

Several studies show encouraging results from simply adding MCT oil to the regular diet for people with mild cognitive impairment or Alzheimer's. Around 2000, Samuel Henderson, had the brilliant idea that the mild ketosis from consuming MCT oil might be beneficial to people with Alzheimer's disease, and he formed the Accera company to test and eventually market a medical food called Axona, in which the only active ingredient is pure tricaprylic acid (C8) MCT oil powder. In their studies, leading to recognition of Axona as a medical food, there was cognitive improvement in nine out of twenty people after just one 40-gram serving of MCT compared to the day they received a placebo. They then performed a long-term study for ninety days with 152 people and had similar results; nearly half of the people tested had sustained cognitive improvements. When they stopped the MCT oil at the end of the study, the improvements disappeared. In both of their studies, people who were negative for the APoE4 gene—which is a major risk factor for Alzheimer's—improved on average; those who carried this gene, on average, did not improve (Reger, 2004; Henderson, 2008).

Finding a press release in 2008 about the results of Accera's first study led me down this whole path to awareness about ketones as an alternative fuel for the brain. Axona was not available yet in 2008, but I learned that it was extracted from coconut oil. As recounted earlier, based on that knowledge, I started giving coconut oil to Steve, who had moderately severe early-onset Alzheimer's disease. He experienced a remarkable improvement from taking just coconut oil and even more with mixing coconut and MCT oil. He took it with each meal and eventually added a bedtime dose. Steve was positive for the ApoE4 gene but responded anyway, and I learned from one of the authors of the Axona studies that some individuals who were ApoE4 positive responded but when they averaged the scores together as a group they did not. In the introduction, I present the story of Steve's struggle with Alzheimer's and how ketosis helped him improve substantially for several years.

After Axona was released and available, researchers conducted a retrospective study, meaning that they looked back at the records of people who were taking the medical food. They found that 80 percent of the fifty-five people they studied were stable or experienced improvement after eighteen months. The case reports were presented in a separate article (Maynard, 2013A and B). The researchers went on to conduct a large study of Axona, but unfortunately, a change in the product's formulation apparently made it non-ketogenic and they did not see positive results. They were not aware that the product did not increase ketone levels until after the study was finished and the data were reviewed.

Other encouraging results come from Japan where an experiment was conducted in a senior care facility for three months with thirty-eight frail elderly patients. One-third of the people continued to eat their regular diet, one-third received a food containing 6 grams of MCT oil, 1.2 grams of leucine (a branched-chain amino acid that can convert to ketones) and vitamin D, and one-third received the same supplement but with long-chain fats instead of MCT oil. After three months, the people taking the supplement with MCT oil had significant improvements in their cognitive testing by 10.6 percent in the mini-mental status exam (increasing from an average of 16.8 to 18.4 points) and by 30.6 percent on the Nishimura geriatric rating scale for mental status (increasing from an average of 24.6 to 32.2 points). The people who were on the regular diet or took the supplement with long-chain fats plus leucine and vitamin D all had worse cognitive scores after three months (Abe, 2017). Abe and his associates published a second report looking at the effects on some physical parameters with this same group of elderly people, and they found that the group who received the supplement with MCT had significantly better muscle strength after three months (improved hand grip by 13.1 percent, speed of walking by 12.5 percent, and a leg open and close test by 68.2 percent) and also had 28.2 percent increase in their peak expiratory flow, a test of lung function (Abe, 2016).

Another study showed improvements in working memory, visual attention, and task switching in nineteen elderly adults without dementia after they received a single "ketogenic meal" with 20 grams of MCT oil (Ota, 2016).

Parkinson's disease is another common condition affecting mainly the elderly and sometimes younger people, and it can often progress to dementia as well. The most obvious symptoms are tremors when the person is at rest, stiffness, a stooped over shuffling gait, and a weak voice. A study of diet in more than 1,000 people with Parkinson's disease showed that people who ate canned fruits and vegetables, other canned foods, and beef; drank soda whether sweetened or diet; and ate fried foods and ice cream seemed to have accelerated progression of their disease; people who ate fresh vegetables and fruits, nuts, fish, turkey, wine, coconut oil, olive oil, eggs, and fresh herbs and spices had slower-than-average rates of progression of Parkinson's disease. A noteworthy point here is that the people who fared better were eating a more whole food diet that is quite similar to the Mediterranean diet.

One group suggests, based on the available evidence, that a "Keto-Mediet" approach using a Mediterranean diet but including coconut oil in place of saturated animal fats, along with exercise could potentially prevent or decrease the rates of Alzheimer's (Perng, 2017).

Suggestions for Seniors

Based on the evidence summarized above, I believe the best approach for seniors who want to try to prevent dementia and any number of other chronic diseases such as diabetes and its complications is to transition toward a whole food, Mediterranean type diet that includes coconut oil and MCT oil, and eliminates as much excessive sugar as possible. While a strict ketogenic diet is possible, it requires great motivation for the long haul, and it may be more feasible to cut down on carbs to somewhere between 50 and 130 grams per day and replace the calories with healthy fats. It is also very important to get adequate protein, about 1 gram for every two pounds you weigh (1.1 grams for each kilogram of body weight), to help maintain muscle mass. The more you cut down on carbohydrates and increase fat, the more likely this diet will be ketogenic. If you have type 2 diabetes, cutting down even more on carbs could be very beneficial.

Adding coconut oil and MCT oil could further support getting into and staying in mild ketosis. Ideally, the carbohydrates would come from mainly low-glycemic-index foods (see Chapter 6) that will not send the blood sugar and insulin levels shooting up. For people who are elderly or have medical conditions, I strongly advise you to get your doctor involved before starting a very-low-carbohydrate diet.

The principles of how to get started on such a diet are covered in Chapter 2, and the finer details are in Chapter 6. Also, I have written another book for this very purpose that you might find helpful called *The Coconut Oil and Low-Carb Solution for Alzheimer's, Parkinson's and Other Diseases.* The plans for eating in this book apply beyond neurologic diseases, and anyone could benefit from making these changes.

Regarding exogenous ketone supplements, such as ketone salts and ketone esters, it is important for seniors to involve the physician for close monitoring. There can be adverse effects with these products, but, on the other hand, there could be great benefits as well. While there are no organized studies published yet for use of exogenous ketone supplements in seniors, many individuals have reported improvements in energy level, mental clarity, memory, focus, sleep, reduced anxiety, and a sense of just feeling better. My own husband, Steve, had a significant reversal of many of his Alzheimer's symptoms while taking the betahydroxybutyrate-butanediol ketone ester as a pilot study of one person that was published in 2015 (Newport, 2015). For some people, the benefits of using ketone salts or ketone esters could outweigh the risks.

Again, if you decide to try ketone salts or a ketone ester, only do so with close monitoring by your physician. Also, take it slow! Packages of ketone salts generally contain about 8 to 11 grams of betahydroxybutyrate per serving but, if you are a senior or have any medical condition, it would be wise to begin with about ¼ of a serving and increase as tolerated. The better results with a ketone salt product would be expected with the D-beta-hydroxybutyrate product from Pruvit called Keto//OS Max than with a 50/50 mixture of D- and L-betahydroxybutyrate. Ideally, carbs would be reduced and healthy fats increased in the diet, but if this is not practical ketone salts could potentially help with memory and cognition. There are anecdotal reports of cognitive improvement in seniors taking ketone salts (see the story of Joe and Carol Prata in Chapter 5) and hopefully clinical trials will be conducted soon to provide more definitive evidence.

The ketone ester is currently being marketed to elite athletes to improve their athletic performance and is not currently recognized as safe (as of early 2018) for use in anyone other than athletes. The dose in one serving is 25 grams, which is quite substantial, and could push the ketone levels into the high range in a matter of thirty to sixty minutes and also cause temporary low blood sugar and mild ketoacidosis. The dose my husband received was about 25 grams three times a day, and his ketone levels were quite high (3.5 to 5 mmol/L) at this dose and he did tolerate it well. His blood sugar dropped every time we tested his levels, regardless of what he ate just after the dose and noting that we were using a concentrated sugar product to make it drinkable. It is important to know that Steve had advanced Alzheimer's with symptoms already for nine years when he started taking the ester and was in his early sixties and otherwise physically in great health.

A big question is whether someone who is trying to prevent Alzheimer's or has memory impairment related to age would need a dose of 25 grams and my belief is they probably would not. The ketone ester is currently quite expensive: $90 to100 for 75 grams, and the jet fuel taste will take your breath away. If you decide to go this route, do it with your physician's approval and help, and begin slowly with perhaps 5 to 10 grams one to three times a day. That could be all you need to see a benefit.

With ketone salts and with ketone esters, if you are diabetic it is important to monitor your blood sugar level very closely since it is likely to drop. There is more information about possible adverse effects from using ketone salts, ketone esters and a strict ketogenic diet in Chapter 10 and on monitoring for healthy and not so healthy people in Chapter 9.

PEOPLE WITH CANCER

Cancer cells thrive on sugar, but most cancers cannot use ketones for fuel. Cancers are so greedy for sugar that some cancer cells take up as much as two hundred times the amount of glucose as a normal cell. The amino acid glutamine is also used by most cancer cells. Evidence is growing that using the ketogenic diet could shrink cancerous tumors and kill small metastases (growths of the cancer in other locations in the body). Studies looking at the ketogenic diet alone or in combination with a ketone ester and/or hyperbaric oxygen are having promising results in animals. The main cancer studied to date is an aggressive brain cancer called glioblastoma. The ketogenic diet can be used in conjunction with "standard of care" treatments for cancer, such as surgery, chemotherapy, and radiation. Potentially the ketogenic diet could shrink a cancerous tumor enough that it will be easier to remove when the time comes for surgery. Numerous human volunteers with cancer have reported a good response, some quite remarkable, to the ketogenic diet and several human clinical trials should be underway by the time this book is in print. See the stories of Dr. Thomas Seyfried and Dr. Angela Poff in Chapter 5 for more specific information about this.

If you have cancer and are considering a ketogenic diet, here are some facts you should know. The first is that the classic ketogenic diet seems to be the most effective approach; it can result in ketone levels well into the therapeutic range of 4 to 6 mmol/L. And lowering blood sugar is critical to the process, probably to less than 60 mg/dL. While most people who are not in ketosis would have symptoms of hypoglycemia when the blood sugar is this low, ketones provide alternative fuel to the brain and other organs, and these tissues can continue to function when ketone levels are elevated in the face of low blood sugar (Page, 2009).

To get it right and have your best chance at controlling the cancer, it is very important that you use the help of a qualified nutritionist or dietician who has experience with the strict ketogenic diet. If you decide to go this route, it should be thought of as a lifelong commitment, since stopping the diet could allow the cancer to take over again. This strategy could buy valuable time for you and your family.

PEOPLE WITH OTHER MEDICAL CONDITIONS

Many middle-aged people already suffer from chronic conditions like diabetes, metabolic syndrome, high blood pressure, and heart disease, often with a long list of medications. Many of these same people could benefit greatly by changing their diet, getting away from excessive sugar intake, and eating more high-quality proteins, fresh vegetables, and healthy fats. Like seniors and every other group we have discussed in this chapter, the same principles apply, whether you plan to try a lower-carb diet or a ketogenic diet, add coconut oil and/or MCT oil to your diet, or try an exogenous ketone supplement like ketone salts or ketone esters. Chapter 9 details monitoring for healthy and not-so-healthy people, and Chapter 10 discusses the common problems that may occur when starting a ketogenic diet or using exogenous ketone supplements. Please read through these carefully before getting started and know that it is imperative to get approval and help from your doctor. It is very possible as time goes on that you might need less of certain medications and may even be able to wean completely off them, however, this should be done only with your doctor's permission.

PETS

It is amazing how much carbohydrate is found in foods for dogs, cats, and other pets. If they were living in the wild without us to feed them, they mainly would be eating meat and would not have access to rice, other grains, or even vegetables. Commercial pet foods tend to be very high in carbohydrate and low in protein and fats, containing grains and fillers. It is no wonder that the same conditions are on the rise in our pets that we are seeing in ourselves, like obesity and diabetes.

Dogs can develop a form of Alzheimer's disease and are sometimes used in studies of the disease. The ketogenic diet is sometimes successfully used in animals to treat epilepsy. One lady reported to me that after she began giving her fourteen-year-old Welsh terrier small amounts of coconut oil, the dog began finding her way to her food bowl again, and she had more energy. Another lady reported that her dog's mastoid tumor virtually shrank away after she placed her pet on a ketogenic diet, and she shared with me the pictures to prove it. Cancer is the leading cause of death in dogs and also affects about one-third of cats. In animal cancer studies, the response to the ketogenic diet is quite impressive. One group, Keto Pet (http://www.ketopetsanctuary.com/), which was founded in 2014 through the Epigenix Foundation, has taken a special interest in treating pets with cancer using the ketogenic diet and other standard treatments. Some pet food companies are beginning to recognize the problem of too much car-bohydrates and are marketing higher quality products. The Internet has an abundance of keto recipes for pets.

Dogs and cats seem to like coconut oil a lot. One of my friends uses coconut oil as a moisturizer when she gets out of the shower and her little Chihuahuas are poised and ready to lick it off as soon as she puts it on her skin. Another friend used coconut oil on her face (lauric acid kills the bacteria that causes acne), and her cat also could not resist licking it off. Others have shared a similar experience with their pets.

Coconut oil is safe to give to animals and is part of the feed for pigs and other animals in parts of the world where coconut oil is a staple in the diet. I suggest starting with a small amount, such as ¼ teaspoon for each 10 pounds that the animal weighs and mixing it into his or her food once or twice a day. Just like humans, pets can have diarrhea if they eat too much coconut oil, so starting slowly is a good idea.

CHAPTER 9

MONITORING FOR HEALTHY AND NOT-SO-HEALTHY PEOPLE

This chapter discusses two different types of monitoring for people on the ketogenic diet. The first involves specifically monitoring ketone levels, and the second covers other parameters that might be monitored depending on one's health status. As with any new diet or nutritional supplement, it is important for elderly people and people with medical conditions to consult with their physician before starting a ketogenic diet and/or using ketone salts or ketone esters.

TO MONITOR OR NOT TO MONITOR KETONE LEVELS

Is ketone-level monitoring necessary? For the average person, probably not, but doing so could provide useful information to help you modify your strategies, as well as offer positive reinforcement and encouragement.

Ketone and glucose monitoring are strongly recommended for someone who is using the classic ketogenic diet for epilepsy or cancer or another serious medical condition; or for someone with diabetes who is attempting to control blood sugar levels through nutritional ketosis; or for someone who is taking a supplemental ketone ester.

Monitoring Ketone Levels

It is not always necessary for healthy people who are transitioning to a low-carb ketogenic diet to measure ketone levels, however, this information could provide positive reinforcement and reassure you that the ketone level is, in fact, elevated. When transitioning from a higher-carb to a low-carb ketogenic type diet, it can take several days to begin to see a significant increase in ketone levels, and the ketone level may continue to rise for two or three weeks before leveling off. The ketone level can fluctuate somewhat throughout the day, often lower in the morning and peaking in the mid afternoon or later and can vary considerably from person to person. You can measure ketone levels in several ways: in the urine, in the blood, or by use of a breath analyzer.

Different methods for achieving a state of ketosis yield different results in terms of measurable ketone levels. If you are not in ketosis, you could expect your blood ketone levels to be no greater than 0.1 mmol/L and a urine test strip to indicate "negative," meaning you are not in ketosis. Using exogenous ketone supplements, such as ketone salts and ketone esters, can give you a jump start on getting into ketosis and increase ketone levels within thirty to sixty minutes of taking the product. Using coconut oil and MCT oil as a regular part of the diet can help increase and sustain a baseline level of ketones. A serving of ketone salts containing 8 to 10 grams of betahydroxybutyrate typically increases the betahydroxybutyrate level by 0.5 to 1 mmol/L. So, if your baseline level is 1 mmol/L, you can expect the betahydroxybutyrate level to increase to 1.5 to 2 mmol/L temporarily. The level will peak somewhere between thirty and sixty minutes and return to baseline within a few hours. Unless you start at a constant baseline level of 6 mmol/L or higher, it is very unlikely you will get into trouble with ketoacidosis with a single serving of ketone salts.

Ketone esters can easily increase ketone levels at least five times higher than ketone salts, depending on the dose. A very high dose, resulting in levels of 7.0 mol/L or higher, could lead to ketoacidosis. So, in the case of taking ketone esters, closely monitoring the ketone level is recommended to determine the dose that works for you and ensure you are not getting into dangerous territory. Once you have established your ideal dose, you may not need to monitor your level as frequently.

Urine Ketone Test Strips

When blood levels of ketones become elevated, excess ketones filter out of the blood into the urine. Urine ketone test strips were originally developed for diabetics to help determine if they are going into diabetic ketoacidosis when the blood sugar is elevated. Many companies sell urine test strips that change color when ketone levels are elevated—usually the deeper the color, the higher the ketone level. If you are not in ketosis, the test strip color will indicate "negative." Most brands have a color code for trace, small, moderate, and large amounts of ketones in the urine. This will not tell you what your actual blood ketone level is, but it can give you a rough idea of whether you are in ketosis or not and how much.

One of the drawbacks to using urine test strips is that they typically measure only the ketone acetoacetate and not betahydroxybutyrate, which tends to be much more elevated than acetoacetate during ketosis. You could have a decent level of betahydroxybutyrate that might not be reflected by the urine test strip. Also, if you drink a lot of fluid, ketones in the urine might be diluted and fall below the levels detected by the urine dipstick.

Some urine ketone test strips state clearly on the package that they measure acetoacetate, and others do not; you might consider contacting the manufacturer directly to find out. (See Photo 9.1.)

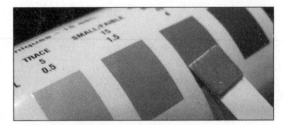

Photo 9.1. Urine ketone strips usually measure acetoacetate but not betahydroxybutyrate.

Blood Ketone Monitoring

A more direct way to measure betahydroxybutyrate is by using a blood glucose/ketone monitor with ketone test strips. These monitors were developed for diabetics and come with a lancet holder and disposable lancets to prick your finger. The ketone test strips require only a small drop of blood and a matter of seconds to get results. The opposite of urine test strips, the ketone test strips do not detect the ketone acetoacetate, but rather D-betahydroxybutyrate. The test strip does not contain the enzyme to detect L-betahydroxybutyrate, so if you are taking a ketone salt or ester that is predominantly L-betahydroxybutyrate or a racemic mixture of the two forms, you could have a higher level of betahydroxybutyrate than the test result indicates. There are several different companies that make blood ketone monitors, including Precision Xtra, NovaMax, and Keto Mojo. All three of these meters are capable of measuring both ketones and glucose but require separate strips to do so. At the time of this writing, the Keto Mojo strips are the least expensive, and the glucose test strip can also measure hemoglobin and hematocrit. All three monitors can be ordered online.

Whenever I test my own blood ketone level, I have a second monitor set up to test my blood sugar at the same time without requiring a second finger prick. It is not easy to run both the ketone and blood glucose test from the same finger prick. I do this to keep an eye on my fasting blood sugar, and I like to document how exogenous ketone supplements affect my blood sugar. A positive health benefit is that fasting blood sugar tends to trend down when transitioning from a higher-carb to a low-carb ketogenic diet and blood sugar also drops shortly after taking MCT oil, ketone salts, and ketone esters. The blood glucose monitors themselves are not very expensive, usually less than $40. At present, ketone test strips cost around $1 to $2 each, and glucose test strips cost much less than that. (See Photo 9.2.)

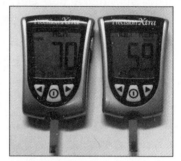

Photo 9.2. Two monitors are set up to test blood glucose and betahydroxybutyrate from the same finger prick.

Ketone Breath Analyzer

Another way to monitor ketosis is by using a ketone breath analyzer, which measures the ketone called acetone. Acetone becomes elevated and is mostly exhaled when you are in ketosis. Like the ketone urine strips, this will give you a rough estimate of how deeply you are into ketosis. The monitor itself is pricey, currently about $190, but it is reusable, and you can monitor your level of ketosis as often as you like throughout the day. This could be very helpful to trend the development of ketosis while you are transitioning from a higher-carb to low-carb diet and to see the before-and-after effects of various ketogenic strategies. (See Photo 9.3.)

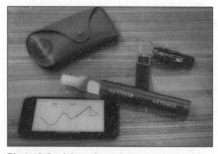

Photo 9.3. A breath analyzer can be used repeatedly throughout the day to detect acetone and can be used to estimate blood ketone levels.

Direct Lab Ketone Testing

The most definitive way to measure ketone levels is also the most expensive way: through direct lab testing of blood. Both betahydroxy-butyrate and acetoacetate can be measured with these techniques. This kind of monitoring would be most useful in ketone research where very precise levels are important. If you are having other lab work done, you could ask your doctor to include a ketone level if you really want to go this route.

MONITORING OTHER HEALTH PARAMETERS

Interest in the ketogenic diet and exogenous ketone supplements is grow-ing rapidly as people experience the benefits for themselves and share this information with others. People of all ages and from many walks of life are already using or want to use ketone salts and ketone esters for themselves or their loved ones, many of whom are very young or elderly or may have one or more chronic medical conditions. It is important for everyone con-sidering these lifestyle changes to be aware that they can include pitfalls (see Chapter 10). But many of these issues can be avoided if care is taken while transitioning to this lifestyle, including consulting your doctor when indicated by age or health and performing appropriate monitoring. What needs to be monitored also will depend on your age and your health status as well as why you are adopting the ketogenic lifestyle.

Basic Monitoring

For everyone starting the ketogenic diet and/or taking exogenous ketones, it is helpful to keep a journal and record the date and some base-line body measurements, particularly if you are trying to lose weight. If you are an athlete and already fit, you may experience changes in your body composition (less fat and more muscle) that could be reflected in these measurements. Many people have reported that their weight has not changed much but that their profile has as they lose body fat. Also, people who are very thin may be worried about losing too much weight, and if you're in this group, changes in these measurements could tip you off that you need to make adjustments in your diet.

Basic measurements could include:

- Weight.
- Height.
- Calculated body mass index (BMI) from height and weight (See side box below.)
- Measurements around chest, waist, hips, as well as around upper and lower arms and the thickest part of legs.
  - According to NIH recommendations, a waist measurement greater than 35 inches for women and greater than 40 inches for men indicates a higher risk of heart disease and type 2 diabetes mellitus. Measure your waist just above the hip bones and after you breathe out.
  - Measuring inches can provide encouragement when there is not much change on the scale. The same volume of muscle weighs more than fat and you could be gaining muscle and losing fat, an ideal scenario.
- Blood pressure and heart rate/pulse. Most electronic blood pressure instruments measure both blood pressure and pulse. You should consult with your physician if your blood pressure is too high (hypertension) or too low (hypotension). See side box, Blood Pressure Status for Adults.
  - Blood pressure guidelines were tightened in recent years. See side box for current guidelines from the NIH.
  - Normal pulse when you have been resting for at least ten minutes is between 60 and 100; generally, a lower number indicates better cardiovascular fitness. People who are very fit may have a heart rate lower than 60.
- Your pulse should be regular (pulsate evenly); if it is irregular, you should consult with your physician right away.
- Optional: If you are very serious about changing your body composition and want to monitor it beyond calculating your BMI, you could request measurements of skin fold thickness, or consider having a more definitive test such as a dual energy X-ray absorptiometry scan (DXA scan) or plethysmography specifically for body composition. Repeat annually or after losing a large amount of weight to make sure you are not losing too much muscle mass.

Body Mass Index (BMI)

The body mass index, or BMI, is a measure of body fat that applies to adults. It is based on height and weight. The ranges are the same for men and women. The main limitations are that the BMI can overestimate body fat for athletes and others who are muscular and can underestimate body fat in people who have lost muscle, such as the elderly.

BMI Categories:

Underweight: Less than 18.5

Normal weight: 18.5 to 24.9

Overweight: 25 to 29.9

Obese: 30 or greater

The actual formula to calculate BMI is complicated. Instead, you can easily plug in your height and weight to calculate your BMI with an online BMI calculator at: https://www.nhlbi.nih.gov/health/educational/lose_wt/BMI/bmicalc.htm

BLOOD PRESSURE STATUS FOR ADULTS

BLOOD PRESSURE STATUS	SYSTOLIC (upper number)	DIASTOLIC (lower number)
Hypotension (low blood pressure)	Less than 90	Less than 60
Normal	Less than 120	Less than 80
Pre-Hypertension*	120 to 139	80 to 89
Hypertension* Stage 1	140 to 159	90 to 99
Hypertension* Stage 2	160 or higher	100 or higher

*Hypertension = High blood pressure

The above values are from https://www.nhlbi.nih.gov/health-topics/high-blood-pressure

For blood pressure values for children see tables at https://www.nhlbi.nih.gov/files/docs/guidelines/child_tbl.pdf

Laboratory Testing

As you begin the ketogenic diet and/or an exogenous ketone supplement, during the first days to weeks, you could experience significant loss of water as well as important electrolytes and minerals, leading to dehydration. You must be careful to replace the fluid adequately and balance electrolytes. Odds are that your fasting blood sugar and insulin levels will drop as well.

Also, ketone salts contain significant amounts of sodium and may contain varying amounts of potassium, calcium and magnesium. This is an important consideration for children, the elderly, and people with medical conditions. People who have had problems with levels of sodium, potassium, calcium, or magnesium that are too low or too high, people who are taking diuretics, or people who need to restrict their sodium intake may not be good candidates for taking ketone salts but could do well with the ketogenic diet or a ketone ester. If you are determined to use ketone salts, your doctor or a nutritionist may be able to help you factor the mineral salts into your diet and adjust, for example, your potassium supplement to account for the amounts in ketone salts. If you have any condition mentioned above as well as heart disease, high blood pressure, diabetes, cancer, hormone abnormalities, kidney or liver disease, take blood thinners for any reason, or have any other chronic medical condition, it is extremely important to involve your doctor before getting started with the ketogenic diet or exogenous ketones.

In addition to the basic measurements mentioned in the previous section, your doctor may wish to check various blood markers before you start a ketogenic program, after three to six weeks from your start, and periodically thereafter, depending on your age and health status. Many of the blood tests listed here can be done as part of two tests called the complete blood count (CBC) and the complete blood panel (CMP), and results might include information on:

- electrolytes (sodium, potassium, chloride, bicarbonate)
- minerals (calcium, phosphorus, magnesium)
- fasting blood glucose

- lipid profile (Total, LDL, HDL, VLDL cholesterol and triglycerides; LDL-P is a newer test that tests cholesterol particle size and may be a better indicator of heart disease risk.)
- kidney function (BUN, creatinine, and GFR)
- liver function (ALT, AST, GGT)
- white blood count, hemoglobin, hematocrit, and platelet count
- hemoglobin A1C (a test for diabetes)
- presence of thyroid disease or other hormone issues (Baseline studies for these may be indicated as well.)

C-reactive protein is a test used to screen for inflammation. This would be helpful to check as a baseline and to follow if it is abnormal. Ketones are anti-inflammatory, and it would be interesting to see whether this test reflects your lifestyle changes over time.

If you are on blood thinners and your doctor allows you to try the ketogenic diet or exogenous ketones, it would be important to check your clotting studies before you get started and within a week or possibly sooner, after starting. Changes in diet can sometimes affect blood clotting for people taking warfarin or other medications.

TAKE THESE GUIDELINES TO YOUR DOCTOR

Ketone salts and ketone esters are so new that most doctors don't know about them yet, much less the potential of ketones to provide alternative fuel to the brain and other organs, reduce inflammation, and burn fat. I suggest that you take the information contained in this book to your doctor for guidance in what needs to be monitored. Your doctor may decide to pass this information on to other patients when they see how a ketogenic diet and/or exogenous ketones have improved your life.

CHAPTER 10

COMMON AND NOT-SO-COMMON PROBLEMS WITH EXOGENOUS KETONES AND THE KETOGENIC DIET

Although adopting a low-carbohydrate ketogenic lifestyle can have very positive health benefits, transitioning abruptly from a high-carb to a low-carb diet can be a challenge and is not without potentially unpleasant side effects. Dehydration, constipation, upset stomach, and electrolyte imbalances are common early on, but these are usually temporary and may be avoidable. In this chapter, we will also discuss the question of whether the ketogenic diet can lead to diabetic ketoacidosis.

KETO-ADAPTATION AND "KETO FLU"

The process of making the transition from a higher-carbohydrate to a low-carb, ketogenic diet is called "keto-adaptation." Basically, while shifting from burning mainly glucose to burning fat, your metabolism will undergo very significant changes.

Human metabolism is very complex and involves hundreds, if not thousands, of chemical reactions. Different chemical reactions, using different enzymes are at play, depending on whether metabolism is driven by glucose or by fatty acids and ketones as fuel. Different transporters are required to ferry glucose, fatty acids, and ketones across cell membranes. More mitochondria are needed to burn fat within cells. As ketone levels increase, blood sugar and insulin levels decrease, which can affect multiple biochemical pathways. All of this takes time to unfold and, in the process, you might feel the effects of these changes. Many people, but not all, develop symptoms that have been called the "keto flu" that can last for days to weeks (Volek, 2015; Volek, 2016). (It's not a true influenza infection, but think of the muscle aches and fatigue that happen when you have the flu.)

This happens for several reasons. Early on, as we transition to a low-carb, low-calorie diet, we tend to lose quite a bit of water, especially from muscle, and the water takes with it important minerals such as sodium, potassium, calcium, and magnesium. If this fluid is not replaced, it is possible to become dehydrated. Also, blood glucose and insulin levels tend to drop, which can cause symptoms as well. For these reasons, it is important for people who are elderly or have medical conditions to work with their doctor when abruptly changing the diet.

The symptoms of keto flu can include fatigue and lethargy, dizziness or light-headedness, trouble focusing, brain fog, headaches, sugar cravings, muscle cramping, irritability, difficulty sleeping, and upset stomach with nausea and diarrhea.

People want quick results when starting a new diet to lose fat. However, one way to avoid keto flu is to cut down gradually on carbs instead of going overnight from a high-carb to a very low-carb diet. Although the results may be slower, there is less chance that keto flu will compel you to abandon the diet altogether. You could start by eliminating obvious sugary drinks, fruit juices, and sweets; begin to increase the fats and oils in the diet; and eat smaller portions of grains and starchy vegetables. Then begin to reduce calories and count carbs, perhaps aiming initially for 50 grams of carbs or less per day and then decrease by 5-gram increments every few days. A strict ketogenic diet could ultimately go as low as 10 to 20 grams of carbs per day, possibly less, mainly as non-starchy vegetables and possibly a few berries or nuts.

Some other things you can do to conquer "keto flu" are:

- Stay well hydrated. Drink plenty of water and/or other clear fluids without added sugar and aim for at least eight to ten 8-ounce servings per day. If you perform heavy exercise or otherwise sweat a lot, drink even more.
- Replace sodium and other minerals. Try bouillon broth or bone broth, coconut water or a sugar free drink with electrolytes; sprinkle sea salt on foods or take an electrolyte supplement.

- Temporarily increase total carbs (such as whole grains or more vegetables, but not sugar!) by 5 or 10 grams per day and/or increase total calories.
- If you have been a couch potato up until now, introduce exercise gradually.
- A short fast, while drinking plenty of fluids to avoid dehydration, can get you into ketosis more quickly and increase availability of ketones to the brain, which could alleviate some symptoms. You could add lemon or lime to water or tea to make the process more pleasant as well as help neutralize ketones, which are acids. You could also try a "fat fast" in which you abstain from food with the exception of eating fats, such as blending coconut oil and/or MCT oil into coffee or tea.
- Taking ketone salts can help get ketone levels higher faster and, at the same time, replace sodium, potassium, magnesium, and calcium that may otherwise be lost while on a ketogenic diet. The Pruvit Ventures company has done a particularly good job at testing and adjusting the balance of minerals in its ketone salts.

Most people get through the keto flu somewhere between a few days to two or three weeks. If you adhere strictly to the ketogenic diet, full keto-adaptation can occur in as little as six to eight weeks, but this process could take months for some people.

Studies of keto-adaptation are few at present, however, in 2016, Jeff Volek and associates reported their study of the metabolic differences between elite endurance athletes who eat a high-carb diet (>55 percent of calories as carbs) versus low-carb diet (<20 percent of calories as carbs and >60 percent as fat; Volek, 2016). The average time the athletes were on a low-carb diet was twenty months and ranged from nine to thirty-six months, so they were well into keto-adaptation. They compared twenty elite ultra-marathoners and ironman distance triathletes who were in the top 10 percent of finalists for their events, with ten in the high-carb and ten in the low-carb groups. On one day, the athletes performed a maximal oxygen consumption test (VO_2max) after fasting for four hours, which consisted of increasing their speed in increments, to determine their peak fat oxidation. They then fasted for ten hours overnight, after which they were given a shake that conformed to whether they were habitually eating a high-carb (50 percent carbs/36 percent fat/14 percent protein) versus a low-carb diet (5 percent carbs/81 percent fat/14 percent protein). Ninety minutes later, they ran for three hours on a treadmill at 64 percent of their maximal oxygen consumption, followed by a two-hour recovery period. Measurements of body composition, height, weight, energy expenditure, muscle glycogen, and numerous metabolites, including blood glucose, ketones, fatty acids, insulin, glycerol, and lactate were performed before and at various points during and after the study.

Peak fat oxidation was on average 2.3 times higher for the low-carb versus the high-carb athletes. A high rate of fat burning (about 1.2 grams of fat per minute) began almost immediately in the low-carb group after they began running on the treadmill and was sustained at about the same level throughout the three-hour run. For the high-carb athletes, fat burning occurred more gradually and never came close to the level of fat burning exhibited by the low-carb group (maximum about 0.8 grams of fat per minute). Instead the high-carb athletes burned glucose at much higher rates than the low-carb athletes, and the rate of burning glucose declined over time during the three-hour run. Muscle glycogen decreased by about the same amounts in both the high-carb and the low-carb athletes at the end of the run and at two hours after the run was over. Also of interest, ketone levels were about double throughout the study for the low-carb athletes compared to the high-carb athletes. The authors concluded that "chronic keto-adaptation in elite ultra-endurance athletes is associated with a robust capacity to increase fat oxidation during exercise while maintaining normal skeletal muscle glycogen concentrations."

What is the advantage for an elite endurance athlete to switch from eating a high-carb to a low-carb diet? We are capable of storing only about 2,000 calories of glucose in our bodies, which can be quickly used up during an endurance event, and so the athlete needs to have a supply of high-carb food or drink available to avoid "hitting the wall" when energy stores run out. The low-carb, keto-adapted athlete has a substantially larger store of fat to burn, on the order of 40,000 calories or more, and does not require replenishment of fat during the event.

CONSTIPATION

Constipation is a common complaint of people on the ketogenic diet and becomes a problem if the stools become hard and difficult to pass. This can be prevented by staying well-hydrated, keeping physically active, increasing fiber in the diet through vegetable choices, adding a fiber supplement or stool softener, and/or taking a magnesium supplement, such as magnesium oxide or magnesium citrate alone or in combination. Also, MCT oil and sometimes coconut oil have a laxative effect for some people. Taking a good probiotic could help keep your bowel movements regular as well. Some high-fiber vegetables include broccoli, cabbage, green beans, kale, spinach, and zucchini, and avocado is particularly high in fiber at 11 grams per medium fruit.

LOW BLOOD SUGAR AND DIABETES

Eating a low-carb diet tends to reduce blood sugar and insulin levels, which is a good thing for most of us. However, taking a ketone supplement, such as ketone salts or ketone esters, could rapidly lower blood sugar, resulting in temporary symptoms such as light-headedness, dizziness, hunger, shakiness, increased heart rate, headaches, and/or irritability. In theory, the increased level of ketones could prevent or reduce these symptoms from occurring, but this might not always be the case, particularly in the early stages of the diet when the baseline ketone level is not very elevated yet. An ounce or two of orange juice or apple juice could help increase the blood sugar enough to alleviate the symptoms.

Low blood sugar, also called hypoglycemia, could be a serious problem for people who are diabetic and are taking insulin and/or oral diabetic medications, since the blood sugar could become dangerously low if precautions are not taken. It is, therefore, extremely important for diabetics to work with their physician to closely monitor their blood sugar and adjust their medications accordingly. Some type 2 diabetics are able to wean off insulin and other diabetic medications in a matter of days to weeks if they restrict carbohydrates to 20 to 25 grams or less per day, and type 1 diabetics may find they need less insulin in short order. Should symptomatic low blood sugar occur, and drinking orange or apple juice does not help, request emergency services immediately.

ELECTROLYTE IMBALANCES

People who are taking diuretics, medications for high blood pressure or heart disease, and/or sodium or potassium supplements need to work closely with their doctor when adopting a low-carb ketogenic diet and/ or taking exogenous ketone supplements. At the beginning of a ketogenic diet, and when taking ketone supplements, considerable water can be lost from the body along with sodium, potassium, calcium, and magnesium. So, it is especially important for people taking medications to stay well-hydrated and to have their electrolyte and mineral levels monitored to ensure that they do not develop an imbalance that could lead to serious symptoms.

LOW BLOOD PRESSURE, HIGH BLOOD PRESSURE

If you are taking blood pressure or other heart medication, check with your doctor before starting the diet. Monitor your blood pressure several times per day and notify your doctor if your blood pressure becomes abnormally high or low, so that adjustments in your medication can be made if necessary. The blood pressure values considered too high or too low will vary from person to person depending on what your usual blood pressure runs on your medications, so your doctor is the best person to advise you what values should be of concern.

Many people with high blood pressure find that even a 10-pound weight loss can significantly lower their blood pressure, and many are able to reduce or even wean off blood pressure medications with their doctor's help.

Some people develop low blood pressure and experience light-headedness, especially when they stand up suddenly (called orthostatic hypotension) due to dehydration and/or loss of too much sodium from the body in the early stages of the ketogenic diet. This can be corrected by drinking plenty of fluids and drinking broth, adding sea salt to water or food, or taking an electrolyte supplement.

Certain people are very sensitive to sodium and taking ketone salts could increase blood pressure to the abnormal range. If this happens, call your doctor immediately and stop taking the ketone salts.

If you do not know what your blood pressure is normally, consider getting a baseline reading before you start the diet or before taking ketone salts and then monitor it periodically. If you do not own a blood-pressure cuff, many pharmacies have a free blood-pressure machine you can use. In general, normal blood pressure is currently considered to be less than 140 for the upper number (systolic) and less than 90 for the lower number (diastolic). The best time to take one's blood pressure is when you are resting and not overly exerting yourself.

There is evidence that a state of ketosis can help with heart disease, specifically congestive heart failure (Sato, 1995; Aubert, 2016; Huynh, 2016).

DIABETIC KETOACIDOSIS VERSUS KETOSIS

A question frequently asked by the general public and by physicians is whether increasing ketone levels through taking oils, such as coconut oil or MCT oil, or using exogenous ketone supplements, such as ketone salts or ketone esters, could cause diabetic ketoacidosis. The answer is of special importance for someone who is diabetic.

Ketones are acids, as are many other substances involved in our metabolism, but the body has natural processes in place to buffer, or neutralize, the acid. This buffering process occurs constantly to keep the pH of our blood within a very narrow range, normally between 7.35 and 7.45. The biochemical reactions in our metabolism are very sensitive to the blood pH and will shut down if the pH deviates too much out of the normal range. If the pH drops to about 7.2 or below, the situation becomes dangerous and potentially life-threatening. If the pH drops below 7.0, risk of death greatly increases unless immediate measures are taken to correct the acidosis.

Diabetic ketoacidosis is a life-threatening condition in which there is an absence of insulin and also extremely high blood sugar; it most often affects people with type 1 diabetes mellitus, or occasionally someone with type 2 diabetes. Glucose cannot get into cells to fuel them due to the lack of insulin, which is required for glucose to enter the cell. The body attempts to put more glucose into the blood through gluconeogenesis, basically making glucose from amino acids from muscle or from lactate or from the glycerol molecule that holds fatty acids together to form a triglyceride. Still, in this case, the gluconeogenesis is not particularly helpful, because insulin is not available to get the new glucose into the cells. Fat begins to break down rapidly, releasing fatty acids to provide alternative fuel, some of which are converted to ketones in the liver. The amount of ketone produced in this scenario can become massive, unless and until insulin is provided. The whole process overwhelms the ability of the body to neutralize the acid, such that the pH will eventually drop to a dangerous level that will halt chemical reactions and the organs will shut down, leading ultimately to death if there is no intervention to correct the problem.

Diabetics, particularly those who require insulin, are instructed to monitor their blood glucose levels closely and to check their ketone levels if the blood glucose is above a certain level. Urine ketone strips, which usually monitor the ketone acetoacetate, were developed to screen for increased ketone levels. They provide a rough estimate rather than an exact level of ketones. Blood ketone monitors, which directly measure the blood level of the ketone betahydroxybutyrate, may provide a better idea of the magnitude of the problem.

When ketone levels are increased as a result of taking coconut oil or MCT oil, overnight fasting, exercise, or moderate reduction in carbohydrates, the levels of ketones are many times lower than ketone levels in diabetic ketoacidosis and the resulting acid is easily buffered to keep the pH in the normal range. The body is even capable of buffering ketone levels that reach significantly higher levels, such as those that occur during starvation, intentional prolonged fasting, use of exogenous ketones in recommended serving sizes and in the classic ketogenic diet for epilepsy, though mild chronic metabolic acidosis has been reported in some people on the classic ketogenic diet. The levels in each of these conditions are still substantially below the levels that occur in diabetic ketoacidosis. Another important point is that a lack of insulin along with an abnormally high blood glucose are not part of the overall picture in nutritional ketosis, but both are required to produce diabetic ketoacidosis. (See Figure 10.1.)

It is conceivable that, if someone is on the edge of developing diabetic ketoacidosis, taking coconut oil, MCT oil, or ketone salts could tip a

```
    KETOGENIC STRATEGY :    KETONE LEVELS mmol/L:
                   Caffeine → 0.2 to 0.3
               Coconut Oil → 0.3 to 0.5
          Vigorous Exercise → 0.3 to 0.5
            Overnight Fast → 0.3 to 0.5
                   MCT Oil → 0.3 to 1.0
   Branched Chain Amino Acids → 0.3 to 1.0
       Ketone Mineral Salts → 0.5 to 1.0
        Classic Ketogenic Diet → 2 to 6
                 Starvation → 2 to 7
      Ketone Esters (Oral or IV) → 2 to 7 or higher
         Diabetic Ketoacidosis → 10 to 25
```

Figure 10.1. Betahydroxybutyrate levels in diabetic ketoacidosis are substantially higher than ketone levels that occur from ketogenic strategies such as diet, exercise, and exogenous supplements in recommended serving sizes.

person over the edge, though this is an extremely unlikely scenario. On the other hand, exogenous ketone esters can elevate ketone levels significantly and very quickly, so, if someone were to take an unusually large amount of a ketone ester (150 to 200 grams or more), the blood pH could drop to abnormally low levels and result in ketoacidosis. A dose of 50 grams in someone who is not already in ketosis could increase the betahydroxybutyrate level to as high as 7 mmol/L, which is equivalent to the expected range after prolonged fasting or starvation of a week or longer. It would be prudent for anyone who takes a ketone ester to monitor their betahydroxybutyrate levels to determine what dose range is appropriate for him or her, and this will likely vary from person to person.

MILD CHRONIC METABOLIC ACIDOSIS

There are reports that some children with epilepsy who are on the classic ketogenic diet, modified Atkins, or MCT oil long term (a year or longer) may experience chronic mild metabolic acidosis (slightly below normal pH that is corrected with more rapid breathing) and this condition may explain certain complications, such as kidney stones, osteopenia (thinning of the bone), fractures, growth retardation and rarely cardiac effects (prolonged QTc on ECG that could result in an abnormal heart rhythm). Use of certain medications, such as diuretics that increase loss of calcium in the urine, could exacerbate this problem. Metabolic acidosis can be confirmed with a lab test called "blood gases," which measures the blood pH, carbon dioxide level, oxygen levels, and bicarbonate level. During metabolic acidosis, the bicarbonate level is low in response to excess acid in the blood. In response, if the metabolism is operating normally, the person will breathe more rapidly, exhaling larger amounts of carbon dioxide. This process will buffer the acid and bring the pH back to normal and would therefore be considered "compensated metabolic acidosis."

A study looking for treatment of the problem of metabolic acidosis, found that use of potassium citrate could help correct this condition and prevent the complications (Sampath, 2007). Potassium citrate is available over the counter, however, taking too much could be dangerous, so you should consult with your doctor to determine the right amount of potassium citrate to take. This is especially important if you are already taking a potassium supplement for a medical condition. A safer alternative might be to take lemon or lime juice every day, which provides citric acid.

In a non-epilepsy population, a study of thirty-nine people by Dr. Yancy and others found that people on a low-carb weight-loss diet had a very slight, temporary decrease from their baseline pH levels (before starting the diet) and in their bicarbonate levels, but the lowest values they documented remained within normal pH range of 7.35 and 7.45 and the bicarbonate was 22 or greater for nearly everyone. Of interest, the people in the higher-carb weight-loss diet group had a slightly larger drop in their pH, compared to the low-carb dieters. No one in either group had a significant metabolic imbalance (Yancy, 2007).

The Acid-Sparing Ketogenic Diet

Yuen and others suggest that an "acidosis-sparing ketogenic" (ASK) diet could help reduce the problem of mild chronic metabolic acidosis and potentially improve seizure control while on the diet for epilepsy (Yuen, 2017). They note that mild chronic metabolic acidosis can also occur in some people eating a typical Western diet and cite several studies that report a higher risk of insulin resistance and diabetes in people who eat an "acidogenic" or acid-producing diet. They note that both ketones and products of fat metabolism are acidic and suggest the following measures to avoid the problem of chronic metabolic acidosis:

- Maintain steady hydration (neither too little nor too much), including a beverage at each meal, between meals, and before bedtime. Suggested beverages: mineral and spring waters high in calcium and bicarbonate and without fluoride, hot and cold infusions of mint, holy basil tea, passionfruit, ginger, lemon, coconut cream, cream shakes or smoothies, meat broths and soups, vegetable juices and vegetable soups.
- Aim for blood betahydroxybutyrate levels around 2 mmol/L or urine ketones at moderate (4 mmol/L) at the beginning of the diet, which can be achieved with 60 percent fat in the diet, and then slowly increase as needed (for example, to improve seizure control).
- Avoid caloric restriction to achieve moderate, but not deep, ketosis.
- Aim for protein intake of roughly 0.5 to 0.55 grams per pound of body weight per day.
- For carbohydrates, include fatty fruits such as avocados and olives; nuts and seeds; lemon and lime; salt-fermented vegetables such as sauerkraut and kimchee. Also include large fixed amounts of low-carbohydrate green vegetables that are high in potassium and bicarbonate and alkaline ash producing. These have a generous alkaline content that will neutralize acid.
- Alkaline vegetables, herbs and spices: alfalfa bean sprouts, artichokes, arugula, asparagus, avocado, bamboo shoots, beet greens, bok choy, broccoli, broccolini, Brussels sprouts, cabbage, cauliflower, celery, chard, collard greens, cucumber, daikon radish, eggplant, escarole, endive, green beans, green bell peppers, green onions, jicama, kale, kohlrabi, leeks, lettuces, mustard greens, okra, pickles, pumpkin, seaweeds, snap peas, snow peas, spinach, Swiss chard, turnips, water chestnuts, watercress, zucchini; basil, chives, cilantro, curry spices, marjoram, oregano, parsley, and thyme.
- Include the juice from a lemon or lime each day to generate bicarbonate (which buffers acid).

- Include a magnesium citrate supplement to help neutralize acid and reduce constipation; when epilepsy is the issue, magnesium itself may provide an anti-seizure effect.
- Avoid acid-producing drugs and supplements (sulfamethoxazole is an example of an acidic antibiotic; excessive vitamin C might be too acidic).
- They suggest using a combination of fats that will mimic the fats in human breast milk, including dairy fat (which contains more than 400 fatty acids), eggs yolks, pork, nuts and seeds as well as fish to obtain the important long-chain omega-3 fats docosahexanoic acid (DHA) and eicosapentanoic acid (EPA) and beef and lamb to provide the important omega-6 fat called arachidonic acid. They do not mention coconut oil and MCT oil, however, these could fit in as well.

Two good books that can serve as references for acidic and alkaline foods are *The Alkaline Diet for Beginners* by Jennifer Koslo and *The Acid Alkaline Food Guide* by Susan E. Brown and Larry Trivieri Jr.

KIDNEY STONES

If you have had kidney stones in the past, or are taking certain medications, you may have a greater risk of developing kidney stones on the ketogenic diet. Medications that may increase risk of kidney stones include, but are not limited to, diuretics like furosemide, acetazolamide, triamterine, hydrochlorothiazide, antacids, steroids such as dexamethasone, theophylline, larger than recommended doses of vitamin C or vitamin D, aspirin, probenecid, acyclovir, and indinavir. If you are taking medications, look for kidney stones in the list of possible side effects.

The measures discussed above under "Mild Chronic Metabolic Acidosis and the Acidosis-Sparing Ketogenic Diet" could help lower the risk of developing kidney stones.

GOUT AND KETONES—MIXED MESSAGE

The bad news about gout is that people who are prone to gout could have a flare up during the early days while transitioning to a ketogenic diet. People with gout tend to have high uric acid levels and uric acid crystals can form in joints, resulting in inflammation and extreme tenderness. The classic location of gout is in the large toe joint, but the entire foot or other joints can be affected as well. During the early weeks of the ketogenic diet, the uric acid level can increase and trigger an episode of gout. Like kidney stones, this could be prevented by taking a potassium citrate supplement. Again, consult with your doctor to determine the right dose of potassium citrate or citric acid for you. This is especially important if you are already taking a potassium supplement. An alternative is to take lemon or lime juice every day, which provides citric acid. Also, the prescription medication allopurinol could reduce the risk of gout but is not normally started during an acute episode. If you develop redness and tenderness in your big toe joint, or any other joint, while on the ketogenic diet, consult with your doctor. Gout can get out of control quickly.

The good news for people with gout is that once you get past the first month or so and ketone levels are elevated, the anti-inflammatory properties of the ketone betahydroxybutyrate appear to relieve gout flare-ups by inhibiting the Nlrp3 inflammasome in very specific cells, called macrophages, that react to the uric acid crystals by bringing on inflammation in the joints. Betahydroxybutyrate also blocks Interleukin-1β, another substance involved in gout inflammation. At the same time, betahydroxybutyrate does not impair the immune system's response to bacterial infection (Goldberg, 2017).

LIPOID ASPIRATION PNEUMONIA

Lipoid aspiration pneumonia occurs when a significant amount of oil, milk, or other fatty food is inhaled directly into the lung, where it can interfere with exchange of oxygen and carbon dioxide and produce serious inflammation. People at risk are those with a medical condition that affects swallowing, such as an infant; someone in the late stages of Parkinson's, Alzheimer's or other neurodegenerative disease; or perhaps someone with epilepsy who is heavily sedated by anticonvulsants. The best way to prevent this is to avoid giving pure oil orally to someone who cannot swallow normally. The oil should be mixed with other foods.

This could also happen in a healthy person who tries to drink oil straight and accidentally inhales the oil, so extra care must be taken if you like to take oil straight or floating on top of your coffee or tea.

RARE DEFECTS IN KETONE METABOLISM AND KETONE TRANSPORT

Several rare defects in ketone body metabolism can affect making ketones, breaking them down, or transporting ketones across cell membranes.

Defects in Ketone Body Synthesis

Two rare inherited defects, called inborn errors of metabolism, can affect the ability to make ketones (ketogenesis). One is a deficiency of mitochondrial HMG-CoA synthase, called mHS deficiency, which results in hypoglycemic (low blood sugar) crises, especially when the person has an intestinal illness, and the liver is enlarged as well. The person is unable to produce ketones normally and has high-free-fatty-acid levels resulting in metabolic acidosis (low blood pH), which sometimes can be quite severe. The extremely low blood sugar can produce brain damage. Ketone levels do not increase during fasting in individuals with this condition, so this can be used as a test to screen for this defect, followed by more specific testing.

Another genetic abnormality in making ketones is a deficiency in HMG-CoA lyase, called HL deficiency, which affects the ability to make ketones from fatty acid oxidation and from leucine, one of the branched-chain amino acids. During crises, the blood sugar can become extremely low along with high free fatty acids, low ketone levels, metabolic acidosis, liver dysfunction, and high ammonia levels in the blood. These two defects can present early in life but sometimes do not become apparent until the teen years or even later in adulthood (Fukao, 2014) (See Figure 10.2).

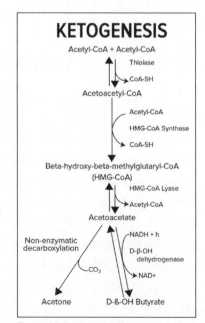

Figure 10.2. Ketogenesis.

Defects in Ketolysis

Two inherited inborn errors of metabolism interfere with breaking down ketones. One is succinyl

CoA:3-oxoacid CoA transferase deficiency, or SCOT deficiency for short. A SCOT deficiency results in episodes of ketoacidosis, in which ketones are very elevated and the blood becomes acidic, usually returning to normal between episodes. Some, but not all, people with SCOT deficiency have a permanent elevation of ketone levels in the blood and urine.

The other error is beta-ketothiolase deficiency, also called T2 deficiency. T2 is also involved in breaking down the branched-chain amino acid isoleucine, which then accumulates to abnormal levels. People with this defect have episodes of metabolic acidosis due to high ketone levels, with normal periods in between (Fukao, 2014) (See Figure 10.3.)

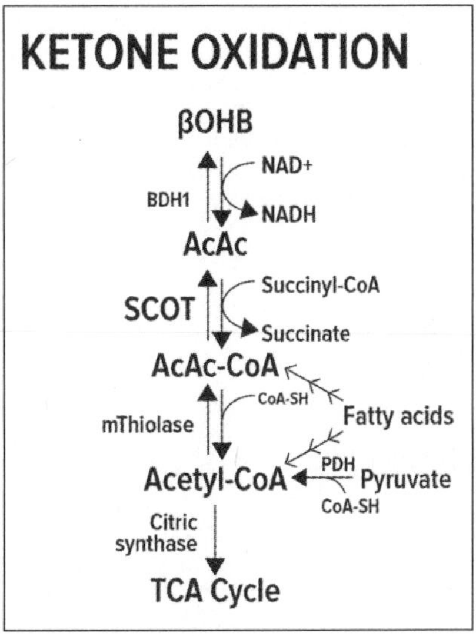

Problems with Ketone Transport

Several genetic mutations can cause a deficiency of monocarbox-ylate transporter 1 (also called MCT

Figure 10.3. Ketolysis.

1, but not to be confused with MCT oil, which is unrelated). Monocarboxylate transporters carry ketones through cell membranes, allowing the ketones to be utilized within the cell. MCT 1 also controls entry of ketones into the brain. If ketones are produced but cannot be transported into organs outside of the liver, a very severe life-threatening ketoacidosis can develop, causing the pH to drop below 7.0. These episodes tend to begin in infancy or early childhood, usually occur in response to poor feeding or infection and can be treated effectively with IV glucose. It is unusual for severe episodes to continue after age seven (Fukao, 2014).

CONTRAINDICATIONS TO THE KETOGENIC DIET

There are a number of medical conditions for which the ketogenic diet may be harmful and for which the ketogenic diet is contraindicated. These are listed on the fifth page of the updated recommendations of the International Ketogenic Diet Study Group published in 2018 (Kossoff, 2018).

CHAPTER 11

THE CONTROVERSY ABOUT SATURATED FAT, CHOLESTEROL, AND YOUR HEART

Periodically, since the early 1960s, the American Heart Association (AHA) has come out with a statement that perpetuates the lipid-heart hypothesis and demonizes saturated fats. (*Lipid* is another word for "fat.") This happened again when they published "Dietary Fats and Cardiovascular Disease: A Presidential Advisory" online in the February 2017 issue of the American Heart Association journal *Circulation* (American Heart Association, 2017). Unfortunately, the media has irresponsibly taken viral a fragment of information purporting that coconut oil may be bad for your heart from a single line opinion in the article. The coconut oil industry on the other side of the world, mainly composed of small farmers, is reeling from the effects of this latest careless media campaign. They have only recently been recovering from the previous advisory put forth by the AHA in the 1980s.

The conclusions of the advisory committee have some serious problems. The four "core studies" this committee relied on were all conducted in the 1950s, were relatively small groups, and included only men in three of the four studies. Further, these four studies were conducted in populations that almost certainly were not consuming coconut oil on any regular basis and were studies comparing diets with animal saturated fats to diets with polyunsaturated fats. Animal and human fat is well known to store hormones, pesticides, antibiotics, and other environmental substances, which could be a factor in heart disease, whereas vegetable fats such as coconut oil would not be so likely to contain these potentially harmful substances.

The authors do not mention whether age and smoking were controlled for in these studies; smoking, which was very prevalent in the 1950s compared to the 2010s is a major contributor to heart disease. The raw numbers of how many people in each group had cardiac events was not presented, making the summaries difficult to evaluate. The clincher in this article is that the authors state on page e13, under the section on coconut oil, *"Clinical trials that compared direct effects on CVD [cardiovascular disease] of coconut oil and other dietary oils have not been reported."* They rely on studies of individual saturated fatty acids that show a miniscule increase in LDL (so called "bad") cholesterol but rationalize away a similar small increase in HDL ("good") cholesterol and an improved LDL to HDL ratio. For example, in the study they cited, lauric acid (50 percent of coconut oil) resulted in a less than 1 mg/dl point increase in both LDL and HDL cholesterol, with typical LDL values ranging from less than 100 to 160 mg/dl. Could a change of less than 1 mg/dl really have that much impact?

In addition, the problem here is that natural fats such as coconut oil and even lard do not come as individual fatty acids but rather combinations of many fatty acids with different properties, which may balance each other out. Completely ignored in this report are the saturated fats in coconut oil known as medium-chain triglycerides that could balance out the longer-chain fats. Coconut oil also contains some mono- and polyunsaturated fats that are touted as healthy by this committee. One of the most important details that the AHA is missing here is that 70 percent of the saturated fats in coconut oil are medium-chain triglycerides (C6 through C12), which are either converted to ketones or burned immediately as fuel by muscle and other organs and not stored as fat. The omission of medium-chain triglycerides from the report is suspicious, since a table in the article on page e4, entitled "Fatty Acid Composition of Fats and Oils" does not contain columns for the medium-chain triglycerides C6, C8, and C10, which are not listed in this table and clearly present in coconut and palm kernel oils. This table also lumps lauric acid (C12) together with C14 and C16, even though lauric acid has many properties of medium-chain triglycerides, as well as some properties of longer-chain fatty acids.

Ketones, as we've discussed throughout this book, come from the breakdown of fat and provide an alternative fuel to the brain and most other organs during starvation or fasting or to cells that are insulin resistant. In a recent study conducted in Japan, lauric acid was found to potently stimulate ketone production in astrocytes in cultures; astrocytes are brain cells that nourish other brain cells (Nonaka, 2016). By comparison to coconut and palm kernel oils, butter, lard and animal fat contain minimal medium-chain triglycerides; nor are medium-chains found in soybean, olive, corn, safflower, and most other oils. There are hundreds of studies of potential benefits of coconut oil; for example, lauric acid, which makes up about 50 percent of coconut oil, is antimicrobial—there are numerous studies showing that lauric acid kills many bacteria, viruses, fungi like candida and protozoa. Lauric acid is not found in any significant amount in soybean, corn, canola and olive oils.

A few small cholesterol studies looking at coconut oil were conducted decades ago in animals and in a few men over a short term of days to weeks and using hydrogenated coconut oil—that is, the coconut oil used in the study wasn't in its natural form but rather had been subjected in a food lab to the hydrogenation process. It is well known that any hydrogenated oil will increase blood cholesterol levels. Furthermore, the diets were deficient in omega-3 fatty acids, a deficiency of which can increase cholesterol levels. By contrast, studies of entire populations for whom coconut oil provides one-third to two-thirds of the diet have shown that the study subjects were of normal height and weight, had normal blood pressure, triglycerides, and cholesterol levels at all ages (Prior, 1981).

In the 2017 article from *Circulation,* the committee surmises—without any proof—that people who eat saturated fats likely have other bad eating habits. These days, many, if not most, of the people who embrace coconut oil are likely embracing healthier foods as well and a healthier lifestyle in general, eating fish and/or taking omega-3 fats, which weren't on the radar in the 1950s when the so-called "core studies" for this report were conducted.

The folks in the AHA and other organizations who perpetuate these myths about coconut oil need to really do their homework and learn more about medium-chain triglycerides and study the other beneficial effects of coconut oil, which they choose to ignore. The point that some people may benefit from eating more polyunsaturated fat in place of animal fat may be very valid. However, coconut oil is not animal fat and, nevertheless, the bottom line that came out of their lengthy report is that "coconut oil is bad for your heart", which has now been perpetuated by media who jumped on this conclusion that was not even based on direct research of coconut oil and heart disease. This message has gone viral worldwide. The impact of this could take a devastating toll on the economies of countries that produce coconut oil, mostly made up of individual farmers and their families trying to make a living. These economies were devastated in the 1960s and again in the 1980s and have been slowly recovering from the initial similar AHA statement on saturated fats in 1961 based on the same four "core studies." It is irresponsible and unconscionable for this advisory committee to make such sweeping claims without direct proof that coconut oil causes heart disease.

OTHER COMMENTS AND SUGGESTED READING AND VIEWING

In my first book, *Alzheimer's Disease: What If There was a Cure? The Story of Ketones* (Second Edition, 2013, Turner Publishing), I dedicated an entire chapter to the questions surrounding saturated fat, cholesterol and statins.

Earlier in this book, there was a discussion of the PURE Study which, among other things, looked at the effects of fat and carbohydrates on heart disease and other conditions. To recap, this was an enormous study, published in *The Lancet* in 2017 that was conducted in eighteen countries on five continents worldwide with 135,335 participants who were studied for an average of 7.4 years. One of their relevant findings is that higher carbohydrate intake was associated with a higher overall risk of total mortality over that period of time. They also found that higher intake of total fat and of each type of fat, including saturated fat, was associated with a *lower than average risk of dying* prematurely and was not associated with a higher risk of heart disease, heart attacks or heart related deaths. Higher saturated fat intake was associated with a lower risk of stroke as well (Dehghan, 2017). This contradicts what the American Heart Association has preached since the 1960s, that we should eat a low-fat diet, which is more often than not a high-carb diet.

I also suggest you watch a YouTube presentation by David Diamond, Ph.D., a neuroscientist at the University of South Florida, who gives an eye-opening presentation on low- versus high-fat diets, saturated fats, cholesterol, and statins that can be viewed at YouTube.com (David Diamond—An Update on Demonization and Deception in Research on Saturated Fat. https://www.youtube.com/watch?v=uc1XsO3mxX8). He is also an author on an article on the same subject in the *British Medical Journal* in 2016 (Ravnskov, 2016).

CHAPTER 12

THE QUESTION: WHY GO KETO? THE ANSWER: WHY NOT?

In this book, we have reviewed the role of ketones in our evolution and how the ability of our brains to easily switch between using glucose and ketones has made it possible for humans to survive as a species. Our ancient ancestors were likely in at least a mild state of ketosis much of the time. Pregnant women, infants, and children develop ketosis more quickly than adult males and non-pregnant women, likely a survival mechanism. Very early in gestation, the fetus is capable of using ketones and the newborn who is breastfed goes into ketosis within hours of birth. Human breast milk is high in fat and contains medium-chain triglycerides, which are partly converted to ketones.

In addition to serving as an alternative fuel for brain cells and cells in other tissues, ketones impact other metabolic pathways, such as those involved with fat accumulation and fat burning, appetite, inflammation, and aging. Studies of fasting and exercise, which result in mild ketosis, show many beneficial effects. Many people who are on a ketogenic diet or using other ketogenic strategies, such as consuming medium-chain triglycerides or exogenous ketone supplements, report improvements in mood, sleep, memory, mental clarity, focus, behavior, improved physical endurance, and performance, as well as a general feeling of well-being.

It is not easy to get into and maintain moderate to high levels of ketones through a true ketogenic diet. This involves careful planning and consistency, with strict calculation and measurement of foods at each meal and snack. For people with epilepsy, cancer and neurodegenerative diseases, as well as endurance athletes, achieving moderate to high levels of ketosis could be rewarding. Adding medium-chain triglycerides to several meals per day can provide a foundation for sustained ketosis, and use of an exogenous ketone supplement, such as ketone salts, can build on this foundation to boost ketone levels higher into the therapeutic range.

The strict forms of the ketogenic diet are not without risk, and when used as a therapeutic for disease, the risks and benefits should be carefully weighed. A qualified nutritionist with experience in implementation of the ketogenic diet can help immensely.

Women who are pregnant or breastfeeding tend to be in ketosis naturally and there are a few reports suggesting that attempting a strict low-carbohydrate or ketogenic diet while pregnant or breastfeeding could result in serious complications, so a better strategy would be to eat a whole food diet with adequate protein, healthy fats, and a moderate amount of carbohydrates, mainly as vegetables and whole grains, and avoid excessive sugar. People with medical conditions, children and the elderly should always seek approval and support through monitoring by their health care provider.

By the same token, with the help of their doctor, people who are overweight or obese, and those with conditions like diabetes, pre-diabetes and metabolic syndrome could benefit enormously by transitioning to a low-carbohydrate, high-fat ketogenic diet. For those of you who are generally healthy but are looking for a lifestyle change to keep you that way, a healthy whole food diet that results in nutritional ketosis could set you off on the pathway to healthier aging. The trends in obesity, diabetes and dementia have been climbing in the wrong direction far too long and appearing at an earlier age, but we don't have to settle for this. By embarking on this journey to healthier eating and encouraging our family and friends to join us, together we can reverse this pattern and provide a healthier outlook for our children and grandchildren. We now have the knowledge and the tools to make this happen.

So in answer to the question, "Why go keto?", my response is, "Why not?"

QUESTIONS AND ANSWERS ABOUT COCONUT OIL, MCT OIL, AND EXOGENOUS KETONE SUPPLEMENTS

COCONUT OIL—QUESTIONS AND ANSWERS

Who Should Try and Who Should Not Try Coconut Oil?

Coconut oil is a healthy fat that can be used by nearly everyone in their everyday diet. It is a staple in the diet of millions who live in tropical parts of the world where coconut palms grow. Coconut oil can be used as part of a ketogenic diet to help sustain the level of ketosis due to the ketogenic medium-chain fatty acids it contains.

Lauric acid is a medium-chain fatty acid that makes up almost half of coconut oil and is a saturated fat. The lauric acid in coconut oil is antimicrobial for many types of bacteria, viruses, fungi, and protozoa and could be used to help control certain infections by eating it, using it on skin or in hair, or swishing it in the mouth. Some examples of organisms killed by lauric acid include the herpes simplex virus type 1, which causes fever blisters, and the bacteria that cause stomach ulcers, dental cavities, and skin acne.

Lauric acid makes up 4 to 6 percent of the fats in human breast milk and is one of the components of human breast milk that helps prevent infection in a newborn. Coconut oil and/or palm kernel oil, which have a similar composition of fats, are added to nearly every infant formula to try to duplicate the important fatty acids, such as lauric acid, found in human breast milk. Coconut oil is considered very safe, and even important, for the human newborn fed with infant formula, so there is every reason to believe it is safe for older children and adults as well.

People who have a neurodegenerative disease that involves decreased glucose uptake in neurons may benefit from taking higher amounts of coconut and/or MCT oil to produce ketones, which may be used by brain cells and other organs as energy. These diseases include Alzheimer's and other dementias, Parkinson's, Lou Gehrig's disease (amyotrophic lateral sclerosis, or ALS), multiple sclerosis, epilepsy, Duchenne muscular dystrophy, autism, Down syndrome, and Huntington's chorea. Some uncommon conditions also involving decreased glucose uptake in the brain or other organs could respond (for a list of the conditions, see Chapter 3 Figures 3.15). Your physician should be able to help you learn if this dietary intervention is appropriate for you or your loved one.

If you are at risk for Alzheimer's disease due to family history or diabetes, it is important to know that changes in the brain related to Alzheimer's begin to appear at least ten to twenty years before symptoms become obvious. You might consider adding coconut oil and/or MCT oil to your diet to try to prevent, or at least delay the onset and lessen the effects of the disease.

Some rare conditions involve a problem of fat metabolism in which the use of coconut oil and/or MCT oil *may not be appropriate and may even worsen the condition.* Therefore, consultation with your physician is very important.

People who are allergic to coconut should not use coconut oil or coconut oil products. Some people who are allergic to coconut oil might do well with MCT oil instead, but you should consult with your physician, who may be able to perform a skin test or other allergy test to make sure.

Should I Eat Coconut Oil if My Gall Bladder Has Been Removed?

The medium-chain fatty acids in coconut oil do not require digestive enzymes to be absorbed from the gut so may be easier to digest than equivalent amounts of other oils. After the gall bladder (where bile is stored) has been removed, the liver continues to make bile, which contains some of the enzymes needed to digest the longer-chain fats in coconut oil. (Some of the digestive enzymes come from the pancreas as well.) It is advisable in people without a gall bladder to begin using coconut oil very slowly and increase as tolerated to avoid indigestion (see *How Much Coconut Oil Should I Take?* below).

What About Someone with Liver Disease Using Coconut Oil?

Using larger amounts of coconut oil in the diet may not be appropriate for someone with liver cirrhosis or liver failure, although MCT oil may provide an alternative. Partially-hydrogenated oils, including partially-hydrogenated coconut oil, along with excessive sugar and/or calorie intake can result in a non-alcohol-related fatty liver (abnormal deposits of fat within the liver). Fatty liver can also be a complication of type 2 diabetes. Therefore, it is important to always use non-hydrogenated coconut oil or any other oil, for that matter, and to avoid excessive sugar intake. At the American Oil Chemists Society 2018 conference, researchers Chaturthi Senanayake and Nimanthi Jayathilaka at University of Kelaniya in Sri Lanka reported very interesting findings relevant to this discussion (Jayathilaka, 2018; Senanayake, 2018). They studied the effects of four different diets on Wistar rats, with each diet containing one of the following fats: soy bean oil, coconut oil, butter, and margarine. They reported that coconut oil resulted in the least amount of fat accumulation in the rat livers and the highest anti-oxidant activity. Coconut oil also resulted in, far and away, the highest HDL (so called "good") and the lowest LDL cholesterol levels and the lowest triglyceride levels. It tied with soy bean oil for the lowest total cholesterol level. The presenters attributed these findings to the predominance of medium-chain fatty acids in coconut oil compared to the other fats.

What if My Loved One with Alzheimer's Is ApoE4+? Should We Bother Trying Coconut or MCT?

Yes! In the Accera studies (the makers of Axona, the prescription powdered form of MCT oil), even though the ApoE4+ people when combined as a group did not show improvement, many of the individuals with that genetic makeup did have improved scores on cognitive testing. This was not noted in the article in which the study results were published, but I learned this in conversation with one of the authors. In addition, Steve is ApoE4+ and responded to treatment with medium-chain fatty acids.

How Much Coconut Oil Should I Take?

If you take too much oil too fast, you may experience indigestion, cramping, or diarrhea. To avoid these symptoms, take coconut oil with food and start with one-half to one teaspoon per meal, increasing slowly as tolerated over a week or longer.

If diarrhea develops, drop back to the previous level and stay at that level for at least a few days before trying to increase again. See more ideas for reducing the problem of diarrhea later in this section.

For most people, the goal is to increase gradually to 4 to 6 tablespoons a day, depending on the size of the person, spread over two to four meals. Not everyone will be able to tolerate this much oil. Steve and other people have reported improvement of their Alzheimer's, Parkinson's and ALS symptoms while taking large amounts (9 tablespoons or more per day) of coconut oil and/or MCT oil.

Mixing MCT oil and coconut oil could provide higher and steadier levels of ketones. One formula is to mix 16 ounces MCT oil plus 12 ounces coconut oil in a quart jar and increase slowly as tolerated, starting with 1 teaspoon. This mixture will stay liquid at room temperature. See more about MCT oil in the next Question and Answer Section.

How Can Coconut Oil Be Used in the Diet?

Coconut oil can be substituted for any solid or liquid oil, lard, butter, or margarine in baking or cooking on the stove, and it can be mixed directly into already prepared foods. Some people take it straight with a spoon, but many people may find it hard to swallow this way and more pleasant to take with food.

Use coconut oil instead of butter on warm vegetables. Use it on toast, English muffins, bagels, grits, corn on the cob, potatoes, sweet potatoes, rice, noodles, and pasta. If adhering to a ketogenic diet, use whole grains and one or two small measured servings of these foods per day. Look for low-carb versions of breads, bagels, pitas, and tortillas. When stir-frying or sautéing on the stove, coconut oil smokes if heated to more than 350°F or medium heat. You can avoid this by adding a little peanut oil. Coconut oil can be used at any temperature in the oven when mixed in foods. Mix coconut oil into your favorite soup, chili, or sauce. It can also be basted onto foods such as fish as long as the oven temperature is 350°F or below.

Coconut oil tends to become hard when exposed to cold foods. For example, if used as a salad dressing, it will turn into hard little chunks if the vegetables in the salad come straight out of the refrigerator. Some people actually like this effect and call them "crunchies." If you do not enjoy that effect, try adding equal amounts of coconut oil to another favorite salad dressing that has been warmed slightly. Also, a mixture of MCT and coconut oil tends to stay liquid and works well in this situation. This also enables you to add it to smoothies, yogurt, or kefir and put it directly on salads without warming first.

For those who cannot handle coconut oil, grated or flaked coconut, coconut milk, and fresh coconut may be good substitutes, as they are digested much more slowly. Caregivers have found many creative ways to get coconut oil into the diet of their loved ones. One of my favorite recipes is for Coconut Fudge (see Keto Friendly Recipe section). Also check the Resources section for cookbooks and websites containing many more great ideas and recipes.

What Is the Nutrient Content of Coconut Oil?

Coconut oil has about 117 to 120 calories per tablespoons, which is about the same as other oils. It contains 57 to 60 percent medium-chain fatty acids, which are absorbed directly from the intestine without the need for digestive enzymes. This portion of the coconut oil is not stored as fat. Coconut oil is about 86 percent saturated fats, most of which are the medium-chain fats that are metabolized differently than animal saturated fats. The oil contains no cholesterol and no trans fat so long as it is non-hydrogenated. An advantage of a saturated fat is that there is nowhere on the molecule for free radicals or oxidants to attach. About 6 percent of coconut oil is monounsaturated fats (the main fat in olive oil) and 2 percent polyunsaturated fats (omega-6). Coconut oil also contains a small amount of phytosterols, which are one of the components of the statins used for lowering cholesterol.

Does Coconut Oil Contain Omega-3 Fatty Acids?

While coconut oil contains a small amount of omega-6 fatty acids, it includes *no* omega-3 fatty acids, so this must be taken in addition to coconut oil. You can obtain all the essential fatty acids required by using just coconut oil and omega-3 fatty acids. You can get this by eating salmon twice a week or taking liquid fish oil or cod liver oil, which also contain significant amounts of vitamins A, D, and E. Some other good sources of omega-3 fatty acids are ground flax meal, chia (a fine grain), walnuts and walnut oil, lingonberry, and purslane. Soybeans, soybean oil, and canola oil contain small amounts of omega-3 fatty acids. It is important to note here that the basic omega-3 fat found in vegetable sources, alpha-linolenic acid (ALA), may not readily convert to the very important docosahexanoic acid (DHA) and eicosapentanoic acid (EPA) omega-3 fatty acids that are also essential. DHA makes up 50 percent of the neuron's plasma membrane, and low levels of DHA have been associated with Alzheimer's disease as well as many other conditions. DHA is so important that very strong consideration should be given to getting this fatty acid directly from a marine source. There are algae forms of DHA available that are marketed to pregnant women and would also be appropriate for vegans. Concentrated DHA supplements are also available usually in capsule form and also in gel form.

What Kind of Coconut Oil Should I Use?

Look for coconut oils that are organic, cold-pressed, also called cold-expeller-pressed, and are non-hydrogenated with no trans fat. Avoid coconut oils that are partially hydrogenated or super-heated because these processes change the chemical structure of the fats. In the United States, food manufacturers are required to state on the product label if a product contains hydrogenated or partially hydrogenated oils and trans fats. One caution is that manufacturers can state on labels that there are no trans fat if a serving contains less than 0.5 grams. This can be deceptive, since the serving size is often adjusted accordingly. Look at the ingredients for the words "hydrogenated" or "partially-hydrogenated" and avoid products with these types of ingredients.

If you like the odor of coconut, look for products labeled "virgin," "extra virgin," "organic," "raw," or "unrefined," which often also read "organic." These products are generally more expensive than "refined," "all natural," or "RBD" (refined, bleached, and deodorized) coconut oils, which do not have an odor. The oil itself is tasteless. Any of these have essentially the same fatty acid composition with about 57 to 60 percent medium-chain fatty acids; however, the more refined products will have fewer of the other nutrients found in the unrefined oils. Refined coconut oil is made from copra (dried coconut flesh), which, in the drying process and transit time to the oil mills, often picks up mold and off-flavors and thus needs to be refined to be palatable. The dried coconut is soaked in bleach and solvents are used to leach out the oils, which are subjected to high temperatures to further purify and liquefy the oils. Refined coconut oils have virtually no coconut taste or aroma. The least expensive brand that I have been able to find so far is the Louanna brand at Walmart. Louanna is not hydrogenated but is manufactured using the RBD process. It will produce the same ketone effect as the unrefined oils but may not carry some of the other important nutrients that are responsible for the other benefits of coconut oil. Some consumers may consider this overly processed; on the other hand, it may be considerably more affordable for those on a low fixed income.

Coconut oil can be found at natural food stores, most Asian markets, and some traditional grocery stores, as well as large department stores with grocery sections. More recently, large 54-ounce containers of organic cold-pressed virgin coconut oil can be purchased at buyers' clubs such as Sam's Club and Costco for less than $16 and organic refined coconut oil for under $11. You can also use the Internet to find other quality brands of coconut oil and at a wide range of prices not available at your local retailer.

Check the Resources section for a listing of websites offering coconut oil and coconut oil products.

What About Using Coconut Oil Capsules?

Using coconut oil capsules is not an efficient way to give the oil since the capsules are relatively expensive and nearly all contain only 1 gram of oil per capsule, whereas a tablespoon of oil has 14 grams. Some products list 4 grams per serving; however, the serving size is four capsules. It would require taking about fourteen capsules to equal 1 tablespoon of coconut oil, so it may not be practical and could be expensive to use capsules. On the other hand, this may be an alternative for people who will not use the oil in liquid form and have no problem with swallowing capsules.

Why Does Coconut Oil Look Cloudy?

Coconut oil is a clear or slightly yellow liquid above 76°F but becomes solid at 76°F and below. If your house is kept right around 76°F, you may even see partly liquid oil with solid clouds floating in it; this is normal. If you generally keep your home at 75°F or below, the oil will tend to be a white or slightly yellow, soft semi-solid, depending on whether it is unrefined or refined.

What Other Coconut Products Contain Coconut Oil?

- Coconut milk is a combination of the oil and the water from the coconut and most of the calories are from the oil. Look for brands with 10 to 13 grams of fat in 2 ounces. Coconut milk also contains some protein and a small amount of carbohydrate, which gives it a slightly sweet taste. Coconut milk can generally be found in natural foods stores, Asian stores, and the Asian and/or Hispanic sections of traditional grocery stores. Look at the fat content closely on the label and be aware that some less-expensive brands are considerably diluted with water. Some of the products in larger milk containers are also very diluted with water with less than ½ tablespoon of oil per 8-ounce cup. You can dilute condensed coconut milk yourself with water, or even better, with coconut water, which is loaded with vitamins and other nutrients. Organic coconut milk products are also available. Some coconut milks are also labeled "light" or "lite." Much of the oil has been removed, so using these lower fat products defeats our purpose of including coconut oil in the diet. Coconut milk blends very well into smoothies and is a tasty substitute for cow's milk on cereal or right out of the glass. Coconut milk can be substituted for some or all of the milk in many recipes.

  Some wonderful ice creams are available in a variety of flavors made with coconut milk as the first ingredient. Coconut milk ice creams are available at Asian markets, many natural food stores, and many traditional grocery stores. There are even some coconut milk ice cream products labeled "gluten free." Coconut ice cream may be one way to encourage coconut oil intake for someone with a sweet tooth or for an otherwise uncooperative loved one.

- Coconut cream is mostly coconut milk, often has added sugar, and comes in liquid and powdered forms.

- Flaked or grated coconut can be purchased unsweetened or sweetened and is a very good source of coconut oil and fiber. Grated coconut has about 15 grams of oil and 3 grams of fiber in ¼ cup; in fact, about 70 percent of the carbohydrate content is fiber. The oil in grated coconut can help with absorption of certain vitamins and other nutrients as well. Flaked or grated coconut can be bought in bulk, usually for less than three dollars per pound, at many natural food stores, and can be added to cold or hot cereals, smoothies, soup, ricotta or cottage cheese, and used as a topper for ice cream. Flaked coconut is often found in trail mix, and some people snack on unsweetened flaked coconut or toasted coconut flakes. Homemade or store-bought macaroons are a delicious source of coconut.

- Frozen or canned coconut meat often has a lot of added sugar and not much oil per serving. Coconut meat can also be found in jars as coconut balls and "coconut sport," which is large strands of coconut. These products are especially nice for adding to fruit salads.

- A fresh coconut can be cut up into pieces and eaten raw. A 2-inch square piece has about 160 calories with 15 grams of oil (equivalent to about one tablespoon oil) and 4 grams of fiber. Removing the meat from the coconut can be quite a challenge, however. In Bruce Fife's *The Coconut Lover's Cookbook* (2008), he suggests heating the whole coconut in an oven for twenty minutes at 400°F after poking two holes in the eyes of the coconut and draining the coconut water. I like to strain off the coconut water, since it has significant nutrients as well. After the coconut cools down, it can be opened with a hammer or whatever tool you can think of. To avoid shattering anything important, we take the coconut outside and crack it open on newspapers covering the garage floor. The meat can usually be pried from the shell with a blunt knife. This is quite a process and can be time-consuming, but some people consider it well worth it. Some Asian stores carry a special tool for removing the coconut meat from the shell. Pieces of coconut meat can be saved for a week or longer in the freezer.

- Coconut water does not usually contain coconut oil but does contain many other nutrients and has other health benefits. The electrolyte composition is similar to human plasma and is useful to prevent or treat dehydration. Coconut water has been used as intravenous fluid in Asia and was even used by our American troops when supplies of standard intravenous fluids were low. Coconut water is coming into its own now as a popular sports drink, plain and flavored.

- MCT oil is part of the coconut oil and can also be purchased in some natural food stores or on the Internet. (Check the Resources section for listings.) This may be useful for people who are on the go and do not have much time to cook. MCT oil can also be mixed with coconut oil as described earlier in this section. MCT oil is used as energy and not stored as fat, so it may be useful for someone who wants to lose weight if it is substituted for some other fats in the diet.

The following coconut foods contain the equivalent of 1 tablespoon of coconut oil:

- Coconut milk (undiluted): 4½ tablespoons
- Coconut meat: 2" x 2" x ½-inch piece
- Coconut grated: ⅓ cup
- Coconut oil capsules (1 gram): 14 capsules

How Should Coconut Products Be Stored?

Coconut oil is extremely stable with a shelf life of at least two years when stored at room temperature. The container should have an expiration date on it. In the refrigerator, coconut oil becomes quite hard, so you may need a chisel to get it out of the jar! If you wish to keep it in the refrigerator, you can measure out one or two tablespoons into each section of a plastic ice cube tray. The coconut oil pops easily out of the tray. Refrigeration is not necessary, but some people may be more comfortable storing it this way.

Coconut milk is mostly coconut oil and can be substituted for the oil in many ways. Coconut milk must be refrigerated after opening and should be used within a few days or tossed out.

Grated or flaked coconut can be stored at room temperature but may last longer if stored in a refrigerator.

A freshly cut coconut can be stored in the refrigerator for a few days or in a freezer for a couple of weeks.

What Other Foods Contain Medium-Chain Fatty Acids?

Please see Chapter 7, Table 7.1, for a list of foods that contain short- and medium-chain fatty acids that are worth mentioning, including human breast milk, whole cow's milk, goat's milk, and cheeses.

Medium-chain fatty acids may be essential fatty acids, not only for adults but also for children. Many people with Alzheimer's have a life-long history of memory problems. Could consuming these fatty acids beginning in childhood lessen this problem? Could there be a connection between autism and deficiency of fats, including medium-chain fats, in the diet?

Are There Any Commercial Products Available That Contain a Mixture of Coconut Oil and MCT Oil?

MCT//143 is a product developed for me by the Pruvit company. It contains the 4:3 ratio of MCT oil to coconut oil that I used to help Steve and have taken myself for ten years. The "143" in the name is text talk that means "I love you" and this product was born out my love for Steve. MCT//143 contains organic virgin coconut oil and MCT oil extracted from coconut oil. I used soy lecithin in Steve's formulation to provide him with brain phospholipids such as phosphatidylcholine, but MCT//143 contains the more-efficient, purified, concentrated phosphatidylcholine. This chemical makes up 40 to 50 percent of cell's membranes and is espe-cially important in the brain, where it helps form the neurotransmitter that is involved in memory and transports important omega-3 fats into the brain.

MCT//143 can be added to many types of foods including coffee and tea, soup or chili, smoothies, milk, yogurt, ricotta, cottage cheese, and vegetables, and it can be drizzled over salad. It can be added directly to Keto//OS to add a keto boost or taken as is. It can be swished in your mouth to help with dental health. It should be started slowly, such as ½ to 1 teaspoon two or three times a day with food and increased every few days. How much you take is up to you, but taking a serving three or four times a day could help maintain a constant baseline level of ketones, which is a great foundation to build on by taking ketone salts and using other strategies, such as intermittent fasting and exercise, to further increase ketone levels and maximize benefits.

This product is available in 15-gram packets, just over 1 tablespoon each, which is very convenient for traveling, taking to work, or—near to my heart—using with people who are in assisted living. (See the next question and answer.) A larger pouch may be available sometime soon.

Can Coconut Oil Be Given to Healthy Children and Children with Medical Conditions?

Yes! Human breast milk includes 10 to 17 percent of its fat as medium-chain triglycerides. To give you an idea of just how important medium-chain fatty acids are to humans, a ten-pound breastfeeding baby gets about 3.12 grams of medium-chain triglycerides per quart of breast milk. Extrapolated to a 150-pound adult, that would be the equivalent of 47 grams of medium-chain triglycerides and would require eating 5½ tablespoons of coconut oil.

To try to duplicate what is in human breast milk, every infant formula manufactured in the United States contains coconut and/or palm kernel oil and formulas for premature newborns and for infants who have trouble with digestion also contain medium-chain triglyceride oil.

When children are weaned from the breast and from infant formulas, the usual next step in the United States is to transition to cow's milk. In recent years, there has been a push to encourage feeding even small children low-fat or fat-free milk and milk products, which would eliminate every potential source of medium-chain triglycerides from the diet of the average child.

I have had many parents of children with autism and Down syndrome (also called trisomy 21) ask about using coconut oil. Several parents have reported improvements when giving coconut oil to their children with autism; these include increased growth, fewer seizures, and improved behavior. Autism is a group of conditions known as autism spectrum disorders that appears to have many different causes, though largely unknown at present. Children with Down syndrome have an extra chromosome (forty-seven instead of the normal forty-six), and the particular chromosome involved (chromosome 21) contains some of the genes that affect the development of Alzheimer's disease. Consequently, people with Down syndrome tend to develop Alzheimer's-type dementia as they enter middle age, with the characteristic plaques and tangles developing much earlier in life.

Studies using PET scans, a unique type of imaging test that helps doctors identify abnormal from normal functioning of organs and tissues, have shown that some children with autism have decreased glucose uptake in certain areas of the brain. This is also true in some children and adults with

Down syndrome, as well as in some children and adults with attention deficit disorders and bipolar disorder. Therefore, ketones could potentially provide alternative fuel to the brains of children and adults with these conditions.

A reasonable amount of coconut oil to give a child would be to start with ¼ teaspoon once or twice a day and gradually work up to ¼ teaspoon of coconut oil for every 10 pounds that the child weighs, three to four times a day, with food or in formula or milk. When that is tolerated, if desired, coconut oil can be further increased as tolerated. The total amount will vary greatly depending on the child's weight and ability to tolerate the oil without having diarrhea. To give an idea of how much oil could be used in the diet for a child, there is a variation of the ketogenic diet, called the MCT oil–modified ketogenic diet, in which 60 percent of the diet's calories are provided in the form of medium-chain triglycerides. This means that for every 1,000 calories, 600 calories come from medium-chain triglycerides, which equates to about 6 tablespoons of MCT oil or the equivalent amount of coconut oil. For parents of children with epilepsy or autism who wish to explore the use of the MCT oil–modified ketogenic diet, I highly recommend contacting The Charlie Foundation (www. charliefoundation.org) or Matthew's Friends (www.matthewsfriends.org) for guidance and referral to a dietitian highly experienced in helping families with ketogenic diets. As with our dietary guidelines here, these organizations generally recommend starting at a much lower percentage of MCT oil and increasing as tolerated to avoid diarrhea.

Also, some children like the taste of coconut milk, in which case the milk can be taken alone or added to other drinks. For coconut milk, I suggest adding 1½ to 2 teaspoons to the diet for every 10 pounds that the child weighs, two or three times a day. If you use coconut milk for a young child, be sure to refrigerate it and toss it after forty-eight hours. Do not add honey to coconut milk for children under one year old due to the risk of contamination with botulism. See the Coconut Milk recipes in the Recipe section for suggested dilutions of canned coconut milk.

There are some very rare medical conditions that interfere with metabolizing fats due to specific enzyme defects. Use of coconut oil should be avoided for a child with liver failure or with an allergy to coconut. For any child with a medical condition, it is important to consult with the child's physician prior to changing the diet drastically, including adding coconut and MCT oil.

Can Someone Who Is in Assisted Living Take Coconut Oil?

If your loved one is in assisted living, the doctor may be willing to prescribe coconut oil or a combination of MCT and coconut oil, such as MCT//143, that staff can give at one or more meals per day. The doctor can add instruction for the oils to be increased gradually as tolerated, such as starting with ½ to 1 teaspoon two or three times a day with food and increasing slowly as tolerated every few days. Many people have reported success in terms of cooperation from their loved one's doctor and the assisted living staff.

I know of one assisted living facility in which the cook was preparing some foods with coconut oil. She said the residents with Alzheimer's seemed more talkative and to have more energy. Two caregivers from an assisted living facility in Taiwan presented me with amazing before and after clock studies in two people with dementia who began to take coconut and MCT oil and they planned to carry out a clinical trial in their facility. Hopefully over time the directors of these facilities will consider allowing staff to cook with coconut oil.

If no such options are possible, another alternative is to ask the person's physician for a prescription for Axona (www.about-axona.com), a powdered form of MCT oil with other inactive ingredients to make it into a drink, manufactured by Accera.

Do I Need to Be Worried About Gaining Weight from the Extra Fat in the Diet?

No and yes! Some studies show that substitution of coconut oil for other fats in the diet can result in weight loss of 10 to 12 pounds in the course of a year because the medium-chain fatty acids are converted directly to energy and not stored as fat. However, if the fat is simply added to the diet and nothing subtracted, you can expect to gain weight. This is an oversimplification, but if you consume more calories than you burn in the course of a day, the net result will be weight gain.

The best way to avoid gaining weight is to *substitute* coconut oil for most other fats and oils in the diet and, if that isn't enough, eliminate or cut back on portion sizes of carbohydrates, such as breads, rice, potatoes, cereals, and other grains. In general, it is a good idea to use whole-milk products, but if weight gain is a problem, you can compensate for some of the new fat in the diet by changing from full-fat to lower-fat dairy products, such as milk, cheese, cottage cheese, and yogurts, as well as to low-fat or fat-free salad dressings, to which you can add coconut and/or oil. By the same token, if you decide to go with low-fat dairy, be aware that you may not absorb as much calcium and vitamin D through the intestine, compared to absorption when using full-fat dairy. Adding coconut or MCT oil directly to the low-fat milk product could overcome this problem.

Also, some people overestimate portions substantially by dipping into the coconut oil jar with a kitchen tablespoon. You can avoid this problem by using a measuring spoon and removing the excess by leveling it off with a knife. This can make a big difference in the number of calories consumed.

Tiny glass measuring cups are available at grocery stores with markings for teaspoons, tablespoons, and milliliters. These little measuring cups are especially useful for combining salad dressing with coconut oil and for measuring out the liquid MCT/coconut oil mixture discussed elsewhere.

Can Coconut Oil Be Given to Animals?

One of the most unexpected emails I received was from a lady who wanted to know if coconut oil might improve cognition in her thirteen-year-old Welsh terrier. It is completely understandable that someone wouldn't want to see his or her beloved elderly pet suffer with dementia any more than another family member. One of the Accera MCT oil studies involved elderly dogs, and the dogs did, in fact, show improved cognition in response to consuming the oil (Studzinski, 2008; Taha, 2009). I relayed this information to her and suggested that she follow the guidelines for children: Give the dog ¼ teaspoon for each 10 pounds of body weight two or three times a day. The dog weighed 20 pounds, so the woman decided to give her ½ teaspoon in her food twice a day. Several weeks later, she reported that her dog was getting up and around more and finding her way to her food bowl, which she was not able to do prior to consuming the oil.

Dogs can also get diarrhea from coconut oil. The lady reported that one of her friends decided to use twice the recommended amount, and her dog developed diarrhea. Apparently, it is a good idea to start with caution and increase gradually with animals as well as people.

As a side note, many pet owners report that their dogs and cats are attracted to the smell of coconut oil when the owner uses it on his or her skin and will try to lick it off!

How Can I Bring Coconut Oil or a Mixture of Coconut and MCT Oil to a Restaurant or Carry It While Traveling?

To bring coconut oil along with you to a restaurant or carry it while traveling, check Trader Joe's. The Trader Joe's stores currently carry their own brand of coconut oil in 15 milliliters (one tablespoon) packets. The small packages tend to be a bit oily on the outside of the packet, so consider placing them in a resealable bag.

MCT//143, a mixture of MCT, coconut oil, and phosphatidyl choline from Pruvit Ventures comes in convenient 15 milliliters (one tablespoon) packets that can be carried in a resealable bag.

These packets of coconut oil and MCT//143 are small enough in volume to be taken through airport security and can be presented to the security agents along with other allowed liquids during the screening process. The coconut packets are clear and unlabeled, so, as a precaution, I cut the front panel off the box of coconut oil packets and place it in the resealable bag to identify what the packets contain.

Can Coconut Oil Be Used as a Deodorant?

The antimicrobial action of the lauric acid in coconut oil may kill bacteria that produce underarm odor. One natural deodorant recipe combines three tablespoons of coconut oil with one tablespoon each of corn powder and baking soda.

Can I Clean My Teeth with Coconut Oil?

The lauric acid in coconut oil kills the bacteria that cause dental cavities and gingivitis (inflammation of the gums) as well as many other disease-causing germs that may be present in the mouth. One way to use coconut oil for oral hygiene is called "oil pulling." Several teaspoons of coconut oil are worked around in the mouth and between the teeth for twenty minutes to effectively kill microorganisms and clean the teeth, reportedly an ancient practice. Instead of swallowing, the accumulated oil and saliva in the mouth should be spit out at the end of the oil pulling session to get rid of the germs. After a week or so of oil pulling, the teeth may feel as slick as they do following a cleaning by a dental hygienist.

Using a toothbrush with coconut oil instead of the oil-pulling method produces surprisingly nice results and saves time. Adding a little baking soda to coconut oil (about 1/8 teaspoon of baking soda to 2 or more ounces of coconut oil) may help whiten teeth as well. If you brush over a sink, run hot water to keep coconut oil from plugging up the drain, or, even better, spit the oil and saliva out into a paper cup or lined garbage container.

For lengthy discussions of these and the many other benefits of coconut oil, I recommend the books *Coconut Cures* (2005), *Oil Pulling Therapy* (2008), *Stop Alzheimer's Now* (2011), and *The Coconut Oil Miracle* (2013), all by Bruce Fife, ND.

MCT OIL—QUESTIONS AND ANSWERS

I knew for several decades that medium-chain triglyceride (MCT) oil existed, since it was in use in newborn intensive care units as early as the 1970s. I assumed it was only available to hospitals, but not long after Steve responded to coconut oil, I learned that it could easily be purchased over the counter. I was surprised to find it in several local natural food stores and to learn that it is commonly used by bodybuilders to increase lean body mass. Numerous companies now sell MCT oil as liquid, powder, and in capsules and even as "liquid coconut cooking oil." Here are the most frequently asked questions I receive about using MCT oil.

What Is Over-the-Counter MCT Oil?

Medium-chain triglyceride oil is derived from coconut oil or palm kernel oil. Most of the products that are readily available over the counter are a mixture of caprylic (C8) and capric (C10) acids, with small amounts of caproic (C6) and lauric acids (C12)—the four medium-chain triglycerides found in coconut oil. Coconut oil is about 60 percent medium-chain fatty acids and contains a much larger proportion of lauric acid compared to

MCT oil. About 70 percent of the saturated fats in coconut oil are medium-chain fatty acids.

Some newer MCT oil products, marketed as "liquid coconut cooking oil," have the heavier long-chain fats removed and contain a combination of lauric acid C12, C10, and C8. For example, in the United States, a Philippine corporation, Chemrez, markets a product called Carrington Farms liquid coconut cooking oil that contains about 31 percent lauric acid and the remainder roughly equal amounts of C8 and C10. It is creamy and great for cooking at medium heat or lower. It is also known as Laurin in Asia and Australia and there is an Alzheimer's clinical trial about to start using this product in 2018 in Australia. I like the idea of the high lauric acid oil since lauric acid is known to be antimicrobial (Dayrit, 2015) and reported to potently stimulate ketone production in astrocytes in the lab. This needs to be confirmed in human brain (Nonaka 2016).

MCT oil can be used as an alternative to coconut oil to produce mild ketosis. The primary differences between using MCT oil and coconut oil are that a smaller volume of MCT oil can be taken without the additional fatty acids found in coconut oil and that the levels of ketones may be higher, although, compared to coconut oil, they leave the circulation after a few hours.

MCT//143 is a mixture of MCT oil, organic virgin coconut oil, and phosphatidylcholine developed with me and marketed by Pruvit Ventures. (See more about this in the section on Coconut Oil above.)

How Much MCT Oil Should I Take?

Diarrhea is a common side effect of using MCT oil, so it is a good idea to start with a small amount, such as ½ or 1 teaspoon and gradually increase to an amount that is tolerated, such as 1 to 2 tablespoons two to four times a day. (More suggestions follow.) At higher levels of MCT oil, most people develop diarrhea, so when this happens, you may want to cut the dose back to the previous level.

How Can I Avoid Diarrhea from Taking MCT Oil?

The most common complaint with MCT oil is the problem of diarrhea, which usually occurs if too much is taken by someone who has not taken it before or if the amount of oil is increased too quickly. MCT oil is more likely than coconut oil to produce this problem, which occurs in about 25 percent of people as they begin taking the oil.

Considering the amount of oil that one might consume in a day's time—upwards of 6 to 8 tablespoons—most people will find the level at which they have diarrhea, which usually occurs within an hour or so of eating the oil. An occasional person will experience diarrhea with just 1 teaspoon, so caution should be exercised with the first dose.

Some strategies to help decrease the likelihood of developing diarrhea are:

1. Start with a small amount of oil, such as ½ to 1 teaspoon (about 2 to 5 grams) once or twice a day and increase slowly as tolerated. Increase by ½ to 1 teaspoon every few days until reaching the desired amount, possibly as much as 2 or more tablespoons three times a day.
2. Always take the oil with other foods.
3. Take the oil slowly during the course of the meal, over twenty to thirty minutes. If the oil is mixed with food, this will be easier to accomplish.
4. Mixing the oil with cottage cheese may decrease the odds that diarrhea will occur, so it might be practical to take the oil with cottage cheese one or more times per day. Cottage cheese is also an excellent source of protein and provides a relatively small amount of carbohydrate.
5. If using even small amounts of oil persists in causing diarrhea, consider trying other coconut products such as coconut milk or even grated coconut, which contains a substantial amount of oil. The oil may be released more slowly during the process of digestion and therefore be less likely to set off diarrhea.
6. Some people tolerate powdered MCT oil more than the liquid form.
7. Another suggestion is to try a mixture of MCT oil and coconut oil, which is described at length in the section earlier in this addendum on coconut oil:
   - *How Much Coconut Oil Should I Take?*
   - *Are There Any Commercial Products Available That Contain a Mixture of Coconut Oil and MCT Oil?*

What Is Axona?

For those who want a method prescribed by their physician, Axona, from the Accera Company, is available in some areas. This is a powdered form of MCT oil mixed with some other nutrients and emulsifiers that dissolve in liquids and can be taken as a drink. The only active ingredient is the medium-chain triglyceride called tricaprylic acid, also known as C8. Current recommendations are to take Axona once a day in the morning. More frequent dosing has not been studied as of this writing, so the company is bound by Food and Drug Administration (FDA) rules to recommend just once-a-day dosing.

A number of other powdered MCT products are available over the counter or easily obtained online but these are usually a combination of C8 and C10.

Why Do You Mix MCT Oil and Coconut Oil?

About two months after starting Steve on coconut oil, after receiving results of his ketone levels, we began experimenting with mixing MCT oil and coconut oil. After Steve took just coconut oil in the morning, his ketone levels peaked at about three hours and were nearly gone after eight to nine hours just before dinner time. Steve's ketone levels with just MCT oil were higher but gone within three hours. I reasoned that a mixture of MCT and coconut oil should result in higher levels and longer-lasting levels, so that some ketones always would be circulating.

Why Not Use Just MCT Oil?

If you decide to take just MCT oil several times a day, the levels fluctuate up and down more than with coconut oil or with a mixture of coconut and MCT oils. Also, some fatty acids in whole coconut oil are not found in MCT oil, and I think they might contribute to the improvements seen in Steve and others. For example, the lauric acid in coconut oil kills bacteria, fungi, protozoa, and certain types of viruses, such as those that cause fever blisters. Several groups of researchers have reported evidence of the herpes simplex virus type 1 that causes fever blisters in the beta-amyloid plaques in the brains of people with Alzheimer's, especially those with the ApoE4 gene like Steve. Taking coconut oil seemed to be working for

Steve in that he had been regularly fighting fever blisters, sometimes for several weeks at a time, before starting the regimen; after, these episodes became much less severe and less frequent, with just four or so episodes over eight years.

Coconut oil is also reported to support the thyroid, and many people with dementia develop hypothyroidism at some point in the disease process. Nearly all people with Down syndrome develop Alzheimer's disease by the time they reach their thirties or forties, and they also have a problem with hypothyroidism. Coconut oil could have a beneficial effect in this regard.

Why Not Use Just Coconut Oil?

Many people have reported to me that they have seen improvements in their loved ones with Alzheimer's using just coconut oil. Steve had a dramatic improvement using just coconut oil for the first two months. I don't know for certain if there is any additional benefit to adding MCT oil, so I see no problem with using just coconut oil for this dietary intervention. One of the reasons to consider adding MCT oil would be to achieve higher levels of ketones. Only part of MCT oil is converted to ketones, so the remaining medium-chain fatty acids could potentially be used by neurons as an alternative fuel. So the more medium-chain fatty acids one can tolerate, the more will be available to brain. Much more needs to be learned about exactly what medium-chain fatty acids do.

Another point to consider is that by mixing MCT and coconut oil in a 4:3 ratio, the long-chain saturated fatty acids are reduced to about 10 percent of the total fat. For those worried about the possible health issues related to saturated fats (read Chapter 11), this offers an alternative to using an equivalent amount of coconut oil.

KETONE SALTS—QUESTIONS AND ANSWERS

What Are Ketone Salts, and Why Do They Contain So Much Salt?

The ketone betahydroxybutyrate is an acid and cannot be taken alone because it would be damaging to the esophagus and stomach lining. It needs to be combined with another compatible substance to be used orally. One way to accomplish this is to combine the naturally occurring ketone betahydroxybutyrate with the mineral salts sodium, potassium, calcium and/or magnesium which can be made into a powder form and reconstituted with water or other liquid. These are called ketone salts.

Where Were Ketone Salts Developed?

A sodium ketone salt has been used in research in Europe and elsewhere in the past. The current ketone salts now widely marketed to the public in the United States and elsewhere were developed and tested at the University of South Florida in Dominic D'Agostino's lab and became widely available in early 2016 through Pruvit Ventures a multilevel network marketing company. A number of other companies now market ketone salt products of varying quality.

What Are the Benefits of Taking Ketone Salts?

Ketone salts are widely used by healthy people and people with a variety of medical conditions. Always consult your physician before using ketone salts if you are very young, elderly, or have a medical condition. Do not use them while pregnant until there is more evidence of safety in this condition. People taking ketone salts report better memory, mental focus, sleep, and mood, as well as more energy and fewer headaches and other aches and pains. These improvements are possible because ketones are anti-inflammatory and provide alternative fuel to the brain and other organs, so could be useful for people suffering from conditions related to inflammation or decreased glucose uptake into the brain and other organs; studies confirming these hypotheses need to be completed. Ketone salts are not currently recognized by the FDA to treat any medical condition, however, the individual components of the ketone salts, including betahydroxybutyrate (a naturally occurring molecule in the body) and the minerals it is attached to, are recognized as safe (GRAS). Many people have reported substantial fat loss, especially when combined with a low-carb diet and without hunger. (Ketones can suppress appetite and encourage fat loss by reducing glucose and insulin levels and stimulating fat breakdown.) World-class athletes and bodybuilders are using ketone salts to enhance physical performance.

Is the Betahydroxybutyrate in Ketone Salts Natural or Synthetic?

The betahydroxybutyrate found in ketone salt products is the same as the naturally occurring betahydroxybutyrate produced from the breakdown of fat in our bodies.

What Is the Difference Between Racemic and Non-Racemic Betahydroxybutyrate Ketone Salts?

Betahydroxybutyrate exists in two forms (D- and L-betahydroxybutyrate) that are mirror images. The "right-handed" form, D-betahydroxybutyrate is the circulating, more bioactive form and more likely to produce the beneficial effects. D-betahydroxybutyrate is considerably more expensive to make than L-betahydroxybutyrate. Most ketone salt products are made with a much-less-expensive racemic mixture, meaning that they are equal mixtures of D- and L-betahydroxybutyrate. The Keto//OS Max products from Pruvit Ventures contains at least 90 percent D-betahydroxybutyrate.

Another important point is that L-betahydroxybutyrate is not detected by the currently available blood ketone test strips, so it is hard to know what impact the racemic ketone salts have on blood ketone levels.

What Kind of Ketone Levels Can I Expect with Ketone Salts?

Most people can expect an increase of 0.5 to 1.0 mmol/L or higher from the baseline ketone level about thirty to sixty minutes after an 8 to 10 gram serving of non-racemic ketone salts. The level will steadily decrease and return to baseline several hours later. This will vary considerably from person to person.

Should I Be Concerned with the High Sodium and Potassium Content in Some Ketone Salt Products?

Ketone salts should not be used by people who are very young or elderly or have medical conditions without the approval of their physician. They also should not be used by people who have been advised to restrict their sodium intake without the approval of their doctor. A dietician could help you factor the sodium and other mineral content of the ketone salts into your diet.

And ketone salts should not be used by people who have high blood pressure related to their sodium intake. In this condition, ketone salts could significantly increase blood pressure. Some seemingly healthy people have high blood pressure and are not aware of this. It is advisable to check your blood pressure prior to using ketone salts and to consult with your physician if your blood pressure is above 140 systolic and/or 90 diastolic.

Certain diuretics cause significant loss of water along with minerals like sodium, potassium, calcium, and magnesium. The ketosis that occurs while taking ketone salts could contribute further to loss of water and minerals, resulting in dehydration and electrolyte imbalances. Most of the commercially available ketone salt products contain between 1,100 milligrams to 1,600 milligrams of sodium per serving (as indicated on the label). Some ketone salt products contain as much as 500 to 1,600 milligrams of potassium per stated serving and people who are taking potassium supplements could develop abnormally high potassium levels, which could be dangerous.

One option to reduce sodium and potassium intake with ketone salts is to use Keto//OS Max, which contains much less sodium per full serving at about 900 milligrams and minimal potassium at 75 milligrams.

How Many Servings per Day of Ketone Salts Can I Safely Take?

The number of servings per day that a person can safely take will be determined by many factors, including age, size, health, and sensitivity to sodium. Most healthy people, without a medical condition, can safely take one or two servings per day. Some people take more than two servings per day without obvious ill effect, but I do not recommend this on a regular basis for anyone. Excessive amounts of any of the minerals used to make the ketone salts could result in serious side effects, such as serious electrolyte imbalances and dehydration, edema (swelling) of the extremities, and potential damage to the kidneys and other organs.

Is It Okay to Use Ketone Salts with Someone Who Is Very Young or Elderly or Who Has a Medical Condition?

For someone who is very young or elderly or who has a medical condition, consult with your physician before starting ketone salts. If your doctor gives you the go ahead, start with 1 to 2 teaspoons of the powder diluted in plenty of water and increase every few days as tolerated (no intestinal or other issues) until reaching one-half to one serving per day. For those who do not tolerate ketone salts or who do not have a doctor's approval to take them, coconut oil and/or MCT oil might be alternatives to achieve the benefits of mild nutritional ketosis. As with ketone salts, check with your doctor.

Will Ketone Salts Affect My Blood Sugar and Insulin Levels? Are Ketone Salts Safe for Diabetics?

Measurements in a number of studies report lower blood glucose and insulin levels after taking ketone salts and ketone esters. Also, people taking ketone salts every day have reported lower fasting blood sugar over time and lower blood sugar lasting for several hours after taking a serving of the product. This is not necessarily a bad thing if you tend to run a high blood sugar and suffer from insulin resistance.

People with diabetes who are taking medications and/or insulin need to be aware that raising ketone levels with ketone salts may result in a significantly lower blood sugar along with a drop in the amount of insulin the body produces. If you are diabetic or prone to low blood sugar levels for another reason, do not begin taking ketone salts without your doctor's approval. To avoid abnormally low blood sugar, monitor your blood sugar closely and work with your doctor to make changes in your medications. On the other hand, many type 2 diabetics report that they are able to reduce their medications, including insulin, rather quickly over days to several weeks, especially if taking ketone salts is combined with a low-carbohydrate diet. Type 1 diabetics could also benefit from combining ketone salts with a low-carb diet, resulting in the need for less insulin but should only go this route with approval and very close monitoring by their physician.

Can Ketone Salts Cause Diabetic Ketoacidosis?

Diabetic ketoacidosis is an abnormal condition that occurs with very elevated blood sugar and inadequate insulin. Levels of ketones are many times (twenty to fifty times higher) than the levels you would get by taking a serving or two per day of ketone salts. The risk of diabetic ketoacidosis from taking ketone salts is very low but could occur in someone on the brink of diabetic ketoacidosis. Blood ketone levels can easily be monitored with a Keto Mojo, Precision Xtra or NovaMax glucose/ketone monitor using ketone strips, available online without a prescription. One or two servings of ketone salts usually produce betahydroxybutyrate levels in the 0.5 to 2 millimole range, compared to 10 to 25 millimole in diabetic ketoacidosis.

Is It Okay to Use Ketone Salts During Pregnancy and While Breastfeeding?

No. Women who are pregnant and breastfeeding are naturally in ketosis and taking ketone salts could result in potentially serious ketoacidosis. There have been some case reports of ketoacidosis (different than diabetic ketoacidosis) in breastfeeding women on a strict ketogenic diet. Also, the high mineral content could affect the electrolyte and mineral balances in the blood and dehydration is a possibility as well. It is not known what effect, if any, ketone salts have on the developing fetus. I do not recommend using ketone salts during pregnancy or while breastfeeding.

How Can I Avoid Diarrhea and/or Cramping When Taking Ketone Salts as a Supplement?

For people with a sensitive bowel, to avoid cramping and/or diarrhea, start with 1 or 2 teaspoons of the powder diluted in plenty of water and increase every few days as tolerated (no intestinal or other issues) until reaching one-half to one serving per day. For those who do not tolerate the use of ketone salts or do not have a doctor's approval to use them, coconut oil and/or MCT oil might be alternatives to achieve the benefits of mild nutritional ketosis. As with ketone salts, check with your doctor and begin with small amounts. (See other sections on coconut oil and MCT Oil in the Addendum.)

How Might Ketone Salts Affect a Person Who Gets Kidney Stones or Gout?

The classic ketogenic diet is known to increase the risk of kidney stones and gout, so it is possible that taking ketone salts could increase the risk of these conditions as well. Taking a supplement to reduce acid in the blood, such as potassium citrate, and eating a low-acid diet could reduce the risk of kidney stones or gout. (See Chapter 10 on the Acidosis Sparing Diet.)

If I Have Eaten Carbohydrates and Drink Ketone Salts Around the Same Time, Which Energy Source Will Take Over? Will One Negate the Other's Effect?

If you eat carbs and drink ketone salts at the same time, your body will use both glucose and ketones as fuel one way or another. Different tissues may prefer one fuel over the other. When both glucose and ketones are available to the brain, ketones are the preferred fuel. In a study of ketone ester for athletic performance conducted at Oxford University by Kieran Clarke, the combination of betahydroxybutyrate ester with a carbohydrate drink produced better results in several experiments than either alone (Cox, 2016).

How can I tell how many grams of ketones I am getting in a serving of ketone Salts?

Companies are not currently required to list the number of grams per serving of betahydroxybutyrate in ketone salts, but some of them list this on their label even so. Contact the company directly to find out how many grams of betahydroxybutyrate a particular product contains. Another good question to ask is what percent of the product is D-betahydroxybutyrate and whether the ketone in the product is a racemic or non-racemic mixture of betahydroxybutyrate. A ketone salt product with 8 grams of non-racemic betahydroxybutyrate per serving could provide more benefit than a product with 10 or 11 grams of racemic betahydroxybutyrate per serving, since it contains a considerably higher percentage of the more bioactive D-betahydroxybutyrate. Please see question *"What Is the Difference Between Racemic and Non-Racemic Betahydroxybutyrate Ketone Salts?"* above for more information.

Can Ketone Salts Be Put into Boiling Water?

It is probably best if ketone salts are not put directly into boiling water to avoid denaturing the ketones and any proteins, amino acids, or other ingredients in the product. The salts should be okay in cold, warm, or hot water below the boiling point. Ketone salts can also be used with sparkling water.

KETONE ESTERS—QUESTIONS AND ANSWERS

What Are Ketone Esters?

The ketone betahydroxybutyrate is an acid and cannot be taken alone because it would be damaging to the esophagus and stomach lining. It needs to be combined with another compatible substance to be used orally. One way to do this is to combine the acid with an alcohol to form a ketone ester. There are several different ketone esters in development, but just one is currently available to the public, technically known as (R)-3-hydroxybutyl (R)-3-hydroxybutyrate, which is a combination of non-racemic betahydroxybutyrate and non-racemic 1, 3-butanediol (BHB/BD). The BHB/BD ketone ester has been developed and studied by Dr. Richard Veech (see his story in Chapter 5) and his associates at the NIH and also studied extensively by Dr. Kieran Clarke and her associates at Oxford University for use in human athletic performance. A betahydroxybutyrate triglyceride ester (glyceride ester) developed by Sami Hashim (see his story in Chapter 5) is also making progress toward market.

The BHB/BD ester is recognized by the FDA as safe in healthy humans when used for athletic performance. Additional studies are underway to determine safety in the general population.

What Are the Benefits of Taking Ketone Esters? Is There an Advantage to Taking Ketone Esters over Ketone Salts?

The BHB/BD ketone ester has just become available to the public for purchase in early 2018. It has not been available long enough to provide a track record of benefits, but anecdotal reports of improvements are beginning to accumulate in people with various medical conditions (though not recognized by the FDA for any medical conditions at present) and in athletes. Most studies of the BHB/BD ester center on human athletic performance (Cox, 2016; Holdsworth, 2017; Vandoorne, 2017; Stubbs, 2017; Clarke 2012), and there is one case report of my husband Steve, who suffered from early onset Alzheimer's disease and had very significant improvement while taking this ketone ester beginning in 2010 (Newport, 2015).

One big advantage of taking ketone esters over taking ketone salts is the much higher level of betahydroxybutyrate that can be achieved with the ester form, which could provide the maximum benefit in certain conditions like epilepsy, Alzheimer's, Parkinson's and cancer that might require higher ketone levels to be most effective. Another advantage is that the ketone esters do not contain the minerals (sodium, potassium, calcium, and magnesium) that may limit the use in the ketone salts in many medical conditions.

Is the Betahydroxybutyrate in Ketone Esters Natural or Synthetic?

The betahydroxybutyrate found in ketone esters of that type are the same as the naturally occurring betahydroxybutyrate produced from the breakdown of fat in our bodies.

Are Ketone Esters Racemic or Non-Racemic Betahydroxybutyrate?

Studies by Richard Veech at the NIH have indicated that the non-racemic form of betahydroxybutyrate is the more bioavailable form and therefore more likely to provide benefit. Both the BHB/BD ester and the Hashim glyceride ester are the non-racemic form.

What Ketone Levels Can I Expect with the Ketone Ester, and How Long Will the Level Stay Elevated?

The BHB/BD ketone ester can easily reach betahydroxybutyrate (BHB) levels of 3 to 6 mmol/L with a 25- to 35-gram dose. The level increases rapidly, peaking somewhere between thirty and sixty minutes for most people, and then tends to drop steadily until the level is back to the pre-dose value at about three to four hours after taking the dose. These results could vary considerably from person to person.

Can Ketone Esters Cause Ketoacidosis or Diabetic Ketoacidosis?

Levels of 7 mmol/L or higher are potentially in the range of ketoacidosis. This means that the blood pH can become abnormally low as a result of the high ketone level because the body is unable to fully buffer the acid when it is released into the bloodstream after digestion. The usual dose marketed to athletes is up to 25 grams, which will put most people at peak levels between 3 and 4 mmol/L. When we were trying to figure out how much ketone ester Steve needed to reach 4 to 5 mmol/L, his BHB level reached 7.0 after taking 50 grams of the ketone ester.

It is advisable to monitor the BHB blood level closely to determine how much of the ester is right for you and keep your BHB level out of ketoacidosis territory. Blood ketone levels can easily be monitored with a Keto Mojo, Precision Xtra, or NovaMax glucose/ketone monitor using ketone strips, which are available online without a prescription. (See Chapter 9.)

Diabetic ketoacidosis is an abnormal condition that occurs with very elevated blood sugar and inadequate insulin and results in ketone levels in the 10 to 25 mmol range. It is unlikely that the BHB/BD ester will result in diabetic ketoacidosis at the recommended dose range, unless you are an insulin dependent diabetic on the verge of diabetic ketoacidosis. However, it is possible that taking several 25- to 35-gram doses too close together or taking a single serving of 100 to 150 grams of BHB/BD ester, could push the BHB level to 10 mmol/L or higher.

Is It Okay to Use Ketone Esters with Someone Who Is Very Young or Elderly or Has a Medical Condition?

For someone who is very young or elderly, or for anyone who has a medical condition, it is recommended to consult a physician before starting ketone esters, which are currently recognized as safe by the FDA only for use in healthy people for athletic performance. Doctors can prescribe treatments "off-label" (for other than their intended purpose), but the overwhelming majority of doctors have not ever heard of ketone esters much less their potential use for medical conditions. Many doctors will likely hear this first from their patients. Likewise, no clinical trials have been completed for use of the ketone ester for any medical condition. The great hope and expectation is that clinical trials studying the ketone esters will show benefit for people with diseases like Alzheimer's, Parkinson's, multiple sclerosis, ALS, autism, epilepsy, traumatic brain injury, and many other conditions in which there is decreased glucose uptake into cells, as well as inflammatory and certain cardiac conditions.

If you are fortunate enough to have your doctor approve your use of a ketone ester, I suggest starting with a small dose, such as 5 grams once or twice a day, and explore what effect that has on you. Monitor the blood BHB level closely. (See Chapter 9.) The dose could be slowly increased to perhaps 10 grams two or three times per day. I would not suggest going much higher than that until the BHB/BD or glyceride esters are approved for use in the general population, and then only with your doctor's approval and only with close blood ketone level monitoring and monitoring of other health parameters. (See Chapter 9.)

For those who do not tolerate ketone esters or have not secured a doctor's approval for their use, coconut oil and/or MCT oil might be alternatives to achieve the benefits of mild nutritional ketosis. As with ketone salts, check with your doctor.

Are Ketone Esters Safe for Diabetics?

Measurements in several studies report significantly lower blood glucose and insulin levels after taking ketone esters. As with ketone salts, people taking a ketone ester may experience a significantly lower blood sugar along with a drop in the insulin level (note that high doses of ketone ester theoretically could stimulate insulin production). If you are diabetic or prone to low blood sugar levels for another reason, do not begin taking ketone esters until obtaining your doctor's approval. To avoid abnormally low blood sugar, monitor your blood sugar closely, and work with your doctor to make changes in your medications. On the other hand, many type 2 diabetics report that they are able to reduce their medications, including insulin, rather quickly over a period of days or several weeks with a combination of ketone salts and a low-carb diet. Some people achieve this result with a low-carb ketogenic diet alone without exogenous ketone supplements; it is quite likely that a ketone ester supplement could enhance the effects of ketogenic diet for diabetics as well. A type 1 diabetic might be able to reduce the dose of insulin with this approach. Again, only go this route with approval and very close monitoring by your physician.

Is It Okay to Use Ketone Esters During Pregnancy and While Breastfeeding?

No. Women who are pregnant and breastfeeding are naturally in ketosis and taking ketone esters potentially could result in significant and serious ketoacidosis. There have been some case reports of very serious ketoacidosis in breastfeeding women on a strict ketogenic diet. It is quite possible that the ketone ester could result in ketoacidosis in a pregnant or breastfeeding woman as well. It is not known what effect, if any, the ketone ester might have on the developing fetus. I do not recommend using ketone esters during pregnancy or while breastfeeding.

How Might Ketone Esters Affect a Person Who Gets Kidney Stones or Gout?

The classic ketogenic diet is known to increase the risk of kidney stones and gout, so it is possible that taking ketone esters could increase the risk of these conditions as well. Taking a supplement to reduce acid in the blood, such as potassium citrate, and eating a low-acid diet could reduce the risk of kidney stones or gout. (See Chapter 10 on the Acidosis Sparing Diet.) Steve had a significant episode of gout while taking the ketone ester; taking a potassium citrate supplement appeared to prevent any further episodes.

Why Is the BHB/BD Ketone Ester So Expensive? How Does the Cost of the Ketone Ester Compare to the Cost of the Ketone Salts?

The process of making non-racemic betahydroxybutyrate is very expensive at present, which explains why both the BHB/BD ester and the non-racemic ketone salts (e.g. Keto//OS Max) cost considerably more than the racemic ketone salts. Millions of dollars have been poured into developing and testing these products as well. A newer method for producing non-racemic betahydroxybutyrate is on the horizon and waiting for the demand to grow for mass production of tons of material to make using this method practical. Once that happens, it is very likely the price will come down.

The actual costs per gram of the BHB/BD ester and non-racemic ketone salts are fairly comparable—currently about 80 cents per gram—before any discounts are applied, although the Keto//OS Max products contain other beneficial ingredients such as fermented ketogenic amino acids and AC-11 (a supplement for DNA repair) that are not found in the ketone esters. There is much more competition among companies producing the racemic mixtures of ketone salts; these are less expensive at 21 to 53 cents per gram. The labels for ketone salts should be studied closely. The least expensive product I could find (from Nutricost) has 13 grams of BHB per serving but also has extremely high levels of potassium (1,665 milligrams per serving) and calcium (1,500 milligrams per serving); this product also has 1,140 milligrams of sodium. These companies only need to adjust their serving size upward (say 28 grams versus 18 grams per serving) to make it appear that their product has more BHB. The trade-off for more BHB is more mineral salts.

Why Do Ketone Esters Taste So Bad?

The ketone esters, due to the nature of their ingredients, taste a lot like jet fuel. The companies marketing these esters are working hard to overcome the unpleasant taste and making some strides by sweetening them with stevia and adding flavor. At present, the taste of the ketone esters has a quality akin to drinking a straight hard liquor such as vodka, even with the recent improvements. People who object to drinking alcohol, a child, or someone with dementia might refuse to take the ketone ester due to the unpleasant and unusual taste. The companies that sell it suggest drinking the dose quickly. The ketone ester also has a heavy lingering after-taste.

I have not had the opportunity to taste the Hashim glyceride ketone ester but have been told the taste has been improved dramatically in the hands of food scientists.

When Steve took the ketone ester, I made a concoction of one part ketone ester, two parts water, and one part Soda Stream or Kool Aid Concentrate (orange, cranberry, and grape worked relatively well). The diet versions of these products made the ester taste more bitter, and the downside of using the sugared version was the sugar. Whenever I measured Steve's ketone level, I measured his blood sugar as well. One remarkable point to mention here is that Steve's blood sugar always dropped after he took the ketone ester even with the sugar in it and even if he ate something at the same time. Another point is that several experiments showed that when the BHB/BD ester was combined with carbohydrate, there were more impressive results in performance athletes than when it was not (Cox, 2016).

What Is the Best Way to Store a Ketone Ester?

The safest way to store the ketone ester is in a glass container or in the packaging provided from the company that makes it. Check the label for storage directions after opening the container. I made large batches of the ketone ester for Steve and stored it in the refrigerator due to the added ingredients. I stored the raw material at room temperature.

Can I Take a Ketone Ester and Ketone Salts at the Same Time?

There is probably no reason to take ketone salts and ketone esters at the same time, and the effect could be additive resulting in excessively high ketone levels. That said, the two different types of products could potentially be taken four or more hours apart.

Should I Continue to Take Coconut Oil and/or MCT Oil While Taking Ketone Salts or Ketone Esters?

There is no reason not to take coconut oil and/or MCT oil while taking ketone salts or ketone esters. To the contrary, coconut oil and MCT oil taken as part of your regular diet several times per day could provide a baseline level of ketosis, a foundation for even higher levels when ketone salts and ketone esters are taken as supplements. Combining this strategy with a high-fat, low-carb ketogenic diet could be a winning plan for achieving the maximum benefits of nutritional ketosis.

REFERENCES BY CHAPTER

Introduction

Bergen SS Jr., SA Hashim, TB VanItallie. "Hyperketonemia induced in man by medium-chain triglyceride." *Diabetes* Vol. 16, No. 10 (1966): 723–725.

Cahill GF Jr., RL Veech. "Ketoacids? Good medicine?" *Transactions of the American Clinical and Climatological Association* Vol. 114 (2003): 149–163.

Clarke K, K Tchabanenko, R Pawlosky, et al. "Kinetics, safety, and tolerability of (R)-3-hydroxybutyl (R)-3-hydroxybutyrate in healthy adult subjects." *Regulatory Toxicology and Pharmacology* Vol. 63 (2012): 401–8.

Cox PJ, T Kirk, T Ashmore, et al. "Nutritional ketosis alters fuel preference and thereby endurance performance in athletes." *Cell Metabolism* Vol. 24 (2016): 1–13.

De la Monte SM, JR Wands. "Review of insulin and insulin-like growth factor expression, signaling, and malfunction in the central nervous system: Relevance to Alzheimer's disease." *Journal of Alzheimer's Disease* Vol. 7 (2005): 45–61.

De la Monte SM, JR Wands. "Alzheimer's disease is type 3 diabetes—evidence reviewed." *Journal of Diabetes Science and Technology* Vol. 2, No. 6 (Nov 2008): 1101–13.

Doody RS, R Raman, M Farlow, et al. "A phase 3 trial of semagacestat for treatment of Alzheimer's disease." *New England Journal of Medicine* Vol. 369 No. 4 (2013): 341–50.

Henderson ST (Inventor). "Combinations of medium-chain triglycerides and therapeutic agents for the treatment and prevention of Alzheimer's disease and other diseases resulting from reduced neuronal metabolism." Available online at: www.freepatentsonline.com United States Patent 20080009467.

Itzhaki RF, MA Wozniak. "Herpes simplex virus type 1 in Alzheimer's disease: the enemy within." *Journal of Alzheimer's Disease* Vol 13 (2008): 393–405.

Kashiwaya Y, T Takeshima, N Mori, et al. "D-β-hydroxybutyrate protects neurons in models of Alzheimer's and Parkinson's disease." *Proceedings of the National Academy of the Sciences of the United States of America* Vol. 97 No. 10 (2000): 5440–44.

Newport MT. "What if there was a cure for Alzheimer's disease and no one knew?" July 2008. Available online at: http://coconutketones.com.

Newport MT, TB VanItallie, Y Kashiwaya, et al. "A new way to produce hyperketonemia: use of ketone ester in a case of Alzheimer's." *Alzheimer's and Dementia.* Vol. 11 No. 1. (2015): 99–103.

Owen OE, AP Morgan, GF Cahill Jr, et al. "Brain metabolism during fasting." *Journal of Clinical Investigation* Vol. 46 (1967): 1589–95.

Reger MA, ST Henderson, C Hale, et al. "Effects of β-hydroxybutyrate on cognition in memory-impaired adults." *Neurobiology of Aging* Vol. 25 (2004): 311–14.

Sato K, Y Kashiwaya, RL Veech, et al. "Insulin, ketone bodies, and mitochondrial energy transduction." *FASEB Journal* Vol. 9 (1995): 651–58.

Scarmeas N, JA Luchsinger, R Mayeux, et al. "Mediterranean diet and Alzheimer's disease mortality." *Neurology.* Vol. 69 (2007): 1084–93.

Simpson IA, KR Shundu, T Davies-Hill, et al. "Decreased concentrations of GLUT1 and GLUT3 glucose transporters in the brains of patients with Alzheimer's disease." *Annals of Neurology* Vol. 35 (1994): 546–51.

VanItallie TB, TH Nufert. "Ketones: metabolism's ugly duckling." *Nutrition Reviews* Vol. 61, No 10 (2003): 327–41.

Veech RL, B Chance, Y Kashiwaya, et al. "Hypothesis paper: ketone bodies, potential therapeutic uses." *IUBMB Life* Vol. 51 (2001): 241–47.

Veech RL. "The therapeutic implications of ketone bodies: the effects of ketone bodies in pathological conditions: ketosis, ketogenic diet, redox states, insulin resistance, and mitochondrial metabolism." *Prostaglandins, Leukotrienes and Essential Fatty Acids* Vol. 70 (2004): 309–19.

Chapter 1

Basu S, P Yoffe, N Hills, et al. "The relationship of sugar to population-level diabetes prevalence: an econometric analysis of repeated cross-sectional data." *PLoS One* Vol. 8 (2013): e57873.

Cahill G F, Jr. "Fuel metabolism in starvation." *Annual Reviews in Nutrition* Vol. 26 (2006): 1–22.

CDC Website (https://www.cdc.gov/diabetes/pdfs/data/statistics/national-diabetes-statistics-report.pdf).

Crane PK, R Walker, RA Hubbard, et al. "Glucose levels and risk of dementia." *New England Journal of Medicine NEJM* Vol. 369 No. 6 (2013): 540–48.

Dashti HM, NS Al-Zaid, TC Mathew, et al. "Long term effects of ketogenic diet in obese subjects with high cholesterol level." *Molecular and Cellular Biochemistry* Vol. 286 (2006): 1–9.

Dehghan M, A Mente, X Zhang, et al. "Associations of fats and carbohydrate intake with cardiovascular disease and mortality in eighteen countries from five continents (PURE): a prospective cohort study." *The Lancet* Vol. 390 No. 10107 (2017): 2050–62.

Feinman RD, WK Pogozelski, A Astrup, et al. "Dietary carbohydrate restriction as the first approach in diabetes management: Critical review and evidence base." *Nutrition* Vol. 31 (2015): 1–13.

Goodman EL, L Breithaupt, HJ Watson, et al. "Sweet taste preference in binge-eating disorder: A preliminary investigation." *Eating Behavior* Vol. 8 (2018): 8–15.

Guyenet, S. "By 2606 the US diet will be 100% sugar." *Whole Health Source: Nutrition and Health Science* www.wholehealthsource.blogspot.com, February 18, 2012.

"Heart Disease and Stroke Statistics—2017 Update: A Report from the American Heart Association." *Circulation* Vol. 135 No. 10 (2017): e146–e603.

Hosley-Moore E. "Sketches in Progress." *St. Petersburg Times* October 28, 2008.

Ivanova EA, VA Myasoedova, AA Melnichenko, et al. "Small Dense Low-Density Lipoprotein as Biomarker for Atherosclerotic Diseases." *Hindawi Oxidative Medicine and Cellular Longevity* Vol. 2017, Article ID 1273042:1–10.

Lennerz BS, A Barton, RK Bernstein, et al. "Management of type 1 diabetes with a very-low-carbohydrate diet." *Pediatrics* Epub ahead of print May 7, 2018.

Lennerz B, JK Lennerz. "Food addiction, high-glycemic-index carbohydrates, and obesity." *Clinical Chemistry* Vol. 64 No. 1 (2018): 64–71.

Makarem N, EV Bandera, Y Lin, et al. "Consumption of sugars, sugary foods and sugary beverages in relation to adiposity-related cancer risk in the framingham offspring cohort (1991–2013)." *Cancer Prevention Research* Epub ahead of print April 19, 2018.

McPherson JD, BH Shilton, DJ Walton. "Role of fructose in glycation and cross-linking of proteins." *Biochemistry*. Vol. 27 No. 6 (1988): 1901–7.

Nebeling LC, F Miraldi, SB Shurin, et al. "Effects of a ketogenic diet on tumor metabolism and nutritional status in pediatric oncology patients: two case reports." *Journal of the American College of Nutrition* Vol. 14 No. 2 (1995): 202–8.

Nohlgren, S. "Twist on Alzheimer's fight." *St. Petersburg Times* August 3, 2009.

Pase MP, JJ Himali, PF Jacques, et al. "Sugary beverage intake and preclinical Alzheimer's disease in the community." *Alzheimer's and Dementia* Vol. 13 No. 9 (2017): 955–64.

Poff AM, C Ari, P Arnold, et al. "Ketone supplementation decreases tumor cell viability and prolongs survival of mice with metastatic cancer." *International Journal of Cancer* Vol. 135 No. 7 (2014): 1711–20.

Scarmeas N, JA Luchsinger, R Mayeux, et al. "Mediterranean diet and Alzheimer's disease mortality." *Neurology* Vol. 69 (2007): 1084–93. Doi: 10.1212/01.wnl.0000277320.50685.7c

Sieri S, V Krogh, C Agnoli, et al. "Dietary glycemic index and glycemic load and risk of colorectal cancer: results from the EPIC-Italy study." *International Journal of Cancer* Vol. 136 No. 12 (2015): 2923–31.

Volek JS, SD Phinney, CE Forsythe, et al. "Carbohydrate restriction has a more favorable impact on the metabolic syndrome than a low-fat diet." *Lipids* Vo. 44 (2009): 297–309.

Zuccoli G, N Marcello, A Pisanello, et al. "Metabolic management of glioblastoma multiforme using standard therapy together with a restricted ketogenic diet: case report." *Nutrition and Metabolism* Vol 7, No 33 (2010): 1–7.

Chapter 2

Guyenet, S. "By 2606 the US diet will be 100% sugar." *Whole Health Source: Nutrition and Health Science* www.wholehealthsource.blogspot.com, February 18, 2012.

Lands, WE. *Fish, Omega-3 and Human Health* AOCS Press, Urbana Illinois, 2nd edition, 2005.

Chapter 3

Cunnane SC, A Courchesne-Loyer, C Vandenberghe, et al. "Can ketones help rescue brain fuel supply in later life? Implications for cognitive health during aging and the treatment of Alzheimer's Disease." *Frontiers in Molecular Neuroscience.* Open Access. Vol. 9 No. 53 (2016): e1–21. doi 10.3389/fnmol.2016.00053

Elamin M, DN Ruskin, SA Masino, et al. "Ketogenic diet modulates NAD+-dependent enzymes and reduces DNA damage in the hippocampus." *Frontiers Cellular Neurosci* Vol. 12 No. 263 (2018):e1-7.

Mattson MP, K Moehl, N Ghena, et al. "Intermittent metabolic switching, neuroplasticity and brain health." *Neuroscience.* Vol. 19 (2018): 63–80. Doi: 10.1038/nrn.2017.156

Mattson M. "Why fasting bolsters brain power: Mark Mattson at TEDxJohnsHopkinsUniversity 2014." https://www.youtube.com/watch?v=4UkZAwKoCP8

Owen OE, AP Morgan, GF Cahill Jr, et al. "Brain metabolism during fasting." *Journal of Clinical Investigation* Vol. 46 (1967): 1589–95.

Puchalska P, P Crawford. "Multi-dimensional roles of ketone bodies in fuel metabolism, signaling, and therapeutics." *Cell Metabolism* Vol. 25 No. 2 (2017): 262–84.

Sato K, Y Kashiwaya, RL Veech, et al. "Insulin, ketone bodies, and mitochondrial energy transduction." *FASEB Journal* Vol. 9 (1995): 651–58.

Veech RL, B Chance, Y Kashiwaya, et al. "Hypothesis paper: ketone bodies, potential therapeutic uses." *IUBMB Life* Vol. 51 (2001): 241–7.

Veech RL, PC Bradshaw, K Clarke, et al. "Ketone bodies mimic the life span extending properties of caloric restriction." *IUBMB Life.* Vol. 69 No. 5 (2017): 305–14.

Xin L, Ö Ipek, M Beaumont, et al. "Nutritional ketosis increases NAD+/NADH ratio in healthy human brain: An *in vivo* study by 31P-MRS." *Frontiers Nutr* Vol. 5 No. 62 (2018):e1-8.

Chapter 4

Abrahams J. Interview with author. February 6, 2018.

Adam PA, N Räihä, EL Rahiala, et al. "Oxidation of glucose and D-B-OH-butyrate by the early human fetal brain." *Acta Paediatrica Scandinavia* Vol. 64 No. 1 (1975): 17–24.

Baker CE , RM Wilder. High-fat diets in epilepsy. *The Clinic Bulletin* Vol. 2 No. 308 (1921): 1.

Banting, W. *Letter on Corpulence, Addressed to the Public.* Harrison, London, 1863.

Batugal P, V Rao, J Oliver, editors. *Coconut Genetic Resources.* 2005. IPGRI - Regional Office for Asia, the Pacific and Oceania, Serdang, Malaysia.

Bourgneres PF, C Lemmel, P Ferre, et al. "Ketone body transport in the human neonate and infant." *Journal of Clinical Investigation* Vol. 77 (1986): 42–8.

Bourgneres PF, L Castano, F Rocchiccioli, et al. "Medium-chain fatty acids increase glucose production in normal and low birth weight newborns." *American Journal of Physiology* Vol. 256 (1989): E692–7.

Cahill GF, Jr. "Fuel metabolism in starvation." *Annual Reviews in Nutrition* Vol. 26 (2006): 1–22.

Castellano C-A, N Paquet, IJ Dionne, et al. A 3-month aerobic training program improves brain energy metabolism in mild Alzheimer's disease: preliminary results from a neuroimaging study. *Journal of Alzheimer's Disease.* Vol. 56 (2017): 1459–69. doi: 10.3233/JAD-161163

CDC Report. "Trends in obesity among participants aged 2–4 years in the special supplemental nutrition program for women, infants, and children—United States, 2000–2014." *Mortality and Morbidity Weekly Report* Vol. 65 No. 45 (2016): 1256–60. PDF at https://www.cdc.gov/mmwr/volumes/65/wr/mm6545a2.htm?s_cid=mm6545a2_w

Cordain L, SB Eaton, JB Miller, et al. "The paradoxical nature of hunter-gatherer diets: meat-based, yet non-atherogenic." *European Journal of Clinical Nutrition.* Vol. 56 No. 1 (2002): 542–52. doi 10.1038/sj/ejcn/1601353.

Cordain L. The Paleo Diet website. https://thepaleodiet.com/what-to-eat-on-the-paleo-diet-paul-vandyken/

Cordain L. *The Paleo Diet* John Wiley & Sons, Revised Edition 2010.

Cunnane SC, CR Menard, SS Likhodil, et al. "Carbon recycling into de novo lipogenesis is a major pathway in neonatal metabolism of linoleate and α-linolenate." *Prostaglandins, Leukotrienes and Essential Fatty Acids.* Vol. 60 No. 5 & 6. (1999): 387–92

Cunnane SC, MA Crawford. "Survival of the fattest: fat babies were the key to evolution of the large human brain." *Comparative Biochem and Physiol Part A.* Vol. 136 (2003): 17–26. doi 10.1016/S1095-6433(03)00048-5

Cunnane, SC. "Human brain evolution: a question of solving key nutritional and metabolic constraints on mammalian brain development." *Human Brain Evolution: The Influence of Freshwater and Marine Food Resources* Chapter 3 (2010): 33–64.

De Boissieu D, F Rocchiccioli, N Kalach, et al. "Ketone body turnover at term and in premature newborns in the first two weeks after birth." *Biology of the Neonate* Vol. 67 No. 2 (1995): 84–93.

De Rooy L, J Hawdon. "Nutritional factors that affect the postnatal metabolic adaptation of full-term and small- and large-for gestational age infants." *Pediatrics*, Vol. 109 No.3 (2002): 1–8.

Densmore, Emmet, M.D. *How Nature Cures—Comprising A New System of Hygiene; Also The Natural Food of Man* 1892. Available on Amazon.

Diamond, David. "David Diamond—an update on demonization and deception in research on saturated fat." https://www.youtube.com/watch?v=uc1XsO3mxX8

Edmondson CH. "Viability of coconut seeds after floating in the sea." *Bernice P. Bishop Museum Occasional Papers* Vol 16 (1941): 293–304.

Food and Agricultural Organization of the United Nations Corporate Document Repository - http://www.fao.org/docrep/005/y4355e/y4355e03.htm

Gibbons A. "Evolution of diet." *National Geographic* published online at (www.nationalgeographic.com/foodfeatures/evolution-of-diet) [date not available online]

Guelpa G, A Marie. "La lutte contre l'épilepsie par la désintoxication et par la rééducation alimentaire." *Revista Ther Medico–Chirurgicale* Vol. 78 (1911): 8–13.

Gunn BF, L Baudouin, KM Olsen. "Independent origins of cultivated coconut (Cocos nucifera L.) in the old world tropics." *PLoS one.* Vol. 6 No. 6 (2011): e21143. doi: 10.1371/journal.pone.0021143

Hamosh M, J Bitman, DL Wood, et al. "Lipids in milk and the first steps in their digestion." *Pediatrics.* Vol. 75 (1985): 146–150.

Hawdon JM, MP W Platt, A Aynsley-Green. "Patterns of metabolic adaptation for preterm and term infants in the first neonatal week." *Archives of Disease in Childhood.* Vol. 67 (1992): 357–65.

Hermanussen M. "Stature of early Europeans." *Hormones.* Vol. 2 No. 3 (2003): 175–8.

Holliday MA. "Metabolic rate and organ size during growth from infancy to maturity and during late gestation and early infancy." *Pediatrics* Vol. 47 No. 1 Suppl. 2 (1971): 169+–

Huttenlocher PR, AJ Wilbourn, JM Signore. "Medium-chain triglycerides as a therapy for intractable childhood epilepsy." *Neurology* Vol. 21 (1971): 1097–1103.

Ijiff DM, D Postulart, DA JE Lambrechts, et al. "Cognitive and behavioral impact of the ketogenic diet in children and adolescents with refractory epilepsy: a randomized controlled trial." *Epilepsy & Behavior.* Vol. 60 (2016): 153–7. Doi: 10.1016/j.yebeh.2016.04.033

Kaplan H, RCG Thompson, BC Trumble, et al. "Coronary atherosclerosis in indigenous South American Tsimane: a cross-sectional cohort study." *The Lancet* Vol. 389 No. 10080 (2017): 1730–9. doi 10.1016/S0140-6736(17)30752-3

Kossoff EH, BA Zupec-Kania, PE Amark, et al. "Optimal clinical management of children receiving the ketogenic diet: Recommendations of the International Ketogenic Diet Study Group." *Epilepsia* Vo. 50 No. 2 (2009): 304–71.

Kossoff, EH, BA Zupec-Kania, S Auvin, et al. Optimal clinical management of children receiving dietary therapies for epilepsy: Updated recommendations of the International Ketogenic Diet Study Group. *Epilepsia Open* Vol. 3 No. 2 (2018):175–192.

Lands, WE. *Fish, omega-3 and human health* AOCS Press, Urbana Illinois, 2nd edition, 2005.

Leith W. "Experiences with the Pennington diet in the management of obesity." *Canadian Medical Association Journal.* Vol. 84 No. 25 (1961): 1411–14.

Lucas A, SR Bloom, A Aynsley-Green. "Metabolic and endocrine events at the time of the first feed of human milk in preterm and term infants." *Archives of Disease in Childhood* Vol. 53 (1978): 731–736.

My Plate for Preschoolers (https://www.choosemyplate.gov/MyPlate).

Pennington AW. "An alternate approach to the problem with obesity." *American Journal of Clinical Nutrition* Vol. 1 No. 2 (1953A): 100–106.

Pennington AW. "Treatment of obesity with calorically unrestricted diets." *The American Journal of Clinical Nutrition* Vol. 1 No. 5 (1953B): 343–8.

Robson SL, B Wood. "Hominim life history: reconstruction and evolution." *Journal of Anatomy* Vol. 212 (2008): 394–425.

Rudolf MCJ, RS Sherwin. "Maternal ketosis and its effects on the fetus." *Clinics in Endocrinology and Metabolis.* Vol. 12 No. 2 (1983): 413–28.

Scarmeas N, J A Luchsinger, R Mayeux, et al. "Mediterranean diet and Alzheimer's disease mortality." *Neurology* Vol. 69 (2007): 1084--93. Doi: 10.1212/01.wnl.0000277320.50685.7c

Tantibhedhyangkul P, SA Hashim. "Clinical and physiologic aspects of medium-chain triglycerides: alleviation of steatorrhea in premature infants." *Bulletin of the New York Academy of Medicine* Vol. 47 No. 1 (1971): 17–33.

VanItallie TB, C Nonas, A Di Rocco, et al. "Treatment of Parkinson disease with diet-induced hyperketonemia: a feasibility study." *Neurology* Vol. 64 (February 2005): 728–30.

Wilder RM. "The effects of ketonemia on the course of epilepsy." *The Clinic Bulletin* Vol. 2 No. 307 (1921): 1.

Wilder RM and GM Randall. *"Diseases of metabolism."* Internal Medicine, 4th Edition, Lea and Febiger, Philadelphia (1945): 1220.

Woodyatt RT. "Objects and method of diet adjustment in diabetics." *Archives of Internal Medicine* Vol. 28 (1921): 125–141.

Wu PYK, J Edmond, N Auestad, et al. "Medium-chain triglycerides in infant formulas and their relation to plasma ketone body concentrations." *Pediatric Research* Vol. 20 No. 4 (1986): 338–41.

Zupec-Kania, B. Interview on January 27, 2018

Chapter 5

Ashmore J, GF Cahill Jr, AB Hastings. "Intracellular ionic environment and enzyme activities; carbohydrate metabolism in liver." *Archives of Biochemistry and Biophysiology* Vol. 65 No. 1 (1956): 78–85.

Bergen SS Jr, SA Hashim, TB VanItallie. "Hyperketonemia induced in man by medium-chain triglyceride." *Diabetes* Vol. 15 (1966): 723–5.

Blesa J, V Jackson-Lewis, N Boaz, S Hashim, et al. "Glyceryl-tris-3-hydroxybutyrate protects dopaminergic neurons in a MPTP model of Parkinson's disease." Society of Neuroscience Annual Meeting Oct 17, 2012. Oral presentation with published abstract and poster. Program/poster # 856.21/G14.

Blurton-Jones M, M Kitazawa, H Martinez-Coria, et al. "Neural stem cells improve cognition via BDNF in a transgenic model of Alzheimer's disease." *Proceedings of the National Academy of the Sciences of the United States of America PNAS* Vol 106, No 32 (Aug 2009): 13594–99.

Cahill GF Jr, MG Herrera, AP Morgan, et al. "Hormone-fuel interrelationships during fasting." *Journal of Clinical Investigation.* Vol. 45 No. 11 (1966): 1751–69.

Cahill GF Jr., RL Veech. "Ketoacids? Good medicine?" *Transactions of the American Clinical and Climatological Association* Vol 114 (2003): 149–63.

Cahill GF Jr, TT Aoki. "Alternate fuel utilization by brain." In *Cerebral Metabolism and Neural Function* by JV Passonneau, RA Hawkins, WD Lust, Welsh FA, Eds. Baltimore, MD: Williams & Wilkins (1980), p. 234–42.

Cahill GF, Jr. "Fuel metabolism in starvation." *Annual Reviews in Nutrition* Vol. 26 (2006): 1–22.

Castellano C-A, N Paquet, IJ Dionne, et al. "A 3-month aerobic training program improves brain energy metabolism in mild Alzheimer's disease: preliminary results from a neuroimaging study." *Journal of Alzheimer's Disease.* Vol. 56 (2017): 1459–69. doi: 10.3233/JAD-161163

Courchesne-Loyer A, E Croteau, C-A Castellano, et al. "Inverse relationship between brain glucose and ketone metabolism in adults during short-term moderate dietary ketosis: A dual tracer quantitative positron emission tomography study." *Journal of Cerebral Blood Flow and Metabolism.* Open Access (2016): E1–9. doi 10.1177/0271678X16669366

Courchesne-Loyer A, M Fortier, J Tremblay-Mercier, et al. "Stimulation of mild, sustained ketonemia by medium-chain triacylglycerols in healthy humans: Estimated potential contribution to brain energy metabolism." *Nutrition.* (2013): 1–6.

Courtice FC, CG Douglas. "The effects of prolonged muscular exercise on the metabolism." *Proceedings of the Royal Society of London* Vol 119B (1936): 381–439.

Croteau E, C-A Castellano, M Fortier, et al. "A cross-sectional comparison of brain glucose and ketone metabolism in cognitively healthy older adults, mild cognitive impairment and early Alzheimer's disease." *Experimental Gerontology* Vol. 107 (2018A): 18–26.

Croteau E, C-A Castellano, MA Richard, et al. "Ketogenic medium-chain triglycerides increase brain energy metabolism in Alzheimer's disease." *Journal of Alzheimer's Disease.*

Cunnane SC, A Courchesne-Loyer, C Vandenberghe, et al. Can ketones help rescue brain fuel supply in later life? Implications for cognitive health during aging and the treatment of Alzheimer's Disease. *Frontiers in Molecular Neuroscience.* Open Access. Vol. 9 No. 53 (2016): e1–21. doi 10.3389/fnmol.2016.00053

Cunnane SC, CR Menard, SS Likhodil, et al. "Carbon recycling into de novo lipogenesis is a major pathway in neonatal metabolism of linoleate and α-linolenate." *Prostaglandins, Leukotrienes and Essential Fatty Acids.* Vol. 60 No. 5 & 6. (1999): 387–92

Cunnane SC, MA Crawford. "Survival of the fattest: fat babies were the key to evolution of the large human brain." *Comparative Biochemistry and Physiology Part A.* Vol. 136 (2003): 17–26. doi 10.1016/S1095-6433(03)00048-5

Cunnane, SC. "Human Brain Evolution: A Question of Solving Key Nutritional and Metabolic Constraints on Mammalian Brain Development. *Human Brain Evolution: The Influence of Freshwater and Marine Food Resources* Chapter 3 (2010): 33–64.

Cunnane SC. "Metabolism of polyunsaturated fatty acids and ketogenesis: an emerging connection." *PLEFA.* Vol. 70 No. 3 (2004): 237–41. Doi: 10.1016/j.plefa.2003.11.002

Cunnane, SC. *Survival of the Fattest: The Key to Human Brain Evolution* (World Scientific, 2005)

Cunnane S. Interview by Mary T. Newport, MD on Nov 5, 2017.

Curtis W. "Guitar before and after drinking coffee concoction for Parkinson's disease." https://www.youtube.com/watch?v=oYaFv-8dv58.

Curtis W. "My Parkinson's treatment with a morning fat filled coffee to release ketones." https://www.youtube.com/watch?v=riGYq5iD2SM

Curtis W. Interview by Mary T. Newport, MD on November 3, 2017.)

D'Agostino DP, R Pilla, HE Held, et al. "Therapeutic ketosis with ketone ester delays central nervous system oxygen toxicity seizures in rats." *American Journal of Physiology-Regulatory Integrative and Comparative Physiology.* Vol. 305 No. 10 (2013): r829–36.

D'Agostino, Dominic. Interview by Mary T. Newport, M.D. on November 19, 2017.

Dayrit FM. "The properties of lauric acid and their significance in coconut oil." *Journal of the American Oil Chemists Society.* Vol. 92 (2015): 1–15.

Fery F, EO Balasse. "Ketone body turnover during and after exercise in overnight-fasted and starved humans." *American Journal of Physiology Endocrinology and Metabolism* Vol 245 (1983): 318–25.

Forssner G. "Über die einwirkung der muskelarbeit auf die acetonkörperausscheiding bei kohlenhydratarmer kost." *Skand Arch Physiol* Vol. 22 (1909): 393–405. Vol. 64 (2018):551-561

Fortier M, C-A Castellano, E Croteau, et al. A ketogenic drink improves brain energy and some measures of cognition in MCI. In press, expected publication in 2019.

Geliebter A, N Torbay, F Bracco, et al. "Overfeeding with medium-chain triglyceride diet results in diminished deposition of fat." *American Journal of Clinical Nutrition.* Vol. 37 (1983): 1–4.

Gracey M, V Burke, CM Anderson. "Medium chain triglycerides in paediatric practice." *Archives of Disease in Childhood.* Vol. 45 (1970): 445–52.

Greene AE, MT Todorova, R McGowan, Seyfried TN. "Caloric restriction inhibits seizure susceptibility in epileptic EL mice by reducing blood glucose." *Epilepsia* Vol. 42 No. 11 (2001): 1371–8.

Hashim SA, RE Clancy, DM Hegsted, et al. "Effect of Mixed Fat Formula Feeding on Serum Cholesterol Level in Man." *American Journal of Clinical Nutrition* Vol. 7 (1959): 30–4.

Hashim SA, TB VanItallie. "Ketone body therapy: from the ketogenic diet to the oral administration of ketone ester." *Journal of Lipid Research.* Vol. 55 (2014): 1818. Doi: 10.1196/jlr.R06599

Hashim S. Interview by Mary T. Newport, M.D. on February 23, 2018.

Hosley-Moore E. "Sketches in Progress." *St. Petersburg Times* October 28, 2008.

Huttenlocher PR, AJ Wilbourn, JM Signore. "Medium-chain triglycerides as a therapy for intractable childhood epilepsy." *Neurology* Vol. 21 (1971):1097–103.

Johnson RH, JL Walton, HA Krebs, et al. "Post-exercise ketosis." *The Lancet* (December 1969): 1383–85.

Kalamian, Miriam. *Keto for Cancer: Ketogenic Metabolic Therapy as a Targeted Nutritional Strategy.* 2017, Chelsea Green Publishing.

Kalamian M. Interview by Mary T. Newport, M.D. on December 9, 2017.

Kashiwaya Y, K Sato, N Tsuchiya, et al. "Control of glucose utilization in working perfused rat heart." *The Journal of Biological Chemistry* Vol. 269, No. 41 (October 1994): 25502–14.

Kashiwaya Y, T King, RL Veech. "Substrate signaling by insulin: A ketone bodies ratio mimics insulin action in heart." *American Journal of Cardiology* Vol. 80, No. 3A (1997): 50A–64A.

Kashiwaya Y, T Takeshima, N Mori, et al. "D-β-hydroxybutyrate protects neurons in models of Alzheimer's and Parkinson's disease." *Proceedings of the National Academy of the Sciences of the United States of America PNAS* Vol. 97, No. 10 (May 2000): 5440–44.

Kashiwaya Y, C Bergman, J-H Lee, et al. "A ketone ester diet exhibits anxiolytic and cognition-sparring properties, and lessens amyloid and tau pathologies in a mouse model of Alzheimer's." *Neurobiology of Aging* Vol. 34 No. 6 (2013): 1530–9.

Kephart WC, PW Mumford, X Mao, et al. "The 1-week and 8-month effects of a ketogenic diet or ketone salt supplementation on multi-organ markers of oxidative stress and mitochondrial function in rats." *Nutrients* Vol. 9 No. 1019 (2017):1–22 1019; doi:10.3390/nu9091019

Koeslag JH, TD Noakes, AW Sloan. "Post-exercise ketosis." *Physiology* Vol. 301 (1980): 79–90.

Lussier DM, EC Woolf, JL Johnson, et al. "Enhanced immunity in a mouse model of malignant glioma is mediated by a therapeutic ketogenic diet." *BMC Cancer* Vol. 16 No. 310 (2016): 1–10.

Lying-Tunell U, BS Lindblad, HO Malmlund, et al. "Cerebral blood flow and metabolic rate of oxygen, glucose, lactate, pyruvate, ketone bodies and amino acids." *Acta Neurologica Scandinavica.* Vol. 63 (1981): 337–50.

Meidenbauer JJ, P Mukherjee, TN Seyfried. "The glucose ketone index calculator: a simple tool to monitor therapeutic efficacy for metabolic management of brain cancer." *Nutrition and Metabolism.* Vol. 12 No. 12 (2015):e1–7. doi: 10.1186/s12986-015-0009-2

Nebeling LC, F Miraldi, SB Shurin, et al. "Effects of a ketogenic diet on tumor metabolism and nutritional status in pediatric oncology patients: two case reports." *Journal of the American College of Nutrition.* Vol. 14 No. 2 (1995): 202–8.

Newport MT. "What if there was a cure for Alzheimer's disease and no one knew?" July 2008. Self-published online at www.coconutketones.com.

Newport MT, TB VanItallie, Y Kashiwaya, et al. "A new way to produce kyperketonemia: use of ketone ester in a case of Alzheimer's." *Alzheimer's and Dementia.* Vol. 11 No. 1. (2015): 99–103. doi: 10.1016/j.jalz2014.01.006

Nugent S, C-A Castellano, P Goffaux, et al. "Glucose hypometabolism is highly localized, but lower cortical thickness and brain atrophy are widespread in cognitively normal older adults." *American Journal of Physiology-Endocrinology and Metabolism.* Vol. 306 (2014): e1315–21. Doi: 10.1152/ajpendo.00067.201

Nugent S, S Tremblay, KW Chen, et al. "Brain glucose and acetoacetate metabolism: a comparison of young and older adults." *Neurobiology of Aging.* Vol. 35 No. 6 (2014): 1386–95. Doi: 10.1016/j.neurobiolaging.2013.11.027

Otto A. "Warburg effect(s)—a biographical sketch of Otto Warburg and his impacts on tumor metabolism." *Cancer & Metabolism* Open Access Vol. 4 No. 5 (2016): e1–8. DOI 10.1186/s40170-016-0145-9

Owen OE, AP Morgan, GF Cahill Jr, et al. "Brain metabolism during fasting." *Journal of Clinical Investigation* Vol. 46 (1967): 1589–95.

Owen OE. "Ketone bodies as a fuel for the brain during starvation." *Biochemistry and Molecular Biology Education* Vol. 33, No. 4 (2005): 246–51.

Passmore R, RE Johnson. "The modification of post-exercise ketosis (the Courtice-Douglas effect) by environmental temperature and water balance." *Experimental Physiology* (1958): 352–61.

Pi-Sunyer FX, SA Hashim, TB VanItallie. "Insulin and ketone responses to ingestion of medium and long-chain triglycerides in man." *Diabetes* Vol. 18 (1969): 96–100].

Plourde M, SC Cunnane. "Extremely limited synthesis of long chain polyunsaturates in adults: implications for their dietary essentiality and use as supplements." *Applied Physiology, Nutrition and Metabolism* Vol. 32 No. 4 (2007): 613–34.

Poff AM, C Ari, P Arnold, et al. "Ketone supplementation decreases tumor cell viability and prolongs survival of mice with metastatic cancer." *International Journal of Cancer* Vol. 135 No. 7 (2014): 1711–20. Doi: 10.1002/ijc.28809

Poff AM, D Kerganis, DP D'Agostino. "Hyperbaric environment: oxygen and cellular damage versus protection." *Comprehensive Physiology.* Vol. 7 No. 1 (2016): 213–34. Doi: 10.1002/cphys.c150032

Poff A. Interview by Mary T. Newport, MD on January 4, 2018.)

Prata C and J. Interview by Mary T Newport, MD on February 7, 2018.)

Preti L. "Die muskelarbeit und deren ketogene wirkung." *Biochemistry Z* Vol 32 (1911): 231–34.

Reger MA, ST Henderson, C Hale, et al. "Effects of β-hydroxybutyrate on cognition in memory impaired adults." *Neurobiology of Aging* Vol. 25 (2004): 311–14.

Rennie MJ, S Jennett, RH Johnson. "The metabolic effects of strenuous exercise: a comparison between untrained subjects and racing cyclists." *Experimental Physiology* Vol. 59 No. 3 (1974): 201–12.

Rho JM, R Sankar. "The ketogenic diet in a pill: is this possible?" *Epilepsia.* Vol. 49 No. 8 (2008): 127-33. Doi: 10.1111/j.1528-1167.2008.01857.x

Sato K, Y Kashiwaya, RL Veech, et al. "Insulin, ketone bodies, and mitochondrial energy transduction." *FASEB Journal* Vol. 9 (1995): 651–58.

Senior J., Editor. *Medium-chain Triglycerides* University of Pennsylvania Press, 1968.

Seyfried TN, P Mukherjee. "Targeting energy metabolism in brain cancer: Review and hypothesis." *Nutrition and Metabolism* Vol. 2, No. 30 (2005): 1–9.

Seyfried T. *Cancer as a Metabolic Disease: On the Origin, Management, and Prevention of Cancer* Hoboken, NY: John Wiley and Sons, Inc. (2012).

Seyfried TN, G Yu, JC Maroon, et al. "Press-pulse: a novel therapeutic strategy for the metabolic management of cancer." *Nutrition and Metabolism* Vol. 14 No. 19 (2017): e1–17. doi: 10.1186/s12986-017-0178-2

Seyfried T. Interview by Mary T. Newport, MD on February 2, 2018

Spindler SR. "Rapid and reversible induction of the longevity, anticancer and genomic effects of caloric restriction." *Mechanisms of Ageing and Development* Vol. 126 No. 9 (2005): 960–6.

Srivastava S, Y Kashiwaya, MT King, et al. "Mitochondrial biogenesis and increased uncoupling protein 1 in brown adipose tissue of mice fed a ketone ester diet." *FASEB Journal* Vol. 1302 (2013): 42–8

Swerdlow R, Marcus DM, Landman J, Harooni M, Freedman ML. "Brain glucose and ketone body metabolism in patients with Alzheimer's disease." *Clinical Research* Vol. 37 No. 461A (1989)

Swerdlow R. Interview by Mary T. Newport, MD on November 5, 2017.

Tantibhedhyangkul P, SA Hashim. "Clinical and physiologic aspects of medium-chain triglycerides: alleviation of steatorrhea in premature infants." *Bulletin of the New York Academy of Medicine* Vol. 47 No. 1 (1971): 17–33.

Taylor MK, DK Sullivan, JD Mahnken, et al. "Feasibility and efficacy data from a ketogenic diet intervention in Alzheimer's disease." *Alzheimer's and Dementia.* (2017): e1–9.

Vandenverghe C, V St.-Pierre, A Courchesne-Loyer, et al. "Caffeine intake increases plasma ketones: an acute metabolic study in humans." *Canadian Journal of Physiology and Pharmacology* (2016): 1–3. doi: 10.1139/cjpp-2016-0338

VanItallie TB, AK Khachadurian. "Rats enriched with odd-carbon fatty acids: maintenance of liver glycogen during starvation." *Science* Vol. 165 No. 3895 (1969): 811–13.

VanItallie TB, TH Nufert. "Ketones: metabolism's ugly duckling." *Nutr Rev* Vol. 61, No. 10 (2003): 327–41.

VanItallie TB, C Nonas, A Di Rocco, et al. "Treatment of Parkinson's disease with diet-induced hyperketonemia: a feasibility study." *Neurology* Vol. 64 (2005): 728–30.

VanItallie TB. Interview by Mary T. Newport, MD on February 8, 2018.

Veech RL, B Chance, Y Kashiwaya, et al. "Hypothesis paper: ketone bodies, potential therapeutic uses." *IUBMB Life* Vol. 51 (2001): 241–47.

Veech RL. "The therapeutic implications of ketone bodies: the effects of ketone bodies in pathological conditions: ketosis, ketogenic diet, redox states, insulin resistance, and mitochondrial metabolism." *Prostaglandins, Leukotrienes and Essential Fatty Acids* Vol. 70 (2004): 309–19.

Veech RL. Interview by Mary T. Newport, MD on November 3, 2017.

Wilson JM, RP Lowery, MD Roberts, et al. "The effects of ketogenic dieting on body composition, strength, power, and hormonal profiles in resistance training males." *Journal of Strength and Conditioning Research* in press (2017).

Wilson J, R Lowery. *The Ketogenic Bible: The Authoritative Guide to Ketosis.* Las Vegas, NV: Victory Belt Publishing (2017).

Yin JX, M Maalouf, P Han, et al. "Ketones block amyloid entry and improve cognition in an Alzheimer's model." *Neurobiology of Aging* Vol. 39 (2016): 25–37.

Yu G. Interview by Mary T. Newport, MD on February 6, 2018.

Zuccoli G, N Marcello, A Pisanello, et al. "Metabolic management of glioblastoma multiforme using standard therapy together with a restricted ketogenic diet: case report." *Nutrition and Metabolism* Vol. 7, No. 33 (2010): 1–7.

Chapter 6

Bergen SS, Jr., SA Hashim, TB VanItallie. "Hyperketonemia induced in man by medium-chain triglyceride." *Diabetes* Vol. 16, No. 10 (1966): 723–25.

Huttenlocher PR, AJ Wilbourn, JM Signore. "Medium-chain triglycerides as a therapy for intractable childhood epilepsy." *Neurology* Vol. 21 (1971): 1097–103.

Jenkins DJA, TMS Wolever, RH Taylor, et al. "Glycemic index of foods: a physiological basis for carbohydrate exchange." *American Journal of Clinical Nutrition* Vol. 34 (1981): 362–66.

Kalamian M. *Keto for Cancer: Ketogenic Metabolic Therapy as a Targeted Nutritional Strategy.* White River Junction, VT: Chelsea Green Publishing, 2017.

Kossoff EH, JR McGogan, RM Bluml, et al. "A modified Atkins diet is effective for the treatment of intractable pediatric epilepsy." *Epilepsia* No. 47 No. 2 (2006): 421–24.

Kossoff EH, JM. Freeman, Z Turner, and JE. Rubenstein. *Ketogenic Diets: Treatments for Epilepsy and Other Disorders.* 5th ed. New York, NY: Demos Medical Publishing, 2011.

Masino SA. *Ketogenic Diet and Metabolic Therapies.* New York, NY: Oxford University Press, 2017.

National Institutes of Health Office of Dietary Supplements, the National Food and Nutrition Board of the Institute of Medicine *Dietary Reference Intakes for Energy, Carbohydrate, Fiber, Fat, Fatty Acids, Cholesterol, Protein, and Amino Acids* (National Academies Press, 2005). Free online at https://ods.od.nih.gov /Health_Information/Dietary_Reference_Intakes.aspx.

Netzer CT. *The Nutribase Complete Book of Food Counts.* 9th ed. New York, New York: Dell, 2017.

Pfeifer HH, A Thiele. "Low-glycemic-index treatment: a liberalized ketogenic diet for treatment of intractable epilepsy." *Neurology* Vol. 65 No. 1810 (2005): 1810–12.

Tantibhedhyangkul P, SA Hashim. "Clinical and physiologic aspects of medium-chain triglycerides: alleviation of steatorrhea in premature infants." *Bulletin of the New York Academy of Medicine* Vol. 47 No. 1 (1971): 17–33.

Wilson, Jacob and Lowery Ryan. *The Ketogenic Bible: The Authoritative Guide to Ketosis,* 2017, Las Vegas, NV: Victory Belt Publishing, 2017.

Zupec Kania B. "KetoCalculator: A web-based calculator for the ketogenic diet." *Epilepsia* Vol. 49 No. 8 (2008): 14–16.

Chapter 7

Bixel MG, B Hamprecht. "Generation of ketone bodies from leucine by cultured astroglial cells." *Journal of Neurochemistry* Vol. 65 No. 6 (1995): 2450–61.

Castellano C-A, N Paquet, IJ Dinne, et al. "A 3-month aerobic training program improves brain energy metabolism in mild Alzheimer's disease: Preliminary results from a neuroimaging study." *J Alzheimer's Disease* Vol. 56 (2017): 1459–68.

Clarke K, K Tchabanenko, R Pawlosky, et al. "Kinetics, safety and tolerability of (R)-3-hydroxybutyl (R)-3-hydroxybutyrate in healthy adult subjects." *Regulatory Toxicology and Pharmacology* Vol. 63 (2012): 401–8.

Cox PJ, T Kirk, T Ashmore, et al. "Nutritional ketosis alters fuel preference and thereby endurance performance in athletes." *Cell Metabolism* Vol. 24 (2016): 1-13

Dayrit FM. "The properties of lauric acid and their significance in coconut oil." *Journal of the American Oil Chemists Society* Vol. 92 (2015): 1–15.

Evangeliou A, M Spilioti, V Douglioglou, et al. "Branched chain amino acids as adjunctive therapy to ketogenic diet in epilepsy: pilot study and hypothesis." *Journal of Child Neurology* Vol. 24 No. 10 (2009): 1268–72. Doi: 10.1177/0883073809336295

Fauser JK, GM Matthews, AG Cummins, et al. "Induction of apoptosis by the medium-chain length fatty acid lauric acid in colon cancer cells due to induction of oxidative stress." *Chemotherapy* Vol. 59 (2013): 214–24.

Hashim S A, T B VanItallie. Ketone body therapy: from the ketogenic diet to the oral administration of ketone ester. *Journal of Lipid Research.* Vol. 55 (2014): 1818–?. Doi: 10.1194/jlr.R046599

Holdsworth DA, PJ Cox, T Kirk, et al. "A ketone ester drink increases post-exercise muscle glycogen synthesis in humans." *Medicine and Science Sports and Exercise.* Vol. 49 No. 9 (2017): 1789–95.

Itzhaki RF, R Lathe, BJ Balin, et al. "Microbes and Alzheimer's disease." *Journal of Alzheimer's Disease* Vol. 51 (2016): 979–84. doi 10.3233/JAD-160152

Kezutyte T, N Desbenoit, A Brunelle, et al. "Studying the penetration of fatty acids into human skin by ex vivo TOF-SIMS imaging." *Biointerphases.* Vol. 8 No. 3 (2013): Open access.

Kondrashova MN, IA Shabanova. "Synthesis of the sodium salt of betahydroxybutyric acid from acetoacetic ester." *Bulletin of Experimental Biology and Medicine* Vol. 51 (1961): 104–5

Lappano R, A Sebastiani, F Cirillo, et al. "The lauric acid-activated signaling prompts apoptosis in cancer cells." *Cell Death Discovery* Vol. 3 No. 17063 (2017): e1–9. doi: 10.1038/cddiscovery.2017.63

Law KS, N Azman, EA Omar, et al. "The effects of virgin coconut oil (VCO) as supplementation on quality of life (QOL) among breast cancer patients." *Lipids in Health and Disease* Vol. 13 No. 139 (2014): e1–7.

Mensink RP, PL Zock, ADM Kester, et al. "Effects of dietary fatty acids and carbohydrates on the ratio of serum total to HDL cholesterol and on serum lipids and apolipoproteins: a meta-analysis of 60 controlled trials." *American Journal of Clinical Nutrition* Vol. 77 (2003): 1146–55.

Newport MT, TB VanItallie, Y Kashiwaya, et al. A new way to produce hyperketonemia: use of ketone ester in a case of Alzheimer's disease. *Alzheimer's and Dementia* Vol. 11 No. 1 (2015): 99–103.

Nonaka Y, T Takagi, M Inai, et al. "Lauric acid stimulates ketone body production in the KT-5 astrocyte cell line." *Journal of Oleo Science* Vol. 65 No. 8 (2016): 693-9. doi: 10.5650/jos.ess16069

Shah C, EB Beall, AMM Frankemolle, et al. "Exercise therapy for Parkinson's disease: Pedaling rate is related to changes in motor connectivity." *Brain Connectivity* Vol. 6 No. 1 (2016): 25–36.

Stubbs BJ, PJ Cox, R Evans, et al. "On the metabolism of exogenous ketones in humans." *Frontiers in Physiology* Vol. 8 No. 848 (2017): 1–13. doi 10.3389 /fphys.2017.00848

Van Hove JLK, S Grünewald, J Jaeken. "D, L-3-hydroxybutyrate treatment of multiple acyl-CoA dehydrogenase deficiency (MADD.)" *The Lancet* Vol. 361 (April 2003): 1433–35.

Vandenberghe C, V St-Pierre, A Courchesne-Loyer, et al. "Caffeine intake increases plasma ketones: an acute metabolic study in humans." *Canadian Journal of Physiology and Pharmacology* Vol. 95 No. 4 (2017): 455–58.

Vandoorne T, S de Smet, M Ramaekers, et al. "Intake of a ketone ester drink during recovery from exercise promotes mTORC1 signaling but not glycogen resynthesis in human muscle." *Front Physiol* Vol. 8 No. 310 (2017): e1–12.

Wozniak MA and RF Itzhaki. "Antiviral agents in Alzheimer's disease: hope for the future?" *Therapeutic Advances in Neurological Disorders* Vol. 3 (2010): 141–52.

Chapter 7: Special References for MCT Oil:

Abe S, O Ezaki, M Suzuki. "Medium-chain triglycerides in combination with leucine and vitamin D benefit cognition in frail elderly adults: A randomized controlled trial." *Journal of Nutrition Science and Vitaminology* Vol. 63 (2017): 133–40.

Abe S, O Ezaki, M Suzuki. "Medium-chain triglycerides in combination with leucine and vitamin D increase muscle strength and function in frail elderly adults in a randomized controlled trial." *Journal of Nutrition* Vol. 146 No. 5 (2016): 1017–26.

Augustin K, A Khabbush, S Williams, et al. Mechanisms of action for the medium-chain triglyceride ketogenic diet in neurological and metabolic disorders. *Lancet Neurol* Vol. 17 (2018):84-93.

Babayan VK. "Medium chain triglycerides and structured lipids." *Lipids* Vol. 22 No. 6 (1987): 417–20.

Bach AC, VK Babayan. "Medium-chain triglycerides: an update." *American Journal of Clinical Nutrition* Vol. 36 No. 5 (1982): 950–62.

Bergen SS, Jr., SA Hashim, TB VanItallie. "Hyperketonemia induced in man by medium-chain triglyceride." *Diabetes* Vol. 16, No. 10 (Oct 1966): 723–25.

Blackburn GL, VK Babayan. "Infant feeding formulas using coconut oil and the medium chain triglycerides." *Journal of the American College of Nutrition* Vol. 8. No. 3 (1989): 253–4.

Castellano C-A, S Nugent, N Paquet , et al. "Lower brain ^{18}F-fluorodeoxyglucose uptake but normal ^{11}C-acetoacetate metabolism in mild Alzheimer's disease dementia." *Journal of Alzheimer's Disease* Vol. 43 No. 4 (2015): 1343–53.

Costantini LC, JL Vogel, LJ Barr, et al. "Clinical efficacy of AC-1202 in mild to moderate Alzheimer's disease." *Proceedings of the 59th Annual Meeting of the American Academy of Neurology Conference*, Apr 28–May 5, 2007.

Costantini LC, LJ Barr, JL Vogel, et al. "Hypometabolism as a therapeutic target in Alzheimer's disease." *BMC Neuroscience* Vol. 9, Suppl. 2 (Dec 2008): S16.

Courchesne-Loyer A, E Croteau, C-A Castellano, et al. "Inverse relationship between brain glucose and ketone metabolism in adults during short-term moderate dietary ketosis: A dual tracer quantitative positron emission tomography study." *Journal of Cerebral Blood Flow and Metabolism* Vol. 37 No. 7 (2017): 2485–93.

Courchesne-Loyer A, M Fortier, J Tremblay-Mercier, et al. "Stimulation of mild, sustained ketonemia by medium-chain triacylglycerols in healthy humans: estimated potential contribution to brain energy metabolism." *Nutrition* Vol. 29 No. 4 (2013): 635–40.

Cunnane SC, A Courschesne-Loyer, C Vandenberghe, et al. "Can ketones help rescue brain fuel supply later in life? Implications for cognitive health during aging and the treatment of Alzheimer's disease." *Frontiers in Molecular Neuroscience* Vol. 9 (2016): 9–53.

Cunnane SC, A Courchesne-Loyer, V St-Pierre, et al. "Can ketones compensate for deteriorating brain glucose uptake during aging? Implications for the risk and treatment of Alzheimer's disease." *Annals of the New York Academy of Science* Vol. 1367 No. 1 (2016): 12–20.

Cunnane S, S Nugent, M Roy, et al. "Brain fuel metabolism, aging, and Alzheimer's disease." *Nutrition* Vol. 27, No. 1 (2011): 3–20.

Das AM, T Lücke, U Meyer, et al. "Glycogen storage disease type 1: impact of medium-chain triglycerides on metabolic control and growth." *Annals of Nutrition and Metabolism* Vol. 56 (2010): 225–232.

Farah BA. "Effects of caprylic triglyceride on cognitive performance and cerebral glucose metabolism in mild Alzheimer's disease: a single-case observation." *Frontiers in Aging Neuroscience* Vol. 6 Article 133 (2014): 1–5.

Fernando WM, IJ Martins, KG Goozee, et al. "The role of dietary coconut for the prevention and treatment of Alzheimer's disease: potential mechanisms of action." *British Journal of Nutrition* Vol. 114 No. 1 (2015): 1–14.

Hashim SA, S Bergen Jr, K Krell, et al. "Intestinal absorption and mode of transport in portal vein of medium-chain fatty acids." *Journal of Clinical Investigation* Vol. 43 (1964): 1238.

Henderson ST (Inventor). "Combinations of medium-chain triglycerides and therapeutic agents for the treatment and prevention of Alzheimer's disease and other diseases resulting from reduced neuronal metabolism." Available online at: www.freepatentsonline.com United States Patent 20080009467.

Henderson ST. "Ketone bodies as a therapeutic for Alzheimer's disease." *Journal of the American Society for Experimental NeuroTherapeutics* Vol. 5 No. 3 (2008): 470–80.

Henderson ST, JL Vogel, LJ Barr, et al. "Study of the ketogenic agent AC-1202 in mild to moderate Alzheimer's disease: a randomized, double-blind, placebo-controlled, multicenter trial." *Nutrition and Metabolism* Vol. 6, No. 31 (Aug 2009): 1–25.

Jayathilaka N. "Effect of fatty acid chain length on regulation of hepatic gene expression by saturated fats." Presentation at American Oil Chemists Society 2018 conference, May 9, 2018.

Mascioli EA, VK Babayan, BR Bistrian, et al. "Novel triglycerides for special medical purposes." *Journal of Parenteral and Enteral Nutrition* Vol. 12, Suppl. 6 (1988): s127s–132s.

Maynard SD and J Gelblum. "Retrospective cohort study of the efficacy of caprylic triglyceride in patients with mild-to-moderate Alzheimer's disease." *Neuropsychiatric Disease and Treatment* Vol. 9 (2013): 1619–27.

Maynard SD and J Gelblum. "Retrospective case studies of the efficacy of caprylic triglyceride in mild-to-moderate Alzheimer's disease." *Neuropsychiatric Disease and Treatment* Vol. 9 (2013): 1629–35.

Mochel F, S Duteil, C Marelli, et al. "Dietary anaplerotic therapy improves peripheral tissue energy metabolism in patients with Huntington's disease." *European Journal of Human Genetics* Vol. 10 (2010): 1–4.

Newport MT, TB VanItallie, Y Kashiwaya, et al. "A new way to produce hyperketonemia: use of ketone ester in a case of Alzheimer's disease." *Alzheimer's and Dementia* Vol. 11 No. 1 (2015): 99–103.

Nonaka Y, T Takagi, M Inai, et al. "Lauric acid stimulates ketone body production in the KT-5 astrocyte cell line." *Journal of Oleo Science* Vol. 65 No. 8 (2016): 693–99.

Owen OE, AP Morgan, HG Kemp et al. "Brain metabolism during fasting." *Journal of Clinical Investigation* Vol. 46, No. 10 (1967): 1589–95.

Page KA, A Williamson, N Yu, et al. "Medium-chain fatty acids improve cognitive function in intensively treated type 1 diabetic patients and support *in vitro* synaptic transmission during acute hypoglycemia." *Diabetes* Vol. 58, No. 5 (2009): 1237–44.

Papamandjaris AA, E MacDougall, PJH Jones. "Medium-chain fatty acid metabolism and energy expenditure: obesity treatment implications." *Life Science* Vol. 62 No. 14 (1998): 1203–15.

Pi-Sunyer FX, SA Hashim, TB VanItallie. "Insulin and ketone responses to ingestion of medium and long-chain triglycerides in man." *Diabetes* Vol. 18, No. 2 (1969): 96–100.

Prior IA, F Davidson, CE Salmond, et al. "Cholesterol, coconuts, and diet on Polynesian atolls: a natural experiment: the Pukapuka and Tokelau island studies." *American Journal of Clinical Nutrition* Vol. 34, No. 8 (1981): 1552–61.

Rebello CJ, JN Kellera, AG Liua, et al. "Pilot feasibility and safety study examining the effect of medium-chain triglyceride supplementation in subjects with mild cognitive impairment: a randomized controlled trial." *Biochimica et Biophysica Acta BBA Clinical* Vol. 3 (2015): 123–125.

Reger MA, ST Henderson, C Hale, et al. "Effects of β-hydroxybutyrate on cognition in memory-impaired adults." *Neurobiology of Aging* Vol. 25 (2004): 311–314.

Schön H, I Lippach, W Gelpke. "Stoffwechsel untersuchungen mit einem mischglycerid der fettsäuren mitlerer kettenlänge. II. Untersuchungen über die veränderungen des ketonkörpergehmaltes von blut and urin nach zufuhr des mischglyderides." *Gasteroenterologia* Vol. 91 (1959): 199.

Senanayake C. "Effect of fatty acid chain length and saturation on the lipid profiles of Wistar rats." Presentation at American Oil Chemists Society 2018 conference, May 7, 2018.

St-Onge MP, A Bosarge, LLT Goree, et al. "Medium-chain triglyceride oil consumption as part of a weight loss diet does not lead to an adverse metabolic profile when compared to olive oil." *Journal of the American College of Nutrition* Vol. 27, No. 5 (2008): 547–52.

Studzinski CM, WA MacKay, TL Beckett, et al. "Induction of ketosis may improve mitochondrial function and decrease steady-state amyloid-β precursor protein (APP) levels in the aged dog." *Brain Research* Vol. 1226 (2008): 209–17.

Taha AY, ST Henderson, WM Burnham. "Dietary enrichment with medium-chain triglycerides (AC-1203) elevates polyunsaturated fatty acids in the parietal cortex of aged dogs: implication for treating age-related cognitive decline." *Neurochemistry Research* Vol. 34, No. 9 (2009): 1619–25.

Tantibhedhyangkul P, SA Hashim. "Clinical and physiologic aspects of medium-chain triglycerides: alleviation of steatorrhea in premature infants." *Bulletin of the New York Academy of Medicine* Vol. 47, No. 1 (1971): 17–33.

Tantibhehyangkul P, SA Hashim. "Medium-chain triglyceride feeding in premature infants: effects on fat and nitrogen absorption." *Pediatrics* Vol. 55 (1975): 359–70.

Turner N, K Hariharan, J TidAng, et al. "Enhancement of muscle mitochondrial oxidative capacity and alterations in insulin action are lipid species dependent: potent tissue-specific effects of medium-chain fatty acids." *Diabetes* Vol. 48 (2009): 2547–54.

Yin JX, M Maalouf, P Han, et al. "Ketones block amyloid entry and improve cognition in an Alzheimer's model." *Neurobiology of Aging* Vol. 39 (2016): 25–37.

Chapter 8

Abe S, E Osamu, M Suzuki. "Medium-chain triglycerides in combination with leucine and vitamin D benefit cognition in frail elderly adults: A randomized controlled trial." *Journal of Nutrition Science and Vitaminology* Vol. 63 (2017): 133–40.

Abe S, O Ezaki, M Suzuki. "Medium-chain triglycerides in combination with leucine and vitamin D increase muscle strength and function in frail elderly adults in a randomized controlled trial." *Journal of Nutrition* Vol. 146 No. 5 (2016): 1017–26.

Cahill GF, Jr. "Fuel metabolism in starvation." *Annual Reviews in Nutrition* Vol. 26 (2006): 1–22.

Croteau E, C-A Castellano, MA Richard, et al. "Ketogenic medium-chain triglycerides increase brain energy metabolism in Alzheimer's disease." *Journal of Alzheimer's Disease* In press May 2018 B.

Dietary Reference Intakes for Energy, Carbohydrate, Fiber, Fat, Fatty Acids, Cholesterol, Protein, and Amino Acids PDF available at https://ods.od.nih.gov/Health_Information/Dietary_Reference_Intakes.aspx.

El-Rashidy O, F El-Baz, Y El-Gendy, et al. "Ketogenic diet versus gluten-free case in free diet in autistic children: a case-control study." *Metabolic Brain Disease* Vol. 32 Nol. 6 (2017): 1935–41

Henderson ST. "Ketone bodies as a therapeutic for Alzheimer's disease." *Journal of the American Society for Experimental NeuroTherapeutics* Vol. 5 No. 3 (2008): 470–80.

Henderson ST, JL Vogel, LJ Barr, et al. "Study of the ketogenic agent AC-1202 in mild to moderate Alzheimer's disease: a randomized, double-blind, placebo-controlled, multicenter trial." *Nutrition and Metabolism* Vol. 6, No. 31 (Aug 2009): 1–25.

Maynard SD and J Gelblum. "Retrospective cohort study of the efficacy of caprylic triglyceride in patients with mild-to-moderate Alzheimer's disease." *Neuropsychiatric Disease and Treatment* Vol. 9 (2013): 1619–27.

Maynard SD and J Gelblum. "Retrospective case studies of the efficacy of caprylic triglyceride in mild-to-moderate Alzheimer's disease." *Neuropsychiatric Disease and Treatment* Vol. 9 (2013): 1629–35.

Newport MT, TB VanItallie, Y Kashiwaya, et al. "A new way to produce hyperketonemia: use of ketone ester in a case of Alzheimer's disease." *Alzheimer's and Dementia* Vol. 11 No. 1 (2015): 99–103.

Ota M, J Matsuo, I Ishida, et al. "Effect of a ketogenic meal on cognitive function in elderly adults: potential for cognitive enhancement." *Psychopharmacology* (*Berlin*) Vol. 233 No. 21-22 (2016): 3797–802.

Page KA, A Williamson, N Yu, et al. "Medium-chain fatty acids improve cognitive function in intensively treated type 1 diabetic patients and support *in vitro* synaptic transmission during acute hypoglycemia." *Diabetes* Vol. 58, No. 5 (May 2009): 1237–44.

Perng BC, M Chen, JC Perng, et al. "A keto-mediet approach with coconut substitution and exercise may delay the onset of Alzheimer's disease among middle-aged." *Journal of Prevention of Alzheimer's Disease* Vol. 4 No. 1 (2017): 51–7. Doi: 10.14283/jpad.2016.104

Reger MA, ST Henderson, C Hale, et al. "Effects of β-hydroxybutyrate on cognition in memory-impaired adults." *Neurobiology of Aging* Vol. 25 (2004): 311–14.

Rudolf M C J, R S Sherwin. "Maternal ketosis and its effects on the fetus." *Clinics in Endocrinology and Metabolism* Vol. 12 No. 2 (1983): 413–28.

Schultz ST, HS Klonoff-Cohen, DL Windgard, et al. "Breastfeeding, infant formula supplementation, and autistic disorder: the results of a parent survey." *International Breastfeeding Journal* Open Access Vol. 1 No. 16 (2006): e1–7.

Sloan G, A Ali, J Webster. "A rare cause of metabolic acidosis: ketoacidosis in a non-diabetic lactating woman." *Endocrinology, Diabetes & Metabolism.* (2017): e1-5.doi: 10.1530/EDM-17-0073

Stubbs BJ, PJ Cox, RD Evans, et al. "On the metabolism of exogenous ketones in humans." *Frontiers in Physiology.* Vol. 8 No. 848 (2017): e1–13. doi 10.3389/fphys.2017.00848

Sussman D, J Germann, M Henkelman. "Gestational ketogenic diet programs brain structure and susceptibility to depression and anxiety in the adult mouse offspring." *Brain and Behavior* Vol. 5 No. 2 (2015): e00300. Doi: 10.1002/brb3.300

Sussman D, M van Eede, MD Wong, et al. "Effects of a ketogenic diet during pregnancy on embryonic growth in the mouse." *BMC Pregnancy and Childbirth* Vol. 13 No. 109 (2013): e1-12.

Van der Louw EJ, TJ Williams, BJ Henry-Barron, et al. "Ketogenic diet therapy for epilepsy during pregnancy: a case series." *Seizure.* Vol. 45 (2016): 198–201.

Von Geijer L, M Ekelund. "Ketoacidosis associated with low-carbohydrate diet in a non-diabetic lactating women: a case report." *Journal of Medical Case Reports* Vol. 9 No. 224 (2015): e1–3. Doi: 10.1186/s13256-015-0709-2

Chapter 10

Aubert G, OJ Martin, JL Horton, et al. "The failing heart relies on ketone bodies as a fuel." *Circulation* Vol. 133 No. 8 (2016): 698–705.

Brown SE, L Trivieri Jr.. *The Acid Alkaline Food Guide.* 2013. Garden City Park, NY: Square One Publishers, 2013.

Fukao T, G Mitchell, JO Sass, et al. "Ketone body metabolism and its defects." *Journal of Inherited Metabolic Diseases* Vol. 37 (2014): 541–51.

Goldberg EL, JL Asher, RD Molony, et al. "β-hydroxybutyrate deactivates neutrophil NLRP3 inflammasome to relieve gout flares." *Cell Repair* Vol. 18 No. 9 (2017): 2077–87. doi 10.1016/j.celrep.2017.02.004

Huynh K. "Ketones as a fuel in heart failure." *Nature Reviews Cardiology* Published online 11 Feb 11, 2016. www.nature.com/nrcardio.

Koslo J.. *The Alkaline Diet for Beginners,* Berkeley, CA: Rockridge Press, 2016.

Kossoff, EH, BA Zupec-Kania, S Auvin, et al. Optimal clinical management of children receiving dietary therapies for epilepsy: Updated recommendations of the International Ketogenic Diet Study Group. *Epilepsia Open* Vol. 3 No. 2 (2018):175–192.

Sampath A, EH Kossoff, SL Furth, et al. "Kidney stones and the ketogenic diet: risk factors and prevention." *Journal of Child Neuro*logy. Vol. 22 No. 4 (2007): 375–378. doi 10.1177/0883073807301926

Sato K, Y Kashiwaya, RL Veech, et al. "Insulin, ketone bodies, and mitochondrial energy transduction." *FASEB Journal* Vol. 9 (1995): 651–658.

Volek JS, DJ Freidenreich, C Saenz, et al. "Metabolic characteristics of keto-adapted ultra-endurance runners." *Metabolism* Vol.65 (2016): 100–10. Doi: 10.1016/j.metabol.2015.10.028

Volek JS, T Noakes, SD Phinney. "Rethinking fat as a fuel for endurance exercise." *European Journal of Sports Science* Vol. 15 No. 1 (2015): 13–20. doi: 10.1080/17461391.2014.959564

Yancy WS Jr, MK Olsen, T Dudley, et al. "Acid-base analysis of individuals following two weight-loss diets." *European Journal of Clinical Nutritio* Vol. 61 No. 12 (2007): 1416–22. doi 10.1038/sj.ejcn.1602661

Yuen AWC, IA Walcutt, JW Sander. "An acidosis-sparing ketogenic (ASK) diet to improve efficacy and reduce adverse effect in the treatment of refractory epilepsy." *Epilepsy & Behavior* Vol. 74 (2017): 15–21. Doi: 10.1016/j.yebeh.2017.05.032

Chapter 11

American Heart Association Presidential Advisory Committee. "Dietary Fats and Cardiovascular Disease: A Presidential Advisory." *Circulation* Vol. 135 No. 3 (2017): e1–e23.

Dehghan M, A Mente, X Zhang, et al. "Associations of fats and carbohydrate intake with cardiovascular disease and mortality in 18 countries from five continents (PURE): a prospective cohort study." *The Lancet* Vol. 390 No. 10107 (2017): 2050–62.

Diamond, David. "David Diamond—An update on demonization and deception in research on saturated fat." https://www.youtube.com/watch?v=uc1XsO3mxX8

Nonaka Y, T Takagi, M Inai, et al. "Lauric acid stimulates ketone body production in the KT-5 astrocyte cell line." *Journal Oleo Science* Vol. 65 No. 8 (2016): 693–9. doi: 10.5650/jos.ess16069

Prior IA, F Davidson, CE Salmond, et al. "Cholesterol, coconuts, and diet on Polynesian atolls: A natural experiment: the Pukapuka and Tokelau island studies." *American Journal Clinical Nutrition* Vol. 34. No. 8. (1981): 1552–61.

Ravnskov U. "The questionable role of saturated and polyunsaturated fatty acids in cardiovascular disease." *Journal of Clinical Epidemiology* Vol 51. No. 6 (1998): 443–60.

Ravnskov U, DM Diamond, L Ham, et al. "Lack of an association or an inverse association between low-density lipoprotein cholesterol and mortality in the elderly: a systematic review." *British Medical Journal BMJ Open* Access Vol. 6 (2016): e1–8. 6:e010401. doi:10.1136/bmjopen-2015-010401

Addendum

Clarke K, K Tchabanenko, R Pawlosky, et al. "Kinetics, safety and tolerability of (R)-3-hydroxybutyl (R)-3-hydroxybutyrate in healthy adult subjects." *Regulatory Toxicology and Pharmacology* Vol. 63 (2012): 401–8.

Cox PJ, T Kirk, T Ashmore, et al. "Nutritional ketosis alters fuel preference and thereby endurance performance in athletes." *Cell Metabolism* Vol. 24 (2016): 1–13.

Dayrit FM. "The properties of lauric acid and their significance in coconut oil." *Journal of the American Oil Chemists Society* Vol. 92 (2015): 1–15.

Holdsworth DA, PJ Cox, T Kirk, et al. "A ketone ester drink increases post-exercise muscle glycogen synthesis in humans." *Medicine and Science Sports and Exercise* (2017): Vol. 49 No. 9 (2017): 1789–95.

Jayathilaka N. "Effect of fatty acid chain length on regulation of hepatic gene expression by saturated fats." Presentation at American Oil Chemists Society 2018 conference, May 9, 2018.

Newport MT, TB VanItallie, Y Kashiwaya, et al. "A new way to produce hyperketonemia: use of ketone ester in a case of Alzheimer's disease." *Alzheimer's and Dementia* Vol. 11 No. 1 (2015): 99–103.

Nonaka Y, T Takagi, M Inai, et al. "Lauric acid stimulates ketone body production in the KT-5 astrocyte cell line." *Journal of Oleo Science.* Vol. 65 No. 8 (2016): 693–9.

Senanayake C. "Effect of fatty acid chain length and saturation on the lipid profiles of Wistar rats." Presentation at American Oil Chemists Society 2018 conference, May 7, 2018.

Stubbs B J, P J Cox, R D Evans, et al. "On the metabolism of exogenous ketones in humans." *Frontiers in Physiology* Vol. 8 No. 848 (2017): 1–13.

Studzinski CM, WA MacKay, TL Beckett, et al. "Induction of ketosis may improve mitochondrial function and decrease steady-state amyloid-β precursor protein (APP) levels in the aged dog." *Brain Research* Vol. 1226 (2008): 209–17.

Taha AY, ST Henderson, WM Burnham. "Dietary enrichment with medium-chain triglycerides (AC-1203) elevates polyunsaturated fatty acids in the parietal cortex of aged dogs: implication for treating age-related cognitive decline." *Neurochemistry Research* Vol. 34, No. 9 (2009): 1619–25.

Vandoorne T, S de Smet, M Ramaekers, et al. "Intake of a ketone ester drink during recovery from exercise promotes mTORC1 signaling but not glycogen resynthesis in human muscle." *Front Physiol* Vol. 8 No. 310 (2017): e1–12.

ADDENDUM
KETO FRIENDLY RECIPES

I found so many brands and variations in quantities when putting together recipes that I have not attempted to calculate the macronutrient content for these recipes. Several recipes from Ketogenic.com include the macronutrient content as on their website. I recommend you do your own calculations for the brands you enjoy and save them for future use.

MCT AND COCONUT OIL MIXTURE

YIELD: 28 ounces

12 ounces coconut oil

16 ounces MCT Oil

DIRECTIONS: Warm coconut oil until completely liquid by placing container in a pan of hot water. Use funnel to add MCT and coconut oil to a glass quart container, such as MCT oil bottle, recap securely, and invert several times to mix the oils now and before each use. Store at room temperature.

OPTIONAL: Add 1 or more tablespoons of liquid soy lethicin to allow for easier mixing with other liquids and provide phospholipids.

COCONUT MILK—THICKER

YIELD: Each 4 ounces gives 15 grams (about one tablespoon) of coconut oil.

**1 can of undiluted full fat coconut milk
(with 11 grams fat per 2 ounces)**

½ can of water or coconut water

10 drops liquid stevia OR 1 to 2 teaspoons of honey, agave syrup, or other sweetener to taste

Pinch of salt

DIRECTIONS: Place ingredients in a container and shake well before use. Store coconut milk in the refrigerator and discard unused portion after four days. When used for children, discard after two days.

VARIATION: Add 1 teaspoon dolomite powder to mixture to add calcium supplementation to diet.

COCONUT MILK—THINNER

YIELD: Each 6.5 ounces gives 15 grams (about one tablespoon) of coconut oil

**1 can of undiluted full fat coconut milk
(with 11 grams fat per 2 ounces)**

1½ cans of water or coconut water

10 drops liquid stevia OR 1 to 2 teaspoons of honey, agave syrup or other sweetener to taste

Pinch of salt

DIRECTIONS: Place ingredients in a container and shake well before use. Store coconut milk in the refrigerator and discard unused portion after four days. When used for children, discard after two days.

VARIATION: Add 1 teaspoon dolomite powder to mixture to add calcium supplementation to diet.

MCT SKIM MILK

4 to 8 ounces skim milk

Your usual serving MCT oil or coconut/MCT mixture

DIRECTIONS: Mix together with wire whisk or blender.

COCONUT MILK QUICK PROTEIN DRINK

YIELD: One 8-ounce serving

2 tablespoons whey, rice, pea, or egg white protein or combination of these

1 cup Thinner Coconut Milk

Extra coconut oil (melted) or MCT/coconut oil (optional)

DIRECTIONS: Add protein powder to coconut milk and mix thoroughly with a wire whisk until dissolved. Add extra coconut oil if desired.

ORANGE-COCONUT MILK

YIELD: One 8 to 10-ounce serving

4 to 6 ounces Thicker or Thinner Coconut Milk (above) or cow or goat milk while gradually increasing your coconut oil intake

4 ounces diet orange soda

Extra coconut oil (melted) or MCT/coconut oil (optional)

DIRECTIONS: Pour coconut milk into a 12-ounce glass. Slowly add the diet orange soda and mix with a spoon. Add extra coconut oil if desired.

VARIATION: Try diet grape soda or root beer instead of orange soda.

COCONUT EGG HIGH-PROTEIN PROBIOTIC SMOOTHIE

YIELD: One 12 to 14 ounce serving

  3 whole eggs hard-boiled or raw

  2 tablespoons vanilla or unflavored whey protein

  10 to 15 drops liquid stevia

  4 ounces plain whole fat kefir

  4 to 6 ounces Thicker or Thinner Coconut Milk (above) or cow or goat milk while gradually increasing your coconut oil intake

  Extra coconut oil (melted) or MCT/coconut oil (optional)

DIRECTIONS: Combine all ingredients, including the extra coconut if using, in a blender. Mix well.

NOTE: For those who are concerned about using raw eggs, microwave the eggs for about 20 seconds to kill bacteria before adding to other ingredients.

VARIATIONS: Add cut up strawberries or blueberries or 2 ounces of fruit or green liquid smoothie or 2 teaspoons of cherry juice concentrate. OR add 1 to 2 tablespoons Earth Balance Coconut and Peanut Spread.

BERRY-COCONUT MILK SMOOTHIE

YIELD: One 14 to 16 ounce serving

½ cup crushed ice

1 cup frozen blueberries or 4 large frozen strawberries

⅓ cup Fiber One Original, Smart Bran cereal, or sliced almonds [lower carb choice]

1 teaspoon honey, agave syrup, or equivalent sweetener such as stevia

1 cup Thicker or Thinner Coconut Milk (above) or cow or goat milk while gradually increasing your coconut oil intake

1 hard-boiled or raw egg

2 tablespoons vanilla or unflavored whey protein powder

Extra coconut oil (melted) or MCT/coconut oil (optional)

DIRECTIONS: Place all ingredients, including the extra coconut if using, in a blender and blend on "liquefy" speed for about 30 seconds. If mixture is too thick, add more coconut milk as needed.

NOTE: For those who are concerned about adding raw egg, microwave the egg for about 20 seconds to kill bacteria before adding to other ingredients.

VARIATIONS: Add ½ banana and 2 large strawberries per serving, or substitute equivalent amount of apple, blueberry, or pomegranate juice for part or all of the milk.

BANANA-PEANUT BUTTER-COCONUT MILK SMOOTHIE

YIELD: One 14- to 16-ounce serving

½ cup crushed ice

1 frozen banana (break into four pieces before freezing)

$1/3$ cup cereal such as Fiber One Original or Smart Bran or sliced almonds [lower carb choice]

1 tablespoon fresh ground or natural peanut or almond butter

1 teaspoon honey, agave syrup, or equivalent stevia or sweetener

1 cup Thicker or Thinner Coconut Milk (above) or cow or goat milk while gradually increasing your coconut oil intake

1 hard-boiled or raw egg

2 tablespoons vanilla or unflavored whey protein powder

Extra coconut oil (melted) or MCT/coconut oil (optional)

DIRECTIONS: Place all ingredients, including the extra coconut oil if desired, in a blender. Blend on "liquefy" speed for about 30 seconds. If mixture is too thick, add more coconut milk as needed.

NOTE: For those who are concerned about using a raw egg, microwave the egg for about 20 seconds to kill bacteria before adding to other ingredients.

GREEN COCONUT SMOOTHIE

YIELD: One 14 to 16 ounce serving

½ cup crushed ice

⅓ sliced almonds

1 cup leafy greens, such as kale, spinach, and/or spring mix

½ cucumber cut up

1 celery stalk cut up

1 tablespoon lemon juice

1 teaspoon honey, agave syrup, or equivalent stevia or sweetener, if desired

1cup Thicker or Thinner Coconut Milk (above) or cow or goat milk while gradually increasing your coconut oil intake

1 hard-boiled or raw egg

2 tablespoons vanilla or unflavored whey protein powder

⅓ cup sliced almonds (optional)

Extra coconut oil (melted) or MCT/coconut oil (optional)

DIRECTIONS: Place all ingredients, including the extra coconut oil if desired, in a blender and blend on "liquefy" speed for about 30 seconds. If mixture is too thick, add more coconut milk.

NOTE: For those who are concerned about using a raw egg, microwave the egg for about 20 seconds to kill bacteria before adding to other ingredients.

KETO MILKSHAKE

With permission from Kira and Ossian Munn

    8 ounces low-carb ice cream, such as Breyer's Carb Smart or Halo Top

    6 ounces coconut milk or almond milk, plus more as needed

    1 packet Keto Kreme or Swiss Cacao Keto//OS Max

    1 tablespoon MCT 1:4:3 or MCT oil (optional)

DIRECTIONS: Blend all ingredients together, including the MCT oil if using. Add more or less coconut or almond milk to bring consistency to your liking.

ORANGE SODA KETO SALTS

YIELD: One 12-ounce serving

    1 packet or one scoop of Pruvit Keto//OS Orange Dream ketone salts

    12 ounces diet orange soda

DIRECTIONS: Combine ketone salts and the soda in a large drinking cup and stir.

CREAMY KETONE SALTS

YIELD: One 13-ounce serving

    1 packet Pruvit Keto//OS or Keto//OS Max, any flavor

    2 tablespoons heavy whipping cream

    12 ounces water

DIRECTIONS: Combine ketone salts, cream, and water in a shaker bottle and shake.

SPARKLING KETONE SALTS

YIELD: One 12-ounce serving

1 packet Pruvit Keto//OS or Keto//OS Max, any flavor

12 ounces sparkling water

DIRECTIONS: Combine ketone salts and sparkling water in a large drinking cup and stir Use a large enough container to allow for considerable foaming.

LOIS'S KETO GELATIN

With permission from Lois Kamp

YIELD: 2 servings

2 packets or two scoops of Pruvit Keto//OS Orange Dream ketone salts

2 cups hot water

1 package sugar-free orange flavored gelatin

DIRECTIONS: In a mixing bowl, add ketone salts to part of hot water. (Water should not be boiling.) Stir to dissolve ketone salts. Add gelatin and remainder of water and mix thoroughly until gelatin and salts are dissolved. Place into a baking dish and cool in refrigerator until gelled.

VARIATIONS: Try with Kira's Whipped Keto Kreme on top. Try alternative flavors of ketone salts with other gelatin flavors.

MARY'S GREEK YOGURT BREAKFAST OR SNACK

YIELD: 1 serving

½ cup plain full fat Greek yogurt

6 to 8 drops liquid stevia

1 tablespoon MCT oil or MCT//143

1 tablespoon unsweetened grated coconut

¼ cup unsalted organic nuts (your choice), crushed or whole

DIRECTIONS: In a small bowl, combine yogurt, stevia, and oil. Mix thoroughly with a spoon. Sprinkle coconut and nuts on top and stir in.

MARY'S RICOTTA CONCOCTION (BREAKFAST OR SNACK)

YIELD: 1 serving

½ cup full fat ricotta

6 to 8 drops stevia

2 ounces coconut milk or 1 tablespoon MCT oil or MCT//143

¼ cup organic unsalted nuts, whole, sliced, or chopped

1 tablespoon unsweetened grated coconut

DIRECTIONS: In a small bowl, combine ricotta, stevia, and coconut milk. Mix thoroughly with a spoon. Add nuts and grated coconut and stir again.

TASTY COTTAGE CHEESE AND OIL MIX

YIELD: One serving

4 ounces cottage cheese

Your serving of MCT oil or coconut/MCT oil mixture

DIRECTIONS: In a small bowl, combine cottage cheese and MCT oil. Mix together with a fork or spoon.

CHEESY SCRAMBLED EGGS

YIELD: Two eggs

1 tablespoon coconut oil

Diced sweet onion (optional)

2 fresh eggs

Pinch of sea salt

2 level tablespoons grated or shredded hard cheese or 2 ounces cream cheese, cut into chunks

DIRECTIONS: In a skillet, melt coconut oil over medium-low heat. If adding onion, sauté for 1 to 2 minutes before adding eggs. Break the yolks and scramble the eggs and coconut milk vigorously with a fork or wire whisk. Add salt and cheese and allow cheese to melt before pouring into the heated skillet. Use a spatula to scrape the cooked egg off the bottom of the skillet, turning the egg over repeatedly until it is no longer liquid but still fluffy and moist.

VARIATIONS: Whisk parsley, spinach, diced green pepper, or green onion into the mixture before adding to the skillet.

MARY'S FAVORITE OMELET

YIELD: One serving

    1 tablespoon coconut oil

    2 or 3 fresh eggs

    2 pinches of salt

    Pepper to taste

    4 cherry tomatoes, cut in half

    6 pitted kalamata olives, cut in half

    1½ ounces shredded cheddar cheese

DIRECTIONS: Heat coconut oil over medium-low heat in a non-stick omelet style skillet. In a separate bowl beat the eggs with a wire whisk, whisk in salt and pepper, and pour evenly into hot skillet. Leave undisturbed for several minutes. When omelet is about ¾ set (some liquid egg still sits on top), carefully flip omelet with a spatula. Evenly distribute the tomato and olive pieces as well as about one ounce of cheese on half of the omelet and use spatula to fold omelet in half covering the vegetables and cheese. Distribute the rest of the cheese evenly over the top of the folded omelet. When cheese on top begins to melt, remove omelet from heat and serve.

VARIATIONS: Make a Greek style omelet by using 2 to 3 large spoonfuls of Greek Salad (see page 403) and feta cheese in place of other vegetables and cheeses.

SPINACH AND FETA OMELET

YIELD: One serving

4 teaspoons coconut oil

1 cup fresh spinach leaves

2 or 3 fresh eggs

2 tablespoons coconut milk

1 pinch of sea salt for each egg

Pepper, as desired

2 ounces feta cheese

DIRECTIONS: Heat 2 teaspoons coconut oil at medium-low heat in a nonstick omelet style skillet. Add spinach and sauté until just wilted; remove from pan and set aside. In a small bowl, beat eggs with a wire whisk and then whisk in coconut milk, salt, and pepper. Add 2 more teaspoons of coconut oil to the skillet and, when heated, pour egg mixture evenly into hot skillet. Leave undisturbed for several minutes. When omelet is about ¾ set (some liquid egg still sits on top), carefully flip omelet with a spatula. Evenly distribute the spinach and feta over half the omelet and, using a spatula, fold omelet in half covering the spinach and cheese. When cheese inside begins to melt, remove omelet from heat and serve.

WHATEVER FRITTATA

YIELD: 4 servings

6 fresh eggs

4 tablespoons coconut oil

About two cups fresh or one bag of frozen vegetables of your choice

Salt and pepper, and/or your favorite spice mix to sprinkle on vegetables

**¾ cup of your choice of shredded cheese
or ½ cup crumbled feta cheese**

Two to three more pinches of salt

1 tablespoon grated Parmesan or Romano cheese

DIRECTIONS: Select an omelet-style skillet that can also be used in the oven. Place oven rack about five inches below broiler and preheat broiler to high temperature. Crack eggs into a bowl. Heat coconut oil in the skillet at medium-low heat. Sauté vegetables in the oil, stirring often, until tender, about 4 to 5 minutes. Add salt and pepper and other spices to vegetables when nearly finished, mix well, and distribute the vegetables evenly around the bottom of the skillet.

In a separate small bowl, beat eggs with a wire whisk while vegetables are cooking. Add salt and shredded cheese to eggs and mix thoroughly. When vegetables are ready, pour egg mixture evenly over the vegetables and then continue to cook undisturbed for 4 to 5 minutes until edges are dry and slightly brown; egg mixture will appear runny on the top. Sprinkle Parmesan or Romano cheese evenly on top of frittata and place under broiler for at least three minutes. Be sure to set a timer to avoid burning. After three minutes, open oven and pull rack out enough to check omelet. With an oven glove on your hand, gently shake skillet handle; if top does not "jiggle" and appears lightly browned, the frittata is set and ready to be removed from the oven. If the top jiggles, replace under broiler for 1 to 2 more minutes, watching closely. Allow to cool for at least five minutes, cut into fourths, and serve.

VARIATION: Add leftover meat, fish, or poultry of any kind. You can add whatever you like!

MARGARITA FRITTATA

YIELD: 4 servings

6 to 8 fresh eggs

4 tablespoons coconut oil

1 tablespoon minced garlic

2 cups fresh spinach leaves

Salt and pepper

8 cherry tomatoes, cut in half

½ teaspoon basil, dry or fresh minced

4 ounces of fresh mozzarella, cut into four slices

DIRECTIONS: Select an omelet-style skillet that can also be used in the oven. Place oven rack about five inches below broiler and preheat broiler to high temperature. Crack eggs into a bowl. Heat coconut oil in the skillet over medium-low heat. Sauté minced garlic in the oil for a few seconds and then add spinach, stirring often, until almost wilted, about 1 to 2 minutes. When nearly finished, sprinkle spinach lightly with salt and pepper and mix well. Distribute the spinach evenly around the bottom of the skillet.

While spinach is cooking, beat eggs with a wire whisk, add a pinch of salt for each egg, and whisk again thoroughly. When spinach is ready, pour egg mixture evenly over the spinach and immediately use a heat-resistant spoon or spatula to swirl spinach into egg mixture. Sprinkle basil and cherry tomato halves evenly over the frittata. Continue to cook undisturbed for about 4 to 5 minutes until edges are dry and slightly brown; egg mixture will appear still runny on the top. Just before removing from stove, place one mozzarella slice flat on top of each quarter of the frittata. Remove from stove and place under broiler for at least three minutes. Be sure to set a timer to avoid burning. After three minutes, open oven and pull rack out enough to check omelet. With an oven glove on your hand, gently shake the skillet handle; if the egg portion does not "jiggle" and appears lightly browned, the frittata is set and ready to be removed from the oven. The now-melted mozzarella might move with this maneuver. If the top jiggles, return pan to oven broil 1 to 2 more minutes and check again. Allow to cool for at least five minutes, cut into fourths, and serve.

JENN'S BREAKFAST SAUSAGE MEATBALLS

With permission from Jenn Rau

YIELD: 24 meatballs

- 16 ounces Italian sausage
- 4 ounces cream cheese room temperature
- ½ cup Parmesan cheese, grated
- ½ cup shredded cheddar cheese
- ½ teaspoon sea salt
- 1 teaspoon garlic powder

DIRECTIONS: Preheat oven to 350°F. Mix all ingredients together and then form mixture into about 24 golf ball–size balls. Place balls on baking sheet lined with parchment. Bake approximately 20 minutes or until no longer pink.

GRILLED CHEESE SANDWICH

YIELD: One sandwich

- 2 to 3 ounces favorite sliced cheese
- 2 slices low-carb whole grain or gluten-free bread
- 2 tablespoons coconut oil

DIRECTIONS: Place cheese between the two slices of bread and spread one tablespoon of coconut oil on the outer surface of both sides of the sandwich. In a skillet, cook over medium-low heat until first side is lightly browned and cheese is beginning to melt. Flip and brown second side.

VARIATION: Place a layer of thinly sliced tomatoes and/or spinach on top of the cheese.

JEN'S SUNFLOWER SEED CRACKERS

With permission from Jenn Rau

YIELD: About 2 dozen crackers

1 cup unsalted sunflower seeds

¾ cup shredded cheddar cheese

½ cup shredded Parmesan cheese

2 tablespoons coconut flour

¼ teaspoon baking powder

1 teaspoon garlic powder

1 teaspoon onion powder

1 tablespoon dried parsley flakes

Pinch of sea salt

2 tablespoons cold butter

2 tablespoons water

DIRECTIONS: Preheat oven to 350° F. Grind sunflower seeds in a food processor until fine.

Add the cheese, coconut flour, baking powder, and seasonings. Blend. Add cold butter and blend again. Add water if needed for dough to form a sticky ball. Turn dough onto a piece of greased parchment paper and slightly flatten with your hands. Top dough with another piece of greased parchment paper and roll out until just under ¼ in thick. Use a pizza cutter to cut into about two dozen cracker shapes. Bake for 25 to 30 minutes or until golden brown. Remove and let cool. They crisp as they cool. Break apart and enjoy.

SIMPLE SALAD DRESSING OR VEGETABLE TOPPING

YIELD: One or two servings

- 1 tablespoon of your favorite salad dressing
- 1 tablespoon MCT oil or coconut/MCT oil mixture

DIRECTIONS: Mix ingredients together with a wire whisk and pour immediately onto salad or vegetables. Toss. Excess can be stored in refrigerator and then rewarmed and remixed before serving.

CAESAR DRESSING

With permission from Ketogenic.com

YIELD: 24 servings

Macronutrients per serving: fat 8.5 grams, protein 0.2 gram, carbs 0.1 gram

- ¼ cup mayonnaise
- 6 anchovy fillets (optional)
- ½ teaspoon Dijon mustard
- 2 tablespoons lemon juice
- 1 teaspoon Worcestershire sauce
- 1 teaspoon garlic powder
- ½ teaspoon salt
- ½ teaspoon pepper

DIRECTIONS: If using anchovies, puree them, and then whisk all ingredients together.

*RECIPE STATEMENT: The macronutrients of your dish will depend on the type and brand of the ingredients you use. This could make your dish different from ours.

SIMPLE TOPPING FOR CHICKEN OR CHICKEN SALAD

YIELD: One serving

   1 tablespoon of honey Dijon or ranch-style salad dressing

   1 tablespoon MCT oil or coconut/MCT oil mixture

DIRECTIONS: Combine ingredients and mix together with a wire whisk. Pour immediately onto chicken or mix into chicken salad.

MANY COLORS SALAD

Yield: About 6 servings

   1 cup broccoli florets

   1 cup cauliflower florets

   1 cup red cherry tomatoes

   ½ to 1 cup yellow sweet or bell peppers, cut up

   2 carrots cut up

   ½ large sweet or purple onion, cut up

   About six cups leafy green and purple spring mix

   1 cup mushrooms, cut up

   1½ cup shredded cheddar cheese

For Simple Salad Dressing:

   6 tablespoons of your favorite salad dressing

   6 tablespoons MCT oil or coconut/MCT oil mixture

DIRECTIONS: Wash vegetables and spring mix thoroughly. Place vegetables and mushrooms in a large salad bowl, add cheese, and toss. Mix together dressing ingredients, whisk, and pour immediately onto salad. Toss again just before serving.

ALTERNATIVE: Toss all vegetables except spring mix together and use for two or three days by storing in refrigerator. At time of serving, add about one cup of vegetable mix to one cup of spring mix and toss with a two-tablespoon serving of Simple Salad Dressing or Vegetable Topping above.

CALIFORNIA SALAD

YIELD: 1 serving

  2 cups mixed colors of salad greens

  10 to 12 dried cherries

  2 heaping tablespoons walnut pieces

  1 ounce Gorgonzola cheese, broken apart

Salad Dressing:

  1 tablespoon MCT/coconut oil mixture

  ½ tablespoon walnut oil

  ¼ to ½ teaspoon raspberry balsamic vinegar plus more as needed

DIRECTIONS: Place salad greens in a medium salad bowl. Sprinkle cherries, walnuts, and cheese on top. Mix dressing ingredients in a small bowl and then pour evenly over salad. Toss before eating.

CHOPPED GREEK SALAD

YIELD: 6 to 8 servings

15-ounce can of garbanzo beans, drained
(for lower carb salad, use an 8-ounce can)

1 large cucumber, chopped

1 large bell pepper, chopped

½ large sweet onion, chopped

1 medium tomato, chopped

About 6 cups leafy green and purple spring mix

25 to 30 kalamata or black olives, for serving

1 to 2 ounces of crumbled feta or goat cheese per serving,
as desired for serving

Salad dressing:

3 tablespoons olive oil

1½ tablespoon lemon juice

¼ teaspoon sea salt

2 teaspoons Greek seasoning
(salt, garlic powder, black pepper, oregano, sage)

Additional salad dressing, per serving:

Your serving MCT or MCT//143

DIRECTIONS: In a large bowl or storage container, combine garbanzo beans, cucumber, bell pepper, onion, and tomato. Toss together with ingredients of salad dressing (except MCT and coconut oil mixture). This can be stored in the refrigerator for 2 to 3 days. When ready to serve, add leafy spring mix to medium-size salad bowls until about half filled. Add 2 to 3 large serving spoons full of chopped vegetable mixture. Evenly distribute 1 to 2 ounces of crumbled cheese over vegetables and four to five olives. Pour MCT mixture evenly over salad and toss.

VARIATION: At time of serving, add fresh cooked or canned beets (not pickled), chopped. If added beforehand, the beets will discolor other vegetables.

TACO DIP

With permission of Ossian and Kira Munn

YIELD: about two pounds of dip

- 16 ounces ground beef
- Salt and black pepper
- 8 ounces cream cheese
- 8 ounces sour cream
- 1 ripe avocado, mashed
- Taco toppers: Choose from shredded lettuce, diced fresh tomatoes, sliced black olives, diced red onion, shredded cheese, and any other topper of your choosing.

DIRECTIONS: Brown the ground beef, drain and set aside. Season with salt and pepper to taste. Mix cream cheese, sour cream and mashed avocado. Layer a deep 9" x 13" pan with cream cheese mixture, ground beef ,and all desired taco toppings. Eat dip by itself or serve with pork rinds or parmesan crisps.

MANY COLORS VEGETABLE SOUP

YIELD: About 6 to 12 servings

- 2 tablespoons minced garlic
- 3 tablespoons coconut oil
- 1 cup broccoli, chopped
- 1 cup cauliflower florets, chopped
- 1 large tomato, chopped
- ½ to 1 cup yellow sweet or bell peppers, chopped
- 1 cup carrot, chopped or shredded
- 1 cup celery, chopped
- ½ large sweet or purple onion, chopped
- 1 cup mushrooms, chopped
- 2 teaspoons sea salt, plus more as needed
- ¼ teaspoon white or black pepper, plus more as needed
- 6 to 9 cups vegetable broth or chicken or beef stock
- For each serving: Your serving coconut oil, MCT oil or MCT//143

DIRECTIONS: Sauté minced garlic for a few seconds in three table-spoons coconut oil over medium-low heat. Then add vegetables and the mushroom and continue to sauté until all are tender. Season to taste with salt and pepper. Add broth and simmer soup over low heat for about one hour. At time of serving, add "your serving" coconut oil. Store remaining soup in the refrigerator.

VARIATION: Add 1 or 2 cups tomato sauce in place of an equal amount of broth.

CHICKEN SALAD

YIELD: 2 to 4 servings

2 cups chicken, cut into chunks

½ cup celery, chopped

½ cup sliced almond or chopped walnuts

¼ cup mayonnaise

2 tablespoons MCT oil or MCT//143

Salt and pepper

DIRECTIONS: Toss chicken, celery, and nuts together. In a separate bowl, use a wire whisk to thoroughly blend mayonnaise and MCT oil and then add to chicken mixture, seasoning with salt and pepper to taste. Toss again until well mixed.

OPTIONAL: Mix additional MCT oil or MCT//143 oil mixture into your serving.

VARIATIONS: Add about 8 ripe black or kalamata olives, cut up.

TUNA SALAD

YIELD: About 2 servings

Two 5-ounce cans of tuna, drained

¼ cup chopped sweet onion

2 tablespoons sweet or dill (lower carb choice) pickle relish

2 tablespoons mayonnaise

1 tablespoon MCT oil or MCT//143

Salt and pepper

DIRECTIONS: In a medium bowl, toss tuna, onion, and relish together. In a separate small bowl, use a wire whisk to thoroughly blend mayonnaise and MCT oil and then add to tuna mixture with salt and pepper to taste. Toss again until well mixed.

OPTIONAL: Mix additional MCT oil or coconut/MCT oil mixture into your serving.

LOIS'S ZUCCHINI BACON BAKE

With permission from Lois Kamp

YIELD: 16 pieces

4 zucchini

8 ounces cream cheese, cut into 16 pieces

8 slices of uncooked bacon

DIRECTIONS: Preheat oven to 375° F. Cut zucchini lengthwise and then across to make 16 pieces. Scoop out part of the seeds to make a well in each piece, fill with cream cheese, and then place on a cookie sheet lined with aluminum. Cut bacon slices in half and place lengthwise over the top of the cream cheese. Bake for 40 to 45 minutes until done to your liking.

SAUTÉED GREENS WITH GARLIC

YIELD: 2 to 3 servings

  1 bunch kale, red or green chard, or beet greens

  2 to 3 tablespoons coconut oil

  1 garlic clove, minced or thinly sliced

  Juice of ½ lemon

  Salt

DIRECTIONS: Rinse and remove stems from greens, cut into ½-inch segments, and set aside. Chop leaves into small pieces. Heat coconut oil in large skillet over medium-low heat and add garlic, sautéing until garlic starts to change color. Add stems and stir occasionally for about two minutes, or until almost tender. Add chopped leaves and continue to cook 3 to 5 minutes more, partially covering skillet with lid. Add lemon juice, sprinkle with salt to taste, and then toss until thoroughly distributed. Remove from skillet and serve.

ALMOND BROCCOLI AND/OR CAULIFLOWER

YIELD: 2 to 3 servings

  1 bunch of broccoli and/or head of cauliflower, cut into bite size pieces

  2 to 3 tablespoons coconut oil

  ¼ teaspoon sea salt

  ¼ cup sliced almonds

DIRECTIONS: Using your favorite steaming method, steam broccoli for 4 to 5 minutes. Place hot broccoli in a bowl, add coconut oil, sprinkle the salt evenly, and add sliced almonds. Toss the ingredients until evenly distributed.

GARLICKY BROCCOLI AND/OR CAULIFLOWER

YIELD: 2 to 3 servings

1 bunch of broccoli and/or head of cauliflower, cut into bite size pieces

2 tablespoons coconut oil

½ teaspoon garlic salt with parsley

DIRECTIONS: Using your favorite steaming method, steam broccoli for about 4 to 5 minutes. Place hot broccoli and/or cauliflower in a bowl and add coconut oil, sprinkle the salt evenly, and add sliced almonds, then toss the ingredients until evenly distributed.

BRUSSEL SPROUTS

YIELD: 3 to 4 servings

2 tablespoons coconut oil

1 pound of small Brussels sprouts

½ teaspoon garlic salt with parsley

DIRECTIONS: Using your favorite steaming method, steam Brussels sprouts for about 4–5 minutes until tender (longer if large Brussels sprouts are used). Place in a bowl and add coconut oil and sprinkle garlic salt evenly over sprouts, then toss until evenly distributed.

GARLICKY SPINACH

YIELD: 2 to 3 servings

　　2 to 3 tablespoons coconut oil

　　Level tablespoon minced garlic

　　1 bunch of fresh spinach

　　¼ teaspoon sea salt

DIRECTIONS: Heat coconut oil in a large skillet at just below medium heat. When heated, add minced garlic and use a spatula to distribute over skillet surface. Add spinach and move around with the spatula until all of the leaves are just moist and slightly wilted but not soggy. Sprinkle with sea salt, stir in quickly, and then remove from the skillet to avoid overcooking.

VARIATIONS: Add a heaping tablespoon of pine nuts along with the garlic.

STIR-FRIED CHICKEN TENDERS

YIELD: 4 servings

　　4 tablespoons coconut oil

　　1 tablespoon peanut or sesame oil

　　1 tablespoon minced garlic

　　1 teaspoon minced peeled fresh ginger

　　2 teaspoons cornstarch

　　2 teaspoons sesame oil

　　12 fresh raw chicken tenders

DIRECTIONS: Preheat coconut and peanut oil in a large wok or skillet on the stove over medium heat. Make a paste with the cornstarch and the 2 teaspoons sesame oil in a large bowl, add the chicken tenders to the bowl, and move the tenders around until completely coated with the paste. Place tenders into hot oil in wok and cook for 3 to 4 minutes on each side until cooked through.

CASHEW CHICKEN

YIELD: 4 servings

Stir-Fry Teriyaki Sauce:

2½ tablespoons teriyaki sauce (preferably low carb or sugar free)

1 teaspoon sesame oil

12 Stir-Fried Chicken Tenders (recipe above)

½ cup cashews

2 cups fresh broccoli florets, cut into small pieces

Salt and black pepper

DIRECTIONS: In a small bowl, combine all ingredients for teriyaki sauce and set aside. When chicken tenders are done, turn heat to low and add stir-fry teriyaki sauce, cashews, and 2 cups broccoli florets. Stir constantly for 1 or 2 minutes more.

STIR-FRIED NAPA CABBAGE WITH CARROTS AND COCONUT

YIELD: 4 servings

Stir-Fry Teriyaki Sauce:

  2½ tablespoons teriyaki sauce

  1 teaspoon sesame oil

  Salt and black pepper to taste

Main ingredients:

  2 tablespoons coconut oil

  1 tablespoon peanut oil

  1 heaping tablespoon minced garlic

  1 tablespoon minced peeled fresh ginger

  2 cups shredded carrots

  ½ cup flaked coconut

  1 medium Napa (also called Chinese) cabbage, thinly sliced

  Minced cilantro or parsley

DIRECTIONS: Combine and stir sauce ingredients well in a small bowl and set aside. In a wok or large skillet, heat coconut and peanut oil to medium-high heat. When hot, add garlic and ginger and stir for several seconds. Add carrots and flaked coconut and stir-fry for about three minutes. Add sliced cabbage and stir-fry for another three more minutes until cabbage is tender. Add the teriyaki mixture and toss with the vegetable mixture until thoroughly coated. Remove from heat to avoid overcooking. Sprinkle with cilantro, toss again, and then serve immediately.

VARIATION: When vegetables are tender, stir in the teriyaki mixture and the already cooked Stir-Fried Chicken Tenders (page 410) and warm together for 1 minute.

SYBIL'S COCONUT CHICKEN TENDERS OR FISH FINGERS

With permission from Sybil Kennedy

YIELD: 4 servings

1 whole egg, beaten

½ cup whole wheat panko or whole wheat Italian bread crumbs

½ cup unsweetened grated coconut

¼ cup grated parmesan cheese

1 teaspoon garlic salt

¼ teaspoon pepper

12 fresh raw chicken tenders or cod fish filets, cut into strips

3 tablespoons coconut oil

1 tablespoon olive or canola oil

DIRECTIONS: Beat egg with a fork in a bowl. Combine all dry ingredients on a large plate and mix thoroughly with a fork. Place tenders in bowl with egg and stir until all pieces are thoroughly coated. Heat coconut and olive oil in a large skillet over medium heat. Roll each tender in dry mix until covered and set aside on another plate. When all tenders are coated, place pieces in hot oil for 3 to 4 minutes on each side until done.

VARIATION: Serve chicken with Simple Topping For Chicken; serve fish fingers with Simple Tartar Sauce, page 414.

SIMPLE TARTAR SAUCE

YIELD: ½ cup

4 tablespoons mayonnaise

2 tablespoons MCT oil or MCT//143

1 teaspoon lemon juice

1 teaspoon prepared yellow mustard

1 tablespoon dill or sweet pickle relish

DIRECTIONS: In a small bowl, use a wire whisk to blend mayonnaise and MCT oil. Blend in lemon juice and yellow mustard, add relish, and mix again.

ROSEMARY'S STUFFED BELL PEPPERS

YIELD: 5 servings

  2 tablespoons olive oil

  5 large bell peppers of various colors

  3 tablespoons coconut oil

  7 cloves garlic, minced

  1 large sweet onion, chopped

  1 pound ground beef or ground turkey

  2 cups tomato sauce

  3 cups chicken broth

  ¾ cup uncooked whole grain rice

  ½ teaspoon sea salt

  ¼ teaspoon black pepper

  1 tablespoon + 1 teaspoon dried peppermint

DIRECTIONS: Preheat oven to 300°F. Cut top off peppers, set aside, and then split body of pepper in half the long way. Spread olive oil on bottom of a 9" x 12" baking pan and lay the peppers—open side facing up—on the pan. Bake in the oven for about 40 minutes while preparing the remaining ingredients. Remove the stems from the pepper tops and chop the remaining pepper pieces. In a large skillet, heat coconut oil over medium-low heat and sauté garlic, chopped onion, and chopped peppers until tender. Add ground beef, breaking it apart and stirring until thoroughly cooked. Add 1 cup tomato sauce (reserve the other cup for later), two cups broth, and rice. With lid in place, simmer over low heat for ½ hour, stirring occasionally. Add salt, pepper, and 1 tablespoon peppermint and stir thoroughly. Remove bell peppers from the oven and increase oven temperature to 375°F. Spoon meat mixture, evenly divided, into the open bell peppers. Spoon remaining 1 cup of tomato sauce over the tops of the meat-stuffed peppers and sprinkle lightly with salt, pepper, and peppermint. Form an aluminum foil tent over top of pan so that foil does not stick to tomato topping. Return peppers to oven and bake for 40 minutes.

CHICKEN POT PIE

With permission from Ketogenic.com

YIELD: 6 servings

  2 teaspoons garlic powder

Pot Pie Filling:

  1 cup frozen mixed vegetables (peas and carrots)

  ¾ cup frozen pearl onions

  1 tablespoon minced garlic

  2 cups chicken broth

  1 cup heavy whipping cream

  ½ pound boneless skinless chicken breasts, cooked and diced

  2 ounces cream cheese

  1 teaspoon pepper

  2 tablespoons dried parsley

Dough:

  ¾ cup mozzarella

  ¾ cup almond flour

  2 tablespoons cream cheese

  1 egg

  1 teaspoon salt

  1 teaspoon dried parsley

DIRECTIONS: Preheat oven to 375° F. Heat a large pan and add the mixed veggies, pearl onions, and garlic. Cook until they begin to soften. Add the chicken broth and bring to a simmer. Add the heavy cream, chicken, and cream cheese. Bring back to a simmer and let the mixture simmer for about 30 minutes until it is thick stirring occasionally. Pour the pot pie mixture into an 8" x 8" glass baking dish and set aside. For the dough, mix the mozzarella cheese and almond flour in a microwave-safe bowl. Add the cream cheese. Microwave on high for 1 minute. Stir the mixture and then microwave again on high for 30 seconds. Remove bowl from microwave and add the egg and salt. Mix until combined. Divide the dough into 16 equal portions. Roll each portion into a ball and place on top of the layers of the pot pie filling. Sprinkle the tops of the fat head dough with parsley. Place in the oven and cook until the dough is golden brown, about 20 to 30 minutes. Remove from the oven, let set for 5 minutes, and then serve.

*RECIPE STATEMENT: The macronutrients of your dish will depend on the type and brand of the ingredients you use. This could make your dish different from ours.

LOIS'S CREAMY CHICKEN BAKE

With permission from Lois Kamp

YIELD: 6 servings

   3 large radishes, chopped

   2 ribs celery, chopped

   ½ cup onions, chopped

   1 stick of butter

   Salt and pepper

   1 pound chicken filets, cut into bite-size pieces

   ¾ cup heavy whipping cream

   1 to 2 teaspoon dry thyme

   1 cup Carbquik Baking Mix

   ⅓ cup water

DIRECTIONS: Preheat oven to 375° F. In a large skillet, sauté vegetables in butter with salt and pepper to taste until vegetables soften. Add chicken and continue to sauté until thoroughly cooked. Use a slotted spoon to remove vegetables and chicken from the skillet and set aside. Add cream and thyme to the butter in the skillet and cook at low heat until mixture thickens to a gravy consistency. Remove from heat, stir chicken and vegetables back into the gravy, and pour into a greased casserole dish. Mix Carbquik dry powder with about ⅓ cup of water to a biscuit consistency and distribute evenly over the top of the chicken and vegetables. Bake for 20 to 25 minutes until done golden brown.

FAT HEAD PIZZA

With permission from Ketogenic.com

YIELD: 8 slices

Macronutrients per slice: fat 20 grams, protein 14 grams, carbs 5 grams

Crust:

- ¾ cup shredded mozzarella
- ¾ cup almond flour
- 2 tablespoons cream cheese
- 1 egg
- 1 teaspoon salt
- 1 teaspoon chopped basil
- 1 teaspoon garlic powder

Toppings:

- ½ cup pizza sauce
- 4 ounces Italian sausage, cooked
- ½ bell pepper, diced
- 10 pepperoni slices
- ½ cup mozzarella
- Chopped basil for garnish

DIRECTIONS: Mix the mozzarella cheese and almond flour in a microwave-safe bowl. Add the cream cheese. Microwave on high for 1 minute. Stir the mixture and then microwave again on high for 30 seconds. Remove bowl from the microwave and add the egg and seasonings. Mix until combined. Place the dough ball on a sheet of parchment paper and place another sheet on top. Using a rolling pin, roll out the crust to about ¼ inch thickness. Remove the top piece of paper and poke with a fork (this will help it cook evenly and avoid bubbles). Put the crust on a baking sheet (bottom parchment paper still there) and bake on 350°F until the crust browns (12 to 15 minutes). Remove the crust from the oven and cover with toppings. Return to the oven and bake until the cheese melts (5 to 8 minutes). Remove and cut into slices and serve.

VARIATIONS: Add or subtract topping ingredients of your choice.

*RECIPE STATEMENT: The macronutrients of your dish will depend on the type and brand of the ingredients you use. This could make your dish different from ours.

SIMPLE SALMON DINNER FOR TWO

YIELD: 2 to 3 servings

10 to 12 ounces salmon fillet, any size

1 bunch fresh asparagus

2 to 3 tablespoons coconut oil, melted

Garlic and herb or other favorite seasoning

DIRECTIONS: Preheat oven to 350°F. Place aluminum foil on a large cookie sheet or spray the cookie sheet with olive oil spray. On one side of the cookie sheet place a salmon fillet, skin side down, and on the other evenly distribute the asparagus spears. Melt about 2 to 3 tablespoons of coconut oil (or more for a very large fillet) and paint the oil onto the salmon and asparagus using a pastry brush. Sprinkle seasoning over fish and asparagus. Bake for 20 minutes. The salmon should be very moist and separate easily with a fork.

CHICKEN BACON BROCCOLI BAKE

With permission from Ketogenic.com

YIELD: 8 servings

*Macronutrients per serving: Fat: 28 grams, protein 21 grams, carbs 7 grams

- 8 ounces cream cheese, softened
- 4 ounces sour cream
- 4 ounces mayonnaise
- ½ tablespoon garlic powder
- ½ yellow onion, diced
- 1 tablespoon Italian seasoning
- 1 teaspoon salt
- ½ teaspoon pepper
- 24 ounces chicken breast, cooked and diced
- 1 pound frozen broccoli, thawed
- 8 ounces shredded cheddar cheese
- 5 slices bacon, crumbled

DIRECTIONS: Preheat oven to 350°F. In a big bowl combine cream cheese, sour cream, mayo, and spices and mix thoroughly. To the cream cheese mixture add the chicken, broccoli, ¾ of the cheese, and the bacon crumbles. Mix well. Dump into an 8" x 8" baking dish sprayed with cooking spray. Sprinkle remaining cheese on top. Bake until hot, about 40 minutes.

*RECIPE STATEMENT: The macronutrients of your dish will depend on the type and brand of the ingredients you use. This could make your dish different from ours.

KIRA'S WHIPPED KETO KREME

With permission from Kira Munn

YIELD: About 8 servings

- **16 ounces heavy whipping cream**
- **1 teaspoon vanilla extract**
- **2 tablespoons Swerve (confectioners) or other sugar substitute**
- **1 packet Keto Kreme (optional)**

DIRECTIONS: Whip heavy whipping cream until firm peaks start to form. Add vanilla extract and Swerve and whip for about 10 seconds. If using, slowly add Keto Kreme to mixture and whip for 30 seconds. When finished, fold the whipped cream. Eat alone or with fresh berries.

OPTIONAL: Add chocolate drizzle.

LOIS'S CREAMY KETO PUDDING POP

With permission from Lois Kamp

YIELD: 4 servings

- **1 package sugar-free pudding, any flavor**
- **½ cup water**
- **½ cup heavy whipping cream**

DIRECTIONS: Whisk pudding with water and cream until fully blended. Pour into four popsicle molds and freeze.

CRISPY PEANUT BUTTER FAT BOMB

With permission from Ketogenic.com

YIELD: 15 servings

Macronutrients per serving: fat 8 grams, protein 2 grams, carbs 3 grams

- 3 ounces unsweetened chocolate, chopped
- 2 ounces unsweetened white chocolate, chopped
- 1 ounce cocoa butter, chopped
- ½ tablespoon unsalted butter
- 1 teaspoon powdered erythritol
- ⅛ tablespoon raw sucralose
- 1 tablespoon peanut butter
- ½ ounce pork rinds

DIRECTIONS: This recipe calls for a silicone mold, but a plastic or silicone ice cube tray could be used instead. Temper chocolate by placing ¾ of chocolate and cocoa butter in a microwave-safe bowl and microwaving on high for 1 to 2 minutes. Stir every 15 seconds until chocolate is melted. Add butter, erythritol, sucralose, and salt to chocolate and stir until combined, checking temperature with a kitchen thermometer after each fifteen seconds of microwaving on high until the temperature is above 115°F and then add remaining chocolate. Stir with a rubber spatula until chocolate is smooth no chunks remain, and temperature is between 88 and 92°F. Once proper temperature is reached, transfer chocolate to a pastry or plastic bag, remove a corner so that chocolate can be "piped," fill half of the silicone mold wells with chocolate, and allow to "set" until firm for about 5 minutes. Mix together peanut butter and pork rinds until a thick paste forms, place a dollop of pork rind mixture on each well of chocolate (about 1 teaspoon), fill remaining mold with chocolate. Place molds in the refrigerator to set for 5 to 10 minutes, remove from mold and store in an airtight container, refrigerated for up to 7 days. [If a plastic or silicone ice cube tray is used, fill each well halfway with the chocolate mixture, add 1 teaspoon of the pork rind mixture, and then fill wells to the top with the remaining chocolate mixture.]

*RECIPE STATEMENT: The macronutrients of your dish will depend on the type and brand of the ingredients you use. This could make your dish different from ours.

LOIS'S CREAMY KETO CUSTARD

With permission from Lois Kamp

YIELD: 6 servings

4 fresh eggs

2 cups heavy whipping cream

25 to 30 drops liquid stevia extract

1 teaspoon vanilla

Nutmeg

DIRECTIONS: Preheat oven to 375ºF. In a mixer, blend all ingredients, except the nutmeg, and pour equally into six custard bowls. Sprinkle nutmeg on top. Fill a baking pan with about 1½ inches of water and place custard bowls into the pan. Bake for 40 to 45 minutes until set. Eat warm or cold.

DUSTIN'S KETO//MAX POPSICLES

With permission from Dustin Schaffer/Schaffer Method

YIELD: Varies with size of mold

  1 can coconut cream

  2 tablespoons cocoa powder

  1 packet of Keto//MAX- Swiss Cacao

  1 packet of MCT 1:4:3

  ½ teaspoon Himalayan sea salt

  ¾ teaspoon vanilla liquid stevia or 2 tablespoons erythritol

  1 teaspoon lemon juice
  or use 1 teaspoon of Keto//MAX Raspberry Lemonade

  1 teaspoon grass-fed gelatin (omit agar for a vegan option)

DIRECTIONS: Whisk first five ingredients together in a bowl or large measuring cup. Adjust sweetness and flavors to taste. Dissolve gelatin in 4 tablespoons boiling water. Whisk gelatin into coconut cream mixture until well combined. Pour into molds of your choice. (Silicone molds of all sorts and sizes work great, especially with the kids. Give the little bunny molds a try.) Freeze for 4 to 6 hours.

DUSTIN'S KETO//KREME CHOCOLATE CHIP CRUNCH COOKIES

With permission from Dustin Schaffer/Schaffer Method

YIELD: Varies with size of cookie

2 cups almond flour (Coconut flour doesn't hold as well.)

½ teaspoon salt

1 packet Keto//KREME

¼ teaspoon baking soda

¼ cup of butter, softened

½ teaspoon vanilla

1 large egg

¾ cup dark chocolate chips
(Lilly's Dark Chocolate Chips or other keto friendly chocolate chips)

DIRECTIONS: Preheat oven to 350°F. In a food processor or with a hand-held electric mixer, mix flour, salt, Keto//KREME, and baking soda. Add the butter, vanilla, and egg and then pulse or mix into the dry ingredients. Stir in chocolate chips by hand. With a tablespoon, ball dough and flatten with your hand. Space the dough out evenly on a cookie sheet and bake for 9 to 10 minutes.

JOANNA'S MERINGUES

With permission from Joanna Newport

YIELD: 25 to 50 meringues, depending on size

2 large egg whites

½ tsp vanilla

¼ tsp cream of tartar

¼ cup Swerve (granulated) or other artificial sugar

DIRECTIONS: Preheat oven to 300°F. Put parchment paper onto a cookie pan. Whip egg whites with vanilla and cream of tartar until stiff peaks form. Add Swerve or other artificial granular type sugar gradually until mixture is glossy with stiff peaks. Place parchment paper on a cookie sheet. Put mixture into piping bag or plastic sandwich bag and cut the tip to pipe ½ to 1½ inch puffs at least ¼ inch apart and about 1 inch tall. Insert into oven and turn off the oven. Set timer for 1 hour to let the meringue dry. Finished product should be hard to the touch but with a light, crispy, puffy texture.

TIP: *Bake with only one cookie sheet at a time as it could affect dry time.*

JENN'S CUT-OUT COOKIES

With permission from Jenn Rau

YIELD: Will depend on size of cookie cutter

Cookies

- 2 sticks butter
- 1 pinch kosher salt
- 1 ⅓ cup granulated Swerve artificial sweetener
- 1 teaspoon vanilla extract
- 2 teaspoons almond extract
- 4 ½ cups almond flour, superfine
- 2 eggs

Frosting (Optional)

- 4 egg whites
- 1 teaspoon cream of tartar
- 4 cups confectioners Swerve
- 3 teaspoons water

DIRECTIONS: For cookies: Beat the butter, salt, and sweetener until fluffy. Add the vanilla and almond extracts and blend well. Add the almond flour and beat until just blended to a stiff dough. Wrap dough in plastic wrap and refrigerate for 2 hours or overnight until stiff. Separate dough into 4 balls. Using parchment paper roll out 1 ball at a time. Use a cookie cutter to cut desired shapes. Place the cut outs on a parchment-lined cookie sheet and bake in a preheated 350°F oven for 15 minutes. Remove and cool before frosting.

FROSTING: Whip the egg whites and cream of tartar. Slowly add in Swerve. Add water until desired consistency is reached. Add the frosting to a piping bag or plastic zip lock. Squeeze out desired amount of frosting to decorate cookies.

KIRA'S CHEESECAKE FRUIT DIP

With permission from Kira Munn

YIELD: About 8 servings

Two 8-ounce blocks cream cheese, softened

1 cup Swerve (granulated) or other sugar substitute

DIRECTIONS: Using a blender or mixer, blend all ingredients together until it is smooth and creamy. Serve with fresh mixed berries. Optional: Add Chocolate Drizzle.

CHOCOLATE DRIZZLE / DIP

With permission from Ossian and Kira Munn

YIELD: About 8 servings

3-ounce Lily's Original Dark Chocolate Bar (or your favorite low-carb or carb-free chocolate)

7 tablespoons heavy cream

DIRECTIONS: Melt chocolate in a double boiler. Slowly add heavy whipping cream one tablespoon at a time until desired consistency is reached. Use as a drizzle or a dip.

COCONUT MACAROONS

YIELD: 18 small cookies

2 egg whites

Pinch of salt

½ teaspoon vanilla, chocolate, or almond extract

¼ cup granulated Swerve

1 cup shredded unsweetened coconut

DIRECTIONS: Beat egg whites with salt and extract until soft peaks form. Gradually add Swerve and beat until stiff. Fold in coconut. Coat a cookie sheet with generous amount of butter. Drop batter by the rounded teaspoon onto cookie sheet. Bake at 325°F for 20 minutes. Each cookie contains approximately 4 grams of coconut oil.

COCONUT FUDGE OR CANDIES

YIELD: About 16 ounces

1 cup coconut oil

8 ounces low-carb or carb-free artificially sweetened solid dark or milk chocolate bar or chips

DIRECTIONS: In a double boiler, melt and thoroughly mix together the oil and chocolate. Divide mixture equally into paper candy cups on a large plate or into a plastic or silicone ice cube tray or mold and place in the refrigerator. Chill until set. In a sixteen-cube tray, each cube will equal one tablespoon of coconut oil and will easily pop out of the tray.

VARIATION: Add about ¼ cup grated coconut to part or all of mixture and/or add nuts or nut pieces for variety. Put some mixture in bottom of candy cups or sections of ice cube, add peanut butter or creamed coconut that has been cut into pieces; then add remainder of mixture over the top of each candy piece. Chill in refrigerator until set. Store in refrigerator or freezer.

COCONUT CHOCOLATE DIP OR TOPPING

YIELD: About 16 ounces

1 cup coconut oil

8 ounces low-carb or carb-free artificially sweetened solid dark or milk chocolate bar or chips

DIRECTIONS: Melt oil and add chocolate at very low heat until melted, mixing thoroughly. Use as topping for ice cream, or dip strawberries or other fruit or nuts into mixture. Can be served immediately or berries can be dipped, placed on a plate and refrigerated for eating later.

RESOURCES

Author's Contact Information

www.coconutketones.com

Facebook: Coconut Oil Helps Alzheimer's, Dementia, ALS, MS
https://www.facebook.com/CoconutOilandAlzheimers/

Facebook: Mary Newport https://www.facebook.com/mary.newport.98

marynewportmd@gmail.com

Books and Special Articles

Dietary Reference Intakes for Energy, Carbohydrate, Fiber, Fat, Fatty Acids, Cholesterol, Protein, and Amino Acids, (National Academies Press, 2005) https://ods.od.nih.gov/Health_Information/Dietary_Reference_Intakes.aspx.

Agatston, Arthur. *The South Beach Diet: The Delicious, Doctor-Designed, Foolproof Plan for Fast and Healthy Weight Loss.* New York, NY: Rodale Inc./St. Martin's Press, 2003.

Agatston, Arthur, and Natalie Geary. *The South Beach Diet Gluten Solution: The Delicious, Doctor-Designed, Gluten-Aware Plan for Losing Weight and Feeling Great—Fast!* New York, NY: Rodale Inc., 2013.

Agatston, Arthur, and Joseph Signorile. *The South Beach Diet Super Charged: Faster Weight Loss and Better Health for Life.* New York, NY: Rodale Inc., 2008.

Allen, K. *Remembering What I Forgot*: Gwen Lee Publishing, 2017.

Atkins, Robert C. *Atkins Comprehensive Carb Counter.*

Atkins, Robert C. *Atkins for Life: The Complete Controlled Carb Program for Permanent Weight Loss and Good Health.* New York, NY: St. Martin's Press, 2003.

Atkins, Robert C., *Dr. Atkins' New Diet Revolution: The Amazing No-Hunger Weight-Loss Plan That Has Helped Millions Lose Weight and Keep It Off.* New York, NY: Avon Books, Inc., 1992.

Banting, William, and Will Meadows. *The Banting Diet: Letter on Corpulence*: Lexington, KY: FCD Publishing, 2015.

Beer, Maggie, and Ralph Martins. *Maggie's Recipe for Life: 200 Delicious Recipes to Help Reduce Your Chances of Alzheimer's & Other Lifestyle Diseases.* Australia: Julie Gibbs/Simon & Schuster (Australia) Pty Ltd, 2017.

Bredesen, Dale E. *The End of Alzheimer's: The First Program to Prevent and Reverse Cognitive Decline.* New York, NY: Avery/Penguin Random House, 2017.

Brown, Susan E., and Larry Trivieri Jr. *The Acid Alkaline Food Guide: A Quick Reference to Foods & Their Effect on pH Levels.* 2nd ed. Garden City Park, NY: Square One Publishers, 2013.

Buckley, Julie A., Lynn Vannucci, and Jenny McCarthy. *Healing Our Autistic Children: A Medical Plan for Restoring Your Child's Health.* New York, NY: Palgrave Macmillan, 2010.

Buettner, Dan. *The Blue Zones: 9 Lessons for Living Longer from the People Who've Lived the Longest.* 2nd ed. Washington, D.C.: National Geographic Society, 2012.

Calbom, Cherie, and John Calbom. *The Coconut Diet: The Secret Ingredient That Helps You Lose Weight While You Eat Your Favorite Foods.* New York, NY: Warner Books, 2005.

Callone, Patricia R., Connie Kudlacek, Barbara C. Vasiloff, Janaan Manternach, D. Min, and Roger A. Brumback. *A Caregiver's Guide to Alzheimer's Disease: 300 Tips for Making Life Easier.* New York, NY: Demos Medical Publishing, 2006.

Chomchalow, Narong, Keith Chapman, and Peyanoot Naka (editors). *Proceedings of the Second International Conference on Coconut Oil (ICCO2017): Theme "Coconut Oil and Downstream Products, Quality and Processing."* Bankok, Thailand: Department of Agriculture, Horticulture Research Institute and Conservation and Development of Coconut Oil Forum of Thailand (CDCOT), 2017.

Cordain, Loren. *The Paleo Diet.* Hoboken, NJ: John Wiley & Sons, Revised Edition 2010.

Cruise, Jorge. *The Belly Fat Cure: Sugar & Carb Counter.* Carlsbad, CA: Hay House, Inc., 2010.

Cunnane, Stephen C. *Survival of the Fattest: The Key to Human Brain Evolution.* Singapore: World Scientific Publishing Ct. Pte. Ltd., 2005.

Dayrit, Conrado S., Fabian M. Dayrit and Bruce Fife. *Coconut Oil from Diet to Therapy.* Philippines: Anvil Publishing, Inc., 2013.

Dietary Reference Intakes for Energy, Carbohydrate, Fiber, Fat, Fatty Acids, Cholesterol, Protein, and Amino Acids (National Academies Press, 2005). Free PDF can be downloaded at https://www.nap.edu/read/10490/chapter/1

Enig, Mary, and Sally Fallon. *Eat Fat Lose Fat.* New York, NY: Plume/Penguin Group, Inc., 2006.

Erasmus, Udo. *Fats That Heal, Fats That Kill.* Summertown, TN: Books Alive, 1993 (first published 1986).

Ferriss, Tim. *Tools of Titans: The Tactics, Routines and Habits of Billionaires, Icons and World-Class Performers.* London: Vermilion/Ebury Publishing/Penguin Random House, 2016.

Fife, Bruce. *The Coconut Ketogenic Diet: Supercharge Your Metabolism, Revitalize Thyroid Function, and Lose Excess Weight.* Colorado Springs, CO: Picadilly Books, Ltd., 2014.

---. *Coconut Lover's Cookbook.* 3rd ed. Colorado Springs, CO: Piccadilly Books, Ltd., 2008.

---. *Eat Fat Look Thin: A Safe and Natural Way to Lose Weight Permanently.* Colorado Springs, CO: Health Wise Publications, 2002.

---. *Oil Pulling Therapy: Detoxifying and Healing the Body Through Oral Cleansing.* Colorado Springs, CO: Piccadilly Books, Ltd., 2008.

---. *Stop Autism Now!: A Parent's Guide to Preventing and Reversing Autism Spectrum Disorders.* Colorado Springs, CO: Piccadilly Books, Ltd., 2012.

---. *Virgin Coconut Oil: Nature's Miracle Medicine.* Colorado Springs, CO: Piccadilly Books, Ltd., 2006.

Fife, Bruce, and Russell L. Blaylock. *Stop Alzheimer's Now!: How to Prevent and Reverse Dementia, Parkinson's, ALS, Multiple Sclerosis, and Other Neurodegenerative Disorders.* Colorado Springs, CO: Piccadilly Books, Ltd., 2011.

Fife, Bruce, and Conrado S. Dayrit. *Coconut Cures: Preventing and Treating Common Health Problems with Coconut.* Colorado Springs, CO: Piccadilly Books, Ltd., 2005.

Frayne, Catherine. *Thoughts of Yesterday.* Galway, Ireland: Book Hub Publishing, 2015..

Graveline, Duane. *Statin Drugs Side Effects and the Misguided War on Cholesterol.* 4th ed: Self-published, 2008.

Graveline, Duane, and Malcolm Kendrick. *The Statin Damage Crisis:* Self-published, 2009.

Greger, Michael,, and Gene Stone. *How Not To Die: Discover the Foods Scientifically Proven to Prevent and Reverse Disease.* New York, NY: Flatiron Books, 2015.

Gursche, Siegfried. *Coconut Oil: Discover the Key to Vibrant Health.* Summertown, TN: Books Alive, 2008.

Guttersen, Connie. *The Sonoma Diet: Trimmer Waist, Better Health in Just 10 Days!* Des Moines, IA: Meredith Books, 2005.

Guyenet, Stephan J. *The Hungry Brain: Outsmarting the Instincts That Make Us Overeat.* New York, NY: Flatiron Books, 2017.

Heimowitz, Colette. *The New Atkins Made Easy: A Faster, Simpler Way to Shed Weight and Feel Greet—Starting Today!.* New York, NY: Touchstone/Simon & Schuster, Inc., 2013.

Heimowitz, Colette. *The New Atkins for a New You Workbook.* New York, NY: Touchstone/Simon & Schuster, Inc., 2012.

Heimowitz, Colette. *The New Atkins for a New You Cookbook: 200 Simple and Delicious Low-Carb Recipes in 30 Minutes or Less.* New York, NY: Touchstone/Simon & Schuster, Inc., 2011.

Heller, Rachael F., and Richard F. *The Carbohydrate Addict's Calorie Counter.* New York, NY: Signet/Penguin Putnam Inc., 2000.

Hermiston, Nyema, and Ian Gawler. *Good News for People with Bad News: Recovery Stories Everyone Must Know About.* Australia: Karuna Publishing, 2014.

Isaacson, Richard S., and Christopher N. Ochner. *The Alzheimer's Diet: A Step-by-Step Nutritional Approach for Memory Loss Prevention & Treatment.* Miami Beach, FL: AD Education Consultants, Inc., 2013.

Johnson, James B., and Donald R. Laur Sr. *The Alternate-Day Diet, The Original Up-Day, Down-Day Eating Plan to Turn on Your "Skinny Gene," Shed the Pounds, and Live a Longer and Healthier Life.* 2nd ed. New York, NY: Perigee/Penguin Group (USA) LLC, 2014.

Kalamian, Miriam, and Thomas N. Seyfried. *Keto for Cancer: Ketogenic Metabolic Therapy as a Targeted Nutritional Strategy.* White River Junction, VT: Chelsea Green Publishing, 2017.

Kendrick, Malcolm. *The Great Cholesterol Con: The Truth About What Really Causes Heart Disease and How to Avoid It.* London, England: John Blake Publishing Ltd., 2007.

Koslo, Jennifer. *The Alkaline Diet for Beginners: Understand pH, Eat Well, Reclaim Your Health.* Berkeley, CA: Rockridge Press, 2016.

Kossoff, Eric H, John M. Freeman, Zahava Turner, and James E. Rubenstein. *Ketogenic Diets: Treatments for Epilepsy and Other Disorders.* 5th ed. New York, NY: Demos Medical Publishing, 2011.

Lands, William E.M. *Fish, Omega-3 and Human Health.* 2nd ed. Urbana, IL: AOCS Press, 2005.

Leblanc, Gary Joseph. *Staying Afloat in a Sea of Forgetfulness: Common Sense Caregiving:* Xlibris Corporation, 2010.

Lipton, Anne M., and Cindy D. Marshall. *The Common Sense Guide to Dementia for Clinicians and Caregivers.* New York, NY: Springer (Science+Business Media LLC), 2013.

London, Jan. *Coconut Cuisine Featuring Stevia.* Summertown, TN: Book Publishing Company, 2006.

Lord, Ethelle. *Alzheimer and Dementia Coaching: Taking a Systems Approach in Creating an Alzheimer's Friendly Healthcare Workforce.* Mustang, OK: Tate Publishing & Enterprises, LLC, 2016.

Masino, Susan A. *Ketogenic Diet and Metabolic Therapies.* New York, NY: Oxford University Press, 2017.

Monk, Arlene, and Marion J. Franz. *Convenience Food Facts: Help for the Healthy Meal Planner.* 2nd ed. Wayzata, MN: Diabetes Center, Inc., 1987.

Moore, Jimmy, and Eric C. Westman. *Keto Clarity: Your Definitive Guide to the Benefits of a Low-Carb, High-Fat Diet.* Las Vegas, NV: Victory Belt Publishing, Inc., 2014.

Nation, Judy, J., Helen Cross, and Ingrid E. Scheffer. *Ketocooking: A Practical Guide to the Ketogenic Diet.* Hertfordshire: The Homewood Press, 2012.

Netzer, Corinne T. *The Complete Book of Food Counts: The Book That Counts It All.* 9th ed. New York, NY: Dell/Random House, Inc., 2012.

Newport, Mary. *Alzheimer's Disease: What If There Was a Cure? The Story of Ketones.* 2nd ed. Laguna Beach, CA: Basic Health Publications, Inc., 2013.

Newport, Mary T. *The Coconut Oil and Low-Carb Solution for Alzheimer's, Parkinson's and Other Diseases,* Laguna Beach, CA: Basic Health Publications, Inc., 2015

Nichols, Lily. *Real Food for Gestational Diabetes.* www.realfoodforGD.com [no other publisher information noted in book]

Nichols, Lily. *Real Food for Pregnancy.* www.realfoodforpregnancy.com [no other publisher information noted in book]

Perlmutter, David, and Kristin Loberg. *The Grain Brain Whole Life Plan.* New York, NY: Little, Brown and Company/Hachette Book Group, Inc., 2016.

Perlmutter, David, and Kristin Loberg. Grain Brain: *The Surprising Truth About Wheat, Carbs, and Sugar—Your Brain's Silent Killers.* New York, NY: Little, Brown and Company/Hachette Book Group, Inc., 2013.

Perlmutter, David, and Kristin Loberg. *Brain Maker: The Power of Gut Microbes to Heal and Protect Your Brain—For Life.* New York, NY: Little, Brown and Company/Hachette Book Group, Inc., 2015.

Price, Weston A. *Nutrition and Physical Degeneration.* 8th ed. La Mesa, CA: Price-Pottenger Nutrition Foundation, 2008 (originally printed in 1939).

Seyfried, Thomas N. *Cancer as a Metabolic Disease: On the Origin, Management, and Prevention of Cancer.* Hoboken, NJ: John Wiley & Sons, Inc., 2012.

Simopoulos, Artemis P., and Jo Robinson. *The Omega Diet: The Lifesaving Nutritional Program Based on the Diet of the Island of Crete (prev. published as "The Omega Plan").* New York, NY: Harper Perennial/HarperCollins Publishers, 1999.

Snyder, Deborah. *Keto Kid: Helping Your Child Succeed on the Ketogenic Diet.* New York, NY: Demos Medical Publishing, 2007.

Stoll, Andrew L. *The Omega-3 Connection: The Groundbreaking Omega-3 Antidepression Diet and Brain Program.* New York, NY: Fireside/Simon & Schuster, Inc., 2001.

Tobin, Alicia, Chris Gursche, and Janelle Murphy. *Keto Genesis: 30 Well Fed Days to a New, Leaner & Healthier You.* New Westminster, BC: Foresight Publishing, 2015.

Vannice, Gretchen. *Improving Omega-3 Nutrition: A New Paradigm for Health, A Guide for Health Professionals.* Santa Cruz, CA: Better Health Books, 2014.

Volek, Jeff S., and Stephen D. Phinney. *The Art and Science of Low Carbohydrate Living: An Expert Guide to Making the Life-Saving Benefits of Carbohydrate Restriction Sustainable and Enjoyable.* Beyond Obesity, LLC, 2011.

Wahls, Terry, and Eve Adamson. *The Wahls Protocol: How I Beat Progressive MS Using Paleo Principles and Functional Medicine.* New York, NY: Avery/Penguin Random House, 2014.

Westman, Eric C., Stephen D. Phinney, and Jeff S. Volek. *The New Atkins for a New You: The Ultimate Diet for Shedding Weight and Feeling Great.* New York, NY: Touchstone/Simon & Schuster, Inc., 2010.

Wilson, Jacob and Ryan Lowery. *The Ketogenic Bible, The Authoritative Guide to Ketosis.* Las Vegas, NV: Victory Belt Publishing, Inc., 2017.

Winters, Nasha, Jess Higgins Kelley, and Kelly Turner. *The Metabolic Approach to Cancer: Integrating Deep Nutrition, the Ketogenic Diet, and Nontoxic Bio-Individualized Therapies.* White River Junction, VT: Chelsea Green Publishing, 2017.

Audiovisual Links

Diamond, David. An update on demonization and deception in research on saturated fat. https://www.youtube.com/watch?v=uc1XsO3mxX8

D'Agostino, Dominic. Episode 14: Dominic D'Agostino discusses the physiological benefits of nutritional ketosis. https://www.ihmc.us/stemtalk/episode-14/

Berry, Ken D. Book Review: Alzheimer's Disease: What If There Was a Cure? by Mary T. Newport, MD.: https://www.youtube.com/watch?v=lJSe5D5HKUU

Ford, Ken. Episode 50: Ken Ford talks about ketosis, optimizing exercise, and the future direction of science, technology, and culture. https://www.ihmc.us/stemtalk/episode-50/

Institute for Human and Machine Cognition—Lecture series: https://www.ihmc.us

Mattson, Mark. Why fasting bolsters brain power: Mark Mattson at TEDx Johns Hopkins University: https://www.youtube.com/watch?v=4UkZAwKoCP8

Newport, Mary T. Coconut Oil Touted as Alzheimer's Remedy - CBN.com: https://www.youtube.com/watch?v=ZZOR-Qd3QSg

Newport, Mary, and Steve Newport with Lori Johnson. Alzheimer's doctors taking note of coconut oil. http://www1.cbn.com/video/alzheimers-doctors-taking-note-of-coconut-oil?show=700club

Newport, Mary and Steve. Interview with Ken Lightburn. https://www.youtube.com/watch?v=lUpADCf5HqQ&list=PLP38DivhF5GsNt2sBDZ8Q11BnbAJhqcDM&index=1

Newport, Mary. Medium-Chain Triglycerides and Ketones: An Alternative Fuel for Alzheimer's: https://www.youtube.com/watch?v=feyydeMFWy4&index=6&list=PLP38DivhF5GsNt2sBDZ8Q11BnbAJhqcDM

Newport, Mary T. Unconventional but Effective Therapy for Alzheimer's Treatment: Dr. Mary T. Newport at TEDxUSF: https://www.youtube.com/watch?v=Dvh3JhsrQ0w

Cunnane, Stephen.—Episode 59: Stephen Cunnane discusses the role of ketones in human evolution and Alzheimer's.: https://www.ihmc.us/stemtalk/episode-59/

Theracycle—Forced Bicycling for Parkinson's: http://www.theracycle.com/articles/parkinsons-bike-study.aspx.

VanItallie, Theodore, with Cecilia Calhoun. Dr. VanItallie Interviews Parts 1-11: Introduction and Background on Ketones https://www.youtube.com/playlist?list=PLQxrx8FHaqT-7C-UYqT0C5qZAc_88BXKD

Curtis, William. "Guitar before and after drinking coffee concoction for Parkinson's disease." https://www.youtube.com/watch?v=oYaFv-8dv58.

Curtis, William. "My Parkinson's treatment with a morning fat-filled coffee to release ketones." https://www.youtube.com/watch?v=riGYq5iD2SM

Resource Organizations and Foundations

The following is a list of organizations and medical websites:

Alzheimer's Association: www.alz.org

Alzheimer's Disease Cooperative Study: www.adcs.org

Alzheimer's Disease International: www.alz.co.uk

Alzheimer's Family Organization: www.alzheimersfamily.org

The Charlie Foundation: https://charliefoundation.org/

Clinical Trials: https://clinicaltrials.gov

Epigenix Foundation: https://epigenixfoundation.org/

Epilepsy Foundation: https://www.epilepsy.com/

> Information on Low Glycemic Index Diet: https://www.epilepsy.com/learn/treating-seizures-and-epilepsy/dietary-therapies/low-glycemic-index-treatment.

> Information on Modified Atkins Diet: https://www.epilepsy.com/learn/treating-seizures-and-epilepsy/dietary-therapies/modified-atkins-diet.)

George W. Yu Foundation for Nutrition and Health, Inc.: www.YuFoundation.org

GLUT1 Deficiency Foundation: http://www.g1dfoundation.org

Ketogenic.Com: https://ketogenic.com

KetoNutrition: https://ketonutrition.org

Ketone Technologies: https://ketonetechnologies.com/

Keto Pet Sanctuary—Help with pet cancers: http://www.ketopetsanctuary.com

Matthews Friends: www.matthewsfriends.org

Michael J. Fox Foundation for Parkinson's Research: www.MichaelJFoxFoundation.org

National Institute on Aging Alzheimer's Disease Education and Referral Center: www.nia.nih.gov/Alzheimers

National Institutes of Health Clinical Trials Registry: www.clinicaltrials.gov

National Institute of Neurologic Disorders and Stroke: www.ninds.nih.gov

Remi Savioz Glut-1 Foundation: www.remisglut1foundation.com

Forums, Websites, Blogs, Foundations, Podcasts and Message Boards

ALS Forums: www.alsforums.com

Alzheimer's Association Message Board: www.alz.org/living_with_alzheimers_message_boards_lwa.asp

Alzheimer's Reading Room: www.alzheimersreadingroom.com

Alzheimer's Research Forum: www.alzforum.org

The Alzheimer's Spouse: www.thealzheimerspouse.com

Coconut Research Center: www.coconutresearchcenter.org

Dementia and Alzheimer's Weekly: www.alzheimersweekly.com

Dr. Dominic D'Agostino's Websites—KetoNutrition: https://ketonutrition.org/ and
   Ketone Technologies: https://ketonetechnologies.com/

Dr. Dominic D'Agostino's Website—KetoNutrition: www.ketonutrition.org

Dr. Mary Newport's Website: www.coconutketones.com

Dr. Mary Newport's Blog: www.coconutketones.blogspot.com

Dr. Mary Newport's Facebook Page; https://www.facebook.com
   /CoconutOilandAlzheimers/?ref=hl. Coconut Oil Helps Alzheimer's,
   Dementia, ALS, MS.

Jimmy Moore's Livin' La Vida Low-Carb: www.livinlavidalowcarb.com

Ketogenic.Com: https://ketogenic.com

Ketogenic Diet Calculator from Beth Zupec-Kania:
   https://www.ketodietcalculator.org

Miriam Kalamian Website: DietaryTherapies.com; Twitter @DietaryTherapy;
   Facebook at Miriam Kalamian.

The Paleo Diet: https://thepaleodiet.com

Winning the Fight—Deanna Protocol for ALS: https://www.winningthefight.org

Sources for Coconut Oil and Medium-Chain Trigylceride Oil

The following websites offer an array of coconut oil and MCT oil products:

Alpha Health Products: www.alphahealth.ca

Amazon.com: www.amazon.com

Barlean's Organic Oils: www.barleans.com

B4 Neuro Restore Coconut Powder and Supplement Mix: www.memorypharmacy.
   com

Carrington Farms—Organic Coconut Oil: https://carringtonfarms.com
   /coconut-oils-ghees/?msclkid=d323e6cac8691f537c05bc78b59e2987&utm_
   source=bing&utm_medium=cpc&utm_campaign=Branded&utm_term=
   carrington%20farm%20coconut%20oil&utm_content=Carrington%20
   Farms%20-%20Coconut%20Oil

Coeurisma Coconut Oil and Chocolate Coconut Oil: www.coeurisma.com

Costco—Organic coconut oil: https://www.costco.com/Kirkland-Signature
   -Organic-Coconut-Oil%2C-84-fl.-oz..product.100381413.html?pageSize=
   96&catalogId=10701&dept=All&langId=-1&keyword=Kirkland+
   Signature+Organic+Coconut+Oil%2C+84+fl.+oz.&storeId=10301

drMCT from Ketoscience, Singapore and elsewhere in Asia: https://mydrmct.com/

Earth Balance: www.earthbalancenatural.com

Dr. Schär in Burgstall, Italy: https://www.drschaer.com

MCT//143—Dr. Mary Newport's MCT/coconut oil/phosphatidylcholine formulation with Pruvit Ventures: marynewport.pruvitnow.com

Nature's Approved: www.naturesapproved.com

Nisshin OilliO Group, Ltd. in Asia: http://www.nisshin-oillio.com/

Niulife: www.niulife.com.au

Nutiva: http://nutiva.com

Parrillo Performance Pure Tricaprylic Acid C8: www.parrillo.com

Sam's Club—Organic coconut oil: https://www.samsclub.com/sams/mm-ev-coconut-oil-56-oz-organic/prod20170548.ip?xid=plp:product:1:1

Spectrum: www.spectrumorganics.com

Swanson Health Products: www.swansonvitamins.com

Tropical Traditions: www.tropicaltraditions.com

True Protein: www.trueprotein.com

Wilderness Family Naturals: www.wildernessfamilynaturals.com

Source for Non-Racemic Ketone Salts

Pruvit Ventures (marynewport.pruvitnow.com)

Sources for Ketone Esters

Ketoneaid: http://ketoneaid.com

HVMN: https://hvmn.com/

Ketone Water (from Ketoneaid): www.ketonewater.com

Ketone Monitoring Devices

Keto Mojo (least expensive ketone test strips) https://keto-mojo.com/

Precision Xtra—Available through Amazon and Walmart and other online stores.

Nova Max—Available through Amazon and Walmart and other online stores.

Ketogenic Diet Apps

KetoDietCalculator.com (The Charlie Foundation)

KetoDiet (https://ketodietapp.com/)—ketogenic diet education, numerous recipes and ability to store planned meals and track progress—available for iPhones, iPads and Android phones.

Low-Carbohydrate Wines

Dry Farm Wines—Organic unsweetened white and red wines:
www.dryfarmswines.com

Ketogenic Foods and Formulas

The following are companies that market specialized prescription or non-prescription ketogenic liquid formulas, powders and other ketogenic foods. Products intended for use as a complete ketogenic diet for infants, children and adults should be consumed only as directed by their physician:

Atkins Nutritionals (www.atkins.com): A complete line of meals, bars, snacks, shakes, and meal kits to help with low-carb and ketogenic diets. Available at many local grocery and online stores.

Betaquik and Carb Zero (Nestle— https://www.nestlehealthscience.co.uk/vitaflo /conditions/ketogenic%20diet/betaquik): Liquid high-fat emulsions with MCT oil.

CarbQuick Complete Baking and Biscuit Mix: Used to make homemade baked goods. Available from Amazon, Walmart, and many other online stores.

Liquigen® (Nutricia: http://www.nutricia.ie/products/view/liquigen): Liquid high-fat emulsions with MCT oil to be used only with medical supervision.

KetoCal (https://www.myketocal.com/default.aspx--a variety of complete liquid or powdered complete ketogenic formulas for use by infants, children and adults.

KetoVie (http://www.ketovie.com/products/ketovie/index.php): Liquid 4:1 ketogenic drinks

Medica Nutrition (http://www.medica-nutrition.com/ketocuisine): KetoCuisine, a 5:1 ketogenic flour for ketogenic home cooking and baking.

Ross Labs RCF® (http://static.abbottnutrition.com/cms-prod/abbottnutrition.com /img/RCF.pdf): Soy-based carbohydrate-free formula, used in milk protein allergy and when carbohydrates must be very limited due to low caloric needs.

Solace Nutrition (https://www.solacenutrition.com/product-category/conditions /conditions-using-ketogenic-diet/): Powdered formulas for specific medical conditions.

Products

Formulas that may be utilized for the ketogenic diet include:

KetoCal® (Nutricia)—KetoCal® 3:1 Powder (Unflavored)—KetoCal® 4:1 Powder (Vanilla Flavored)—KetoCal® 4:1 LQ Liquid (Flavored and Unflavored)

RCF® (Abbott)—Ross Carbohydrate Free Formula—soy-based carbohydrate free formula—Used in milk protein allergy—Used when carbohydrates must be very limited due to low caloric needs

KetoVolve™ (Nutr-e-volultion)—Bland flavored powder

KetoVie™ 4:1 (Cambrooke)—Available in chocolate and vanilla flavors—Ready-to-feed liquid

Modular Products

A variety of modular products may need to be added to ensure nutrient needs are met and ketogenic ratios are correct.

Lipid S

Microlipid® (Nestle)—safflower oil emulsion at 4.5 kcal/mL o MCT Oil® (Nestle)—fractionated coconut oil at 7.7 kcal/mL o Liquigen® (Nutricia)—MCT emulsion at 4.5 kcal/mL o Betaquik™ (Vitaflo)—MCT emulsion at 1.89 kcal/mL of Carb-zero™ (Vitaflo)—LCT emulsion at 1.8 kcal/mL o Retail Oils (Olive oil, coconut oil)—variable caloric density

Carbohydrate o Solcarb® powder (Medica Nutrition)—carbohydrate powder—maltodextrin—3.75 kcal/g • Polycal™ powder (Nutricia)—carbohydrate powder—maltodextrin—3.84 kcal/g

Protein • Beneprotein® (Nestle)—whey protein powder—6 gm protein in 7 gm powder o Complete Amino Acid Mix (Nutricia)—100% amino acid powder—8.2 g protein in 10 g powder

Baking Mixes/Flours

CarbQuik™ (Tova Industries, LLC) • KetoCuisine™ (Medica Nutrition) • KetoCal® (Nutricia) • Almond flour • Coconut flour

INDEX

ABOUT THE AUTHOR

Mary T. Newport, MD, grew up in Cincinnati, Ohio, and was educated at Xavier University and University of Cincinnati College of Medicine, both in Cincinnati, Ohio. She is board certified in pediatrics and neonatology and completed her training at Children's Hospital Medical Center in Cincinnati and Medical University Hospital in Charleston, South Carolina. She practiced neonatology in Florida for thirty years and was founding medical director of two newborn intensive care units

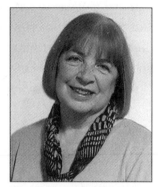

Mary T. Newport, MD

in the Tampa Bay area. Dr. Newport then practiced for three years at the opposite end of the spectrum, providing hospice care in the Tampa Bay area of Florida. She makes home visits to people with chronic illnesses, writes and speaks at home and around the world on ketones as an alternative fuel for the brain for Alzheimer's and other disorders.

Dr. Newport was caregiver for fifteen years for her husband of forty-three years, Steven Jerry Newport, who suffered from early-onset Alzheimer's disease and died in January 2016. They have two daughters and a grandson. She is author of *Alzheimer's Disease: What if There Was a Cure? The Story of Ketones,*

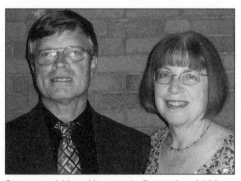

Steven and Mary Newport in December 2008.

now in its second edition, with multiple foreign language translations, and *The Coconut Oil and Low Carb Solution for Alzheimer's, Parkinson's and Other Diseases.* Dr. Newport has been an invited speaker on this subject for symposia and conferences throughout the United States, Australia, Canada, China, France, Greece, Germany, India, Italy, Japan, The Philippines, Singapore, and Thailand, and, specifically, for University of South Florida, American College of Nutrition, Institute for Human and Machine Cognition, Fellowship in Anti-Aging and Regenerative Medicine, International College of Integrative Medicine, Weston A. Price Foundation, and has given numerous lectures for university students and for the public. For more information, view her website and blog at http://coconut-ketones.com and follow her on Facebook at https://www.facebook.com/CoconutOilandAlzheimers/?ref=hl.